British Social Welfare

British Social Welfare

Past, present and future

Edited by

David Gladstone
University of Bristol

UCL
PRESS

First published in 1995 by UCL Press.

UCL Press Limited
University College London
Gower Street
London WC1E 6BT

The name of University College London (UCL) is a registered
trade mark used by UCL Press with the consent of the owner.

ISBN: 1-85728-198-5 PB

British Library Cataloguing-in-Publication Data
A CIP catalogue record for this book is available from the British Library.

Library of Congress Cataloging-in-Publication Data are available.

Typeset in Baskerville.
Printed and bound by
Page Bros (Norwich) Ltd, England.

Contents

CONTENTS

Preface

David Gladstone

This text faces in two directions. It is first of all a retrospective examination of the services of the classic British welfare state. It is now 50 years since legislation passed between 1944 and 1948, by the wartime Coalition government and the post-war Labour government in Britain, brought about the transition from a "social service state" to a more comprehensive and solidaristic welfare state. Traditionally half centuries constitute a significant milestone, a time for reflection and reassessment. That is the task undertaken by the authors of the first nine chapters in this collection, each of whom was asked to address the main directions of policy change over the last 50 years and the factors which had shaped it. Those chapters are narrative and analysis; accounts of change and continuity in specific service sectors of the British welfare state. Inevitably certain common themes recur: the end of the expansionary state in the mid 1970s, for example, and the dynamic of the new more market oriented discourse on welfare that characterized the 1980s. Those of us who have lived through the experiences which these chapters narrate can identify with the strength of Peter Hennessy's recent observation (1993):

> The choices made, or funked, during the first six years after the war, were genuinely formative. Those that were later reversed – by our going into Europe instead of keeping out, by our dropping the full employment pledge as the political and social aspiration, shedding universality of welfare provision, the health service apart, as the principle of welfare across the board – each of these benchmarks when crossed proved both difficult and painful, as the still protracted and ever-raging arguments around them demonstrate.

But this text faces also towards the future. If half-centuries create recollection, the approach of a millennium stimulates a looking forward. The final four chapters in this collection are part of that process. From different party political standpoints, alternative visions of the future of welfare are set out in Chapters 10 and 11, while the final two chapters 12 and 13 address issues of empowerment and quality which, emerging in the very recent past, seem likely to be part of the British welfare future, irrespective of party political considerations.

Like many other books with "British" in their title, this one too focuses almost entirely on England and Wales. As one who has researched and written on nineteenth-century Scottish social policy, I offer apologies in advance to those who have come to this book expecting more than they will receive!

Many people have assisted in the production of this book, most obviously those who agreed to write individual chapters, often in the midst of busy schedules. I am grateful to them all; and also to Zaheda Anwar, Wendy Dear, Helen Bush, Carrie Hughes and Judith Roberts who have provided much appreciated practical help in the final stages of preparing the manuscript for the publishers. At UCL Press, Justin Vaughan and his colleagues have been helpful and forbearing. Students, colleagues, family and friends have all good naturedly put up with my recent absorption in *British social welfare: past, present and future*. It will, I hope, both inform about the past and stimulate discussion about the future responsibilities of state and citizen in the pursuit of welfare.

University of Bristol
June 1994

Contributors

Judith Allsop is Professor of Health Policy at South Bank University. She has written a number of books and articles on health policy including *Health policy and the NHS, Changing primary care* and, with Annabelle May, the *Emperor's new clothes, FPCs in the 1980s*. She is a member of a health authority in London and served on the NHS Complaints Review team.

John Barnes lectures in government at the London School of Economics and is the Director of the Centre for Educational Research. He is the co-author (with Dr Nicholas Barr) of *Strategies for higher education. The alternative white paper* (Aberdeen University Press 1988) and of various articles on the funding of education. He chaired the Kent Education Committee 1977–82 and was a Member of the Council for National Academic Awards and the School Examinations and Assessment Council. He serves currently on the National Council for Vocational Qualifications.

Paul Burton trained and worked as a planner in London before joining the University of Bristol in 1980 where he has carried out research in a wide variety of policy areas including inner cities, homelessness, drugs prevention, children's play and equal employment opportunities. In addition to teaching comparative and urban policy he edits the journal *Policy and Politics*.

Eamonn Butler is Director of the Adam Smith Institute, an independent, non-profit and influential think tank which explores new ways of introducing choice, competition and market disciplines into public services. He has lectured and written extensively on health and welfare policy.

Alan Deacon is Professor of Social Policy at the University of Leeds. He is the author of several books and numerous articles on social security and the history of social policy, including *Reserved for the poor* (with Jonathan Bradshaw 1983). He was editor of the *Journal of Social Policy* between 1986 and 1991, and is currently co-director of research on the delivery of social security benefits to black communities.

Lucy Gaster's concern for quality arose directly from her experiences as a frontline manager in a London Borough neighbourhood office in the 1980s and, before that, through her involvement in local community groups. She has been a Research Fellow at the University of Bristol's School for Advanced Urban Studies since 1990, where she has been researching and teaching a variety of aspects of public service delivery, including service quality, local democracy and decentralization.

David Gladstone previously worked in the Scottish Office and the University of Exeter before taking up his present appointment at the University of Bristol in 1990. A historian by training, his main interests are in British government and welfare policies in the nineteenth and twentieth centuries. He has produced a considerable number of articles, chapters in edited collections, and papers and reports on aspects of welfare past and present, and has held several visiting appointments, especially in the USA.

Robin Means is a Senior Lecturer at the School for Advanced Urban Studies, University of Bristol. He has written extensively on community care issues as well as more generally on public policies and older people. He is co-author with Randall Smith of *The development of welfare services for elderly people* (Croom Helm 1985) and *Community care policy and practice* (Macmillan 1994) and co-editor with Peter Malpass of *Implementing housing policy* (Open University Press 1993).

Alan Murie is Professor of Urban and Regional Studies at the University of Birmingham and Director of the Centre for Urban and Regional Studies. He was previously Professor of Planning and Housing at Heriot-Watt University. He has published widely on housing issues, and books include *Housing inequality and deprivation* (Heinemann 1983) and *Housing policy and practice* (Macmillan 1994), now in its fourth edition. He is also editor of *Housing Studies*.

Roy Parker is Emeritus Professor of Social Policy at the University of Bristol. He has a long-standing interest in policies for children and has published extensively in that area. He was a member of the Seebohm Committee and has advised government on matters of child care policy and research over a number of years.

Sally Sainsbury is a Senior Lecturer specializing in the personal social services at the London School of Economics, where she has spent most of her career. Her research has focused mainly on disability and includes recent studies of deafness, residential care, the war pensions and industrial injuries schemes. She is currently participating in a study of the implementation of the 1990 NHS and Community Care Act.

John Stewart is Professor of Local Government Studies at the University of Birmingham. He was appointed to the Institute in 1966 and was its Director from 1976 to 1983. Until recently he was Head of the School of Public Policy which includes the Institute and other departments concerned with the public sector at home and overseas. He has written extensively on the case for local government and on its management.

Marilyn Taylor is Lecturer in the Management of Health and Social Care at the School for Advanced Urban Studies, University of Bristol. She has had 25 years experience of the voluntary sector, as a researcher, as a community activist and has served on voluntary management committees. She has recently worked with voluntary organizations in Eastern and Central Europe. She has written widely for a policy, practice and academic audience on voluntary and community activity and the policy challenges they face, and on voluntary–statutory relationships.

Noel Whiteside is Reader in Social Policy at the University of Bristol. Among other books, she is the author of *Bad times: unemployment in British social and political history* (Faber & Faber 1991) and co-author (with Gordon Philips) of *Casual labour* (OUP 1985). She has also published a number of articles on labour market policies in a range of historical journals, both in the UK and Europe. She is currently working on an ESRC-funded research project, in co-operation with a CNRS group in Paris, on comparative developments in French and British labour markets since the 1930s.

Malcolm Wicks became Labour MP for Croydon North West in 1992. He is a member of the Social Security Select Committee. He was Founder Director of the Family Policy Studies Centre (1983–92) and was previously lecturer in social administration at Brunel University; a member of the Home Office Urban Deprivation Unit; and Research Director and Secretary of the Study Commission on the Family. His publications include *Old and cold: hypothermia and social policy* (1978) and *A future for all: do we need a welfare state?* (1987). He is also co-author of *A new agenda* (1993) and *The active society: defending welfare* (1995).

Introduction:
change, continuity and welfare

David Gladstone

The future pattern of Britain's welfare state is very firmly on the political agenda. The present (1994) Conservative government has ordered a fundamental review of the programmes of its spending departments; and social expenditure is a major part of government spending. Currently, the social security budget, for example, accounts for one third of all public expenditure, or £13 for each working person for every working day. The Chief Secretary to the Treasury, who is in charge of the government's spending review, has argued "Throughout the public sector it is right to question whether existing spending patterns and levels are appropriate; to give serious thought to the fundamental question of the government's proper role" (Portillo 1993). Central to the government's analysis is that Britain can no longer afford the kind of welfare state – universal and solidaristic – that was fashioned in the 1940s and the immediately following decades; that welfare services need increasingly to be targeted to ensure that, whether especially by means of financial benefits but also services in kind, help really reaches those who need it. Meanwhile the Labour party's Commission on Social Justice, established by John Smith when Labour party leader, is also considering the future shape of Britain's welfare system. Whereas 50 years ago, in the conditions of wartime Britain, William Beveridge evoked the image of the Five Giants – of Idleness, Want, Disease, Ignorance and Squalor – standing athwart the road to post-war reconstruction, the Commission on Social Justice, in one of its early reports, identified "the five great opportunities that will in the years ahead be the basis of social cohesion and economic security. These opportunities – for life-long learning, work, good health, a safe environment and financial independence are today's political and moral frontier" (Commission on Social Justice 1993). In this book, the chapters by

Butler and Wicks propose two alternative scenarios for the future of welfare: the former based on the development of alternatives to state supply; the other, emphasizing the positive role for government in the construction of the active society. Whichever model of the future commands political support, it is unlikely that the welfare state will remain unchanged.

Change and the welfare state have, indeed, been almost inseparably bound together over the past 50 years. The chapters in the first part of this book address the issue of change in relation to specific service sectors. What have been the elements of change since the 1940s in health and housing, education and employment, income maintenance, urban policy and the non-statutory sector, for example? What have been the factors or agents promoting change in welfare policies and arrangements over that half century? And what has been the outcome of those changes on access to welfare and the distribution of life chances between different sectors of the population? Changes in the boundaries between public and private sectors of welfare, in the relationship between the state and the citizen, in family structures and employment patterns, in popular and political support for the institutions of the collectivist welfare state, are all integral to any analysis of the past 50 years.

But in that period there have also been continuities. The contemporary concern with the costs of welfare is nothing new to those familiar with the debates of the 1950s. And far from being constrained by economic factors a recent study (Hills 1993) has suggested that "the sort of welfare state we have in future can be a matter not just of bowing to inevitable forces but of making real choices and exercising political will". Professional power, much highlighted in the public choice critique, is another continuity in welfare. There is indeed a significant relationship between the development of the welfare state and the rise of professional society. The expanding welfare state has created considerable new job opportunities for those in the white collar or white blouse occupations that have characterized the change in the British labour market over the past half century. Over the same period "clients" may have been redesignated "consumers" or "users" but how far has their position of dependency altered in the welfare relationship? Much political attention too has focused on the restructuring of welfare state institutions. In the recent past this has included the possibility of "opt outs" and "quasi-markets" for schools and hospitals and the development, under certain conditions, of fundholding for general practitioners. A similar concern for more efficient working and improved management of welfare in the 1960s created the conditions for significant organizational change at that time, which mainly resulted in new and larger government departments. In its present form, of course, it increasingly represents a move beyond the institutions and agencies of state welfare into the private market (often with tax subsidies) and other sectors.

One of the paradoxes of that process of apparent diversification and the increasingly centralized concentration of power is the re-establishment, almost on the nineteenth-century model, of agencies of regulation, inspection and control. As a consequence, issues of public accountability and quality become more central to the emerging agenda in welfare. Both the chapters in this book where these issues are explored indicate that they are contested concepts. In that, they enter an arena where once apparently established values are being redefined, and many assumptions, taken for granted in the post-war world, are being questioned. Interestingly, though the critique is now more sophisticated, the discourse is structured in ways that would have been familiar to critics, both on the left and the right, in the 1940s. But in the mid 1990s there is on each side of the political spectrum a recognition that it is inappropriate to call up the remembrance of things past as a guide to planning the future. Not only the institutions of welfare, but the social, political and economic world in which they were embedded has changed. The issue for the future, therefore, is much more about the political choices that will be made in fashioning a new welfare settlement and the economic conditions, both for individuals and collectively, which will sustain it.

CHAPTER 1
The welfare state and the state of welfare

David Gladstone

Fifty years on, the essential features of the classic welfare state as created in Britain in the 1940s are still visible. But that period has also been marked by challenge, crisis and change:
- challenge from the political left and right to the principles and practices of the welfare state;
- crisis created principally by changing economic circumstances from the early 1970s that undermined the precarious political legitimacy of the post-war welfare consensus;
- change in the management and organization of welfare state services as well as in social and economic priorities.

A recent vision of the future contends that "The pressures of continuing economic difficulty, the demand for more flexible services and the wide-spread dissatisfaction with state bureaucracies suggest[s] that the process of restructuring will continue into the next millennium, whichever party is in power" (Taylor-Gooby & Lawson 1993).

Against that background, the purpose of this chapter is to provide a narrative of change in the welfare state over the past 50 years. This it does by reference to three historical debates concerning the relationship between war and welfare, the existence and nature of the post-war consensus and the impact of Thatcherism on the welfare state. Interspersed between each of these narrative sections is a discussion of the relationship between the welfare state and the social relationships of class, race and gender. But underlying both the narrative and analysis is the view that the development of welfare over the past 50 years is "a story of the complexity of political, economic and social forces, of pressures both internal and international, all subject to conflict and change" (Williams 1993).

1

War and welfare

The debate

Richard Titmuss (1950) argued that the specific experiences of the Second World War created the conditions conducive to the implementation of a range of more solidaristic and statist welfare policies. Subsequent writers have challenged aspects of the Titmuss thesis and Corelli Barnett has attributed much of Britain's declining fortunes to the "New Jerusalemitis" represented by the welfare state.

There is general agreement that Britain's classic welfare state was established between 1944 and 1948: a period spanned politically by the Churchill-led coalition government and the Labour government with Clement Attlee as Prime Minister that was returned to power with an overwhelming majority at the General Election in 1945. Between those years "to a greater or lesser extent, liberal opinion converged upon the belief that the welfare of the people is ultimately a collective responsibility of the state" (Morgan & Evans 1993). For such a society a new designation became appropriate: that of a welfare state, a society in which "organized power [is] deliberately used to modify the play of market forces" (Briggs 1961).

This welfare state had two dimensions, full employment and an extensive range of public services. The coalition government's commitment to "a high and stable level of employment after the war" (Cmd 6527) provides the economic underpinning for the welfare state in general and for its system of social security in particular. There was little political agreement on the means by which this objective would be attained. Keynesian demand management was favoured by the centre and the centre left, while the right wing of the Conservative party looked to a recovery of markets and foreign trade. In spite of such differences, "the maintenance of full employment was both a direct contribution to individual welfare and an essential support for other welfare services, because it simultaneously maximised revenue and minimised demand for them" (Lowe 1993).

A range of social legislation passed between 1944 and 1948 constitutes the second dimension of the welfare state and forms the starting point for several chapters in this book. It, too, divides into two parts. The first is legislation concerning cash benefits: the introduction of a series of financial benefits available "from the cradle to the grave" for those who were members of the National Insurance scheme, and below it the "safety net" of National Assistance. The final measure offering a "new deal" in financial security was the introduction of a system of family allowances: a cash benefit paid to mothers in respect of second and subsequent children. The second form of social legislation concerned services in kind and includes the 1944 Education Act and the National Health Service which, like the major social security reforms, came into effect on 5 July 1948.

As a result both of its economic objective of full employment and its raft of social legislation, "the government . . . had assumed and developed a measure of direct concern for the health and well-being of the population which, by contrast with the role of government in the 1930s, was little short of remarkable" (Stevenson 1984). It appeared to be Britain's "new deal" in welfare; and its achievement was that "for over a decade it delivered a remarkable combination of full employment, low inflation and economic growth" (Morgan & Evans 1993).

But would such a "new deal" have occurred without the catalyst of the Second World War? Beveridge, whose report – *Social insurance and allied services* (Cmd 6404) – was the basis for much wartime optimism about what could be achieved by social planning was in no doubt. In the conditions of national unity created by war it was much easier to achieve recognition of the fact that "the prevention of Want and the diminution of disease are . . . a common interest of all citizens" (Cmd 6404).

The sense of solidarity created by wartime conditions and experiences was also central to Titmuss's analysis (1950) in his volume on social policy for the official *History of the Second World War*. "Titmuss believed that public attitudes became more egalitarian during the Second World War and maintained that this led directly to dramatic changes in social policy" (Smith 1986).

More recent historical research has developed a significant critique of the Titmuss thesis. It has questioned, first, his interpretation of wartime solidarity. Wartime experiences such as the rationing of food and clothing and indiscriminate bombing, "may have democratised hardship, fostering a greater sense of social cohesion . . . but the strength of class attitudes and the existence of social divisions should not be under estimated" (Digby 1989). There was a world of difference between those dining in well-known London hotels and the population seeking refuge in its underground stations. Similarly the existence of a vigorous wartime black market also calls into question the solidarity that Titmuss identified. Nor it seems did the process of evacuation of women and children from urban to rural areas, which was central to Titmuss's thesis, provide an unequivocal shock to public consciousness and a new commitment to right the inter-war experiences of children reared amid conditions of financial poverty, ill health and unemployment. A more recent assessment has concluded that "heightened social awareness among some

3

sections of the middle classes clearly did not exclude the sharpening of prejudice in others" (Calder 1991).

Secondly, more recent writing has emphasized the continuities between the welfare state legislation and earlier developments.

> Almost all the ideas and proposals for reform in social security and education, for example, had been long discussed in the 1920s and 1930s. The new structures built on or simplified many of the systems that preceded them. In many cases they extended to a national scale experiments which had been introduced by some local authorities. (Glennerster 1990a)

Health care provides another example. During the 1930s both the British Medical Association and the Socialist Medical Association set out proposals designed to extend the health care coverage of the population, the former advocating an extension of the insurance scheme introduced in 1911, the latter local authority control.

But, thirdly, in their attempt to explain the increased role of government in welfare and the development of more comprehensive universal services, recent writers have suggested both the variety and the interrelationship of several other factors than those that Titmuss identified. ". . . by inviting the Labour and Liberal parties to join the coalition, Churchill broke the Conservative political hegemony of the inter war years" (Kavanagh & Morris 1989). It is generally agreed that while Churchill devoted himself to war objectives, matters of domestic policy were left in the hands of Labour members of the coalition, with Attlee as Deputy Prime Minister. That, and their perceived warmer welcome for the Beveridge proposals, may help to explain Labour's election victory in 1945. But Churchill, although apparently less interested in domestic affairs, unwittingly gave shape to the ideology of reform. In nationalistic terms, Churchill's rhetoric emphasized "a 'common people' united in a common cause": their shared determination to win the war. "No longer were British workers seen as the idle, intractable troublemakers of pre-war years", as soldiers and civilians they were "called to the centre of the national stage . . . in a patriotic struggle for justice, liberty, equality against oppression" (Morgan & Evans 1993) and in the process performed many acts of courage and heroism in their daily struggle. The people's war in a sense necessitated the people's peace.

In many of its features that peacetime world had been presaged in the inter-war planning movement that had commanded some measure of support across the political spectrum and with progressive opinion. In early 1941 a celebrated issue of the popular magazine *Picture Post* "produced a forty page prospectus for 'a new Britain' ". Well known writers and thinkers set out "proposals for a fresh employment strategy, social security, town planning, architecture, the countryside, education, health, the medical services and leisure" (Stevenson 1986). Wartime conditions were to prove propitious for developing the legitimacy of its programme. Wartime controls, increased taxation and the necessity of a more interventionist state had already created a changed relationship between the state and the citizen. But the exigencies of war had also brought into government a cadre of "reforming liberal academics from the universities", such as Keynes and Beveridge, who had espoused the principles of the inter-war planning movement. As a result, the nature of political discourse changed: "promises, programmes and planning had become the norm; those who questioned their validity now occupied the eccentric minority position" (Harris 1990).

The consequence of that process has been controversially discussed by Corelli Barnett (1986) who argues that the British victory in the Second World War was lost to social rather than to economic and industrial change. In the light of knowledge available to ministers and civil servants that Britain would face an economic emergency once the war was over, Barnett argues that the principal priority of the coalition government should have been the reconstruction of British industry. Instead, it planned for a New Jerusalem with the creation of the welfare state; a movement Barnett identifies as "inspired by soggy liberal idealism, a lofty disdain for industry and the means by which wealth was created" (Addison 1987). Barnett's interpretation has itself been subject to critical review (Addison 1987, Harris 1991) but it serves to remind us how much the development of social citizenship was inextricably linked to Britain's economic performance.

Class and the welfare state

At the end of the 1940s, T. H. Marshall, Professor of Sociology at the London School of Economics, delivered a series of lectures at Cambridge. Although his analysis has been criticized (Ferris 1985, Held 1989, Turner 1986) as "Anglocentric, evolutionary and historicist" (Pierson 1991), his social democratic perspective has remained an important point of departure for any assessment of the relationship between the welfare state and the system of social stratification. For Marshall, the creation of the welfare state in the 1940s was the latest stage in Britain's evolving history of expanding citizenship. Progressively through the eighteenth to the twentieth centuries, he argued, British citizenship was extended, first of all, to incorporate legal rights – equality before the law; then political rights, achieved by means of the extension of the franchise and the introduction of the secret ballot; and finally social rights specifically as a result of the welfare state legislation. In general the extension and establishment of citizenship rights "reduces the authority and power of previously dominant groups in society" (King 1987). Specifically, the social rights embodied in the welfare state legislation promote "an equality of status helping counterweigh disparities of income and class" (Baldwin 1990). As one recent commentator has observed

> Marshall's formulation caught the aspirations embodied in the Welfare [State] better than any other. The rich man and the poor man would collect the same pensions from the post office counter, and sit next to each other in the same doctor's waiting room. They would be no less rich or poor for doing so, but they would be that much more citizens of one community. (Marquand 1988)

Entitlement would thus create an equality of status which, in its turn, would be the means of securing social cohesion, integration and solidarity. In these terms, the welfare state was the fulfilment of fraternity, the creation of community.

But in those terms, it had its immediate critics. Some on the political right saw the welfare state as a threat to the existing system of social differentiation, especially to the position of the middle class, and as a harbinger of a totalitarian state regime.

> Education, other than that provided in State aided schools becomes more and more costly, while some politicians would abolish it altogether. Medical attention is being "equalized" and those who wish to obtain it outside the NHS must pay twice . . . Finally, not only are legacies taxed, but keen socialists broadcast their longing to abolish completely the transmission of wealth in any form. (Lewis & Maude 1949)

Nor was there unanimity on the political left that what had been accomplished in the welfare state legislation represented the establishment of socialism. This issue was central to the second phase of Labour's post-war period in power. After 1948, there was increasing recognition that Labour needed a new vision. But opinion differed as to what form such a vision should take. *Tribune* called for "a socialist philosophy based on a fresh and unprejudiced analysis of the difficulties that confront us", while Michael Young and others, critical of the statist tendencies in the post-war economic and social settlement, sought "to set socialism in the context of freedom and democracy" (Brooke 1992). Morgan's (1984) judicious conclusion at the end of his study of *Labour in power 1945–1951* is that while the Attlee Government "brought the British Labour movement to the zenith of its achievement as a political instrument for humanitarian reform . . . it did so by evading, rather than resolving, those dilemmas inherent in the potent, beguiling vision of socialism in our time".

Much subsequent analysis has called into question the central features of Marshall's paradigm. In place of the integrating force of the "hyphenated society" of social-democratic welfare capitalism, much more attention has been paid to their incompatibility.

> If capitalism entails a system of allocating power and resources according to the ownership of private property, welfare services entail a system of allocating society's resources according to the right of all citizens to share in the common wealth of the society according to their needs. (Dearlove & Saunders 1991)

There is, in this sense, a "fundamental logical contradiction" between capitalism and welfare that calls into question the more optimistic assumptions of Marshall's analysis.

That conclusion is attested by a whole genre of writing and research in social policy. Three elements of it will briefly be considered here: the distribution of payments and benefits; the middle class welfare state and the experience of public welfare. Any assessment of the distributional impact of the welfare state involves not only an assessment of who consumes its services and the duration of their consumption but how, and by whom, the services are paid for. Changes in the nature and level of taxation (such as the switch from direct taxes on income to indirect taxes such as VAT on fuel) need to feature alongside changing entitlements to financial benefits as well as the use of services in kind such as education. Le Grand's (1982) conclusion "that the strategy of promoting equality through public expenditure on the social services has failed" was refined by Hindess (1987). Emphasizing the centrality of incremental change in governments' programmes, he concluded, "far

7

from showing that 'the strategy of equality' has been tried and failed, the record shows that it has played at most a limited role in the development of British social services". Hills (1993) has recently concluded that for most people in the income maintenance sector the welfare state acts as a savings bank; far less does it undertake or achieve redistribution between social classes.

Considering distributional aspects in relation only to the public sector of welfare, however, is misplaced. One of Titmuss's perceptive observations directed attention, in addition, to the contribution to welfare produced by occupational schemes (the "perks" of the job) and the fiscal benefits that accrued through the tax system. Had he been writing in the 1980s it is likely that he would have extended his analysis of the divisions of welfare to include the more recent issues of the "hidden costs" of personal tending care and the public subsidy of private welfare that occurred in that period. When it was originally presented in the mid 1950s, however, his analysis challenged the stereotypical image of an all pervasive welfare state for the working classes. In addition to the welfare state-established universal benefits (such as health care and education) the middle classes were also the beneficiaries of other states of welfare, with each sector operating independently of the others. In that respect, they reinforced the pattern of class based inequalities rather than promoted the cohesion of social-democratic welfare capitalism.

This aspect became more established in subsequent discussions of the welfare state. Not only as consumers of its universal services but also as employees in the expanding welfare sector the middle classes appeared disproportionately to be the beneficiaries of its existence (Abel-Smith 1958). Meanwhile the greater reliance on means tested National Assistance benefits in social security created a situation in which the receipt of welfare was a demeaning experience. Studies began to identify "the casualties of the welfare state", (Harvey 1960) and, most famously, "the rediscovery of poverty" (Abel-Smith & Townsend 1965). "The giant of want turned out to be far too protean a creature for Beveridge's net to catch. 'Doles' duly reappeared, only faintly disguised; and the promise of equal citizenship was denied by the very mechanism which had been designed to make it a reality" (Marquand 1988).

In its 1940s manifestation, the welfare state served the interests of both capital and labour. To the latter it offered the promise of improved material conditions in line with their wartime aspirations; to the former a healthy, trained and educated workforce as well as the potential of increased markets. That coalition of interests supported the welfare state with varying com-

8

mitment to the mid 1970s. Then a combination of factors were to splinter that fragile commitment to the communality of values and equality of status that for Marshall was the hallmark of the social rights of citizenship: the slowdown of economic growth; increasing diversification in the labour market, a working class many of whom had moved from austerity to affluence and who were accustomed increasingly to consumer choice in other aspects of their lives. Meanwhile business interests were becoming increasingly globalized, rendering continuing support for national institutions such as the welfare state less important. But perhaps it was more the 1940s than the mid 1970s that were to blame for the decline in support for the solidaristic welfare state. Post-war Britain, as one assessment concludes (Williamson 1990) "was reconstructed by a Labour government possessed of a much clearer image of what it sought to avoid from the past than what it wished to realise in the future".

The welfare consensus

The debate

Did a high level of agreement exist between the two political parties to maintain the social and economic objectives of the post-war settlement? Recent research has suggested that while a certain measure of unanimity existed, there were also differences of emphasis between the parties that can be traced back to the coalition government itself.

The existence of a post-war consensus concerning welfare has been expressed figuratively in a variety of ways. First, in the personalities of Beveridge, Bevan and Butler, respectively Liberal, Labour and Conservative, yet each responsible for three key features of the welfare state settlement. Secondly, in the term "Butskellism", a term perjoratively coined by *The Economist* in 1954 to emphasize the difficulty of distinguishing between the economic policies of the Conservative Chancellor of the Exchequer R. A. Butler and Hugh Gaitskell his opposite number in the Labour party. Thirdly, the names of Keynes and Beveridge have been linked representing the fusion of social and economic objectives and attempts to "reconcile interventionism with liberalism" (Marquand 1988).

But Pimlott (1988) has suggested that consensus may not so much describe as distort a period of Britain's recent past. It has ideological rather than descriptive powers. For some on the left it represents a lost golden age, while in Mrs Thatcher's period as Prime Minister it came to symbolize a period from which some Conservatives desired to break free into a new style of leadership and a commitment to a more radical political programme. Whether or not such a period of bipartisan consensus existed depends upon two factors: the meaning of the term and the period to which it is thought to apply. So far as the period is concerned, there is considerable – but not total – agreement that it characterizes the years 1951 to 1976. This section will also examine the 1940s, arguing that many later differences have their origin in that decade. But even if the whole period cannot be considered consensual it may be possible to identify periods within it that were. That could apply, for example, to both parties' commitment to economic growth (maybe for different reasons, however) and the management of the public sector that occurred in the 1960s. It was at exactly that time when American commentators began to write of "the end of ideology" suggesting that "there is today a rough consensus among intellectuals on political issues: the acceptance of a welfare state, . . . a system of mixed economy and of political pluralism" (Bell 1960).

This, of course, raises the issue of the meaning that attaches to consensus. Seldon lists its five main aspects: "a commitment to full employment; an acceptance of the right of trade unions to consultation by government; the mixed economy; the welfare state; and a commitment to equality, in an attempt to mitigate the worst aspects of inegality" (Seldon 1991). For Kavanagh & Morris (1989) it is "a set of parameters which bounded the site of policy options regarded by senior politicians and civil servants as administratively practicable, economically affordable and politically acceptable". Yet while such policy convergence occurred between 1951 and 1976 there was also "far less homogeneity in views and policies than is usually believed" (Deakin 1988). That divergency has increasingly been traced back to the coalition government itself. It is now well known that it deferred detailed discussion of social policy reform in order to avoid fracturing and splintering the agreement that existed between its members on achieving war-based objectives.

> In practical as well as ideological terms differences between the parties remained profound . . . The Labour Party was able to sharpen its commitment to economic planning and welfare as the political tide ran in its direction. By contrast, mainstream Conservative opinion had grave doubts about both the feasibility and desirability of the New Jerusalem. (Jeffreys 1991)

Addison (1993) has suggested that had Churchill been the victor in the 1945 general election, it is likely that his equation of wartime controls with socialism and his own growing libertarianism would have led him to a return to market forces but tempered by a national minimum standard of welfare. It is paradoxical, therefore, that although Churchill continued as party leader there was no significant attack on the framework of the welfare state with the exception of the NHS where, as Minister of Health, Bevan moved considerably beyond the arrangements that had been reached by the end of the war. Indeed, as Sullivan (1992) shows, Conservative party conferences in the late 1940s ratified and endorsed and claimed as their own the institutions of the welfare state. Even though they were outside mainstream Conservatism, however, there were voices of opposition who saw in the welfare state a threat to the British class structure, and in the taxation on which it was based the removal of the individual's right to dispose of their income as they wished. Towards the end of its period in government there was also more public evidence of the factionalism within the Labour party. Those who saw Labour's role as consolidating the welfare state reforms were countered by those who wished to extend the impetus to change. Issues of defence and NHS expenditure gave public expression to the dispute that resulted in the resignation in 1950 of three ministers, including the Minister of Health, Aneurin Bevan.

> This dispute was effectively about choices between the democratic socialist policies (as represented by the Bevanite wing of the party) and the new politics of social democracy which were adopted by Gaitskell and others [and which] accepted that the pace and nature of social policy development would be determined by political decisions about the economy. (Sullivan 1992)

If both the main political parties had their wings of dissent, how far is it accurate to identify some sort of "Butskellite" consensus existing between the major parts of the Conservative and Labour parties? Writing in 1962 the Labour politician Anthony Crosland suggested that:

> . . . deep differences exist between the two parties about the priority to be accorded to social welfare. This is not because Conservatives are less humanitarian but because they hold particular views as to the proper role of the state, the desirable level of taxation and the importance of private as opposed to collective responsibility. Their

> willingness for social expenditure is circumscribed by these views;
> and the consequence is a quite different order of priorities. (Crosland
> 1962)

There were differences between the parties on issues of taxation, public spending and the principles that should govern the supply of services. "A high level of personal taxation, including a stiffly graduated income tax and death duties" (Morgan 1984) were the methods Labour used between 1945 and 1951 as the means of realizing their social objectives. In government in the 1960s and 1970s their commitment was to blocking the main loopholes of tax avoidance and in 1974 they produced proposals for a wealth tax, although it was never implemented. This failure provided to one contemporary commentator "more disconcerting evidence of unwillingness to develop a framework of planning to bring about a significant reduction in inequality" (Townsend 1980). By contrast, the "burden" of taxation was one of the issues on which the Conservatives began to harass the Labour government from 1948: an issue especially popular with those sections of the middle class who had uncharacteristically voted Labour in 1945. For them the "opportunity state" offered enhanced possibilities; but the commitment to lower taxation was also much advocated and approved by business and banking interests. For Conservatives high levels of taxation discouraged incentives and were providing benefits for many who, because of the advent of full employment, were no longer in need of them. But, most importantly, they were perceived to be unnecessary because, in their post-war move to the right, Conservatives affirmed their belief that "individual welfare was best maximised by private initiative and that the state's role was to ensure the efficient working of the market, not the direct provision of services" (Lowe 1990).

Public expenditure was a second area of difference. For Labour, committed to a high level of provision of universal services, public spending was an integral element of their programme. " . . . a vote for Labour was at once a vote for the New Jerusalem and a vote for the party which the electors believed could be trusted – unlike the Conservatives – to deliver it" (Barnett 1986). It is, therefore, paradoxical that it was the Labour government who in 1976 effectively abandoned the commitment to the post-war settlement. "The decision to reduce public expenditure and the acceptance that such a decision was likely to result in increased unemployment confirmed the beginnings of the departure within the Treasury from the principles of Keynesian demand management" (Mullard 1993). In social policy "deprived of the protection of additional resources, politicians entered a world where priorities meant choices between programmes not for expansion but for cuts" (Deakin 1989).

Throughout the 1950s, although "the Conservatives largely acquiesced in the maintenance of the social programmes put in place during the late 1940s [they] spent hardly a shilling more than was required by the exigencies of politics and the growing demand for services" (Cronin 1991). To have done otherwise would have called into question their commitment to reduce taxation. Hence the review of NHS expenditure carried out between 1953 and 1956, and that concerned with the financial provisions for old age; the attempt to find savings in public spending programmes such as education; and, ultimately in 1957, the resignation of Thorneycroft as Chancellor of the Exchequer when the Cabinet failed to agree his proposals for economies in spending programmes, cuts in family allowances and increased charges in the NHS.

After the "stop-go" economic policies of the 1950s, Macmillan's rediscovered commitment to planning, modernization and the achievement of sustained growth without inflation represented an altogether new direction with much popular support. "So many different groups in society saw growth and what it would bring as the best way to realise their highest hopes" (Williamson 1990). Out of growth would come increased government revenue that could avoid the need to reduce and limit welfare services; while "Labour also hoped that economic growth would disguise the growing incidence of taxation" (Lowe 1990). If a period of bipartisan consensus existed it was probably during the 1960s. Government departments commissioned research, the new cadre of social science academics generated "a continuous flow of proposals" (Banting 1979) around which political debate revolved, and interest groups and professional associations established links with major spending departments. Optimism and expansion, however, were shortlived. The performance of the economy was, at best, indifferent. Administrative reforms in health and personal welfare, in local government and the civil service seemed to be the high point of consensus.

The final difference is in relation to specific services of the welfare state. Housing and education provide examples, but more broadly these raise the question of universalist and selective or targeted services. Housebuilding under Labour in the immediate post-war period was limited by licence to the public sector. In the 1950s the Conservatives' commitment to an active housing policy was to be achieved by both the public and the private sectors, although increasingly from the middle of the decade the role of the public sector was reduced. "Local authorities were increasingly exposed to market s, while the private sector was boosted by a series of tax concessions" (Lowe 1993). From the late 1950s the Conservatives sought to expand education as part of its new found commitment to economic growth. But whereas Conservatives sought to maintain the institutional status quo of the school system, Labour were already committed to the introduction of multilateral or comprehensive schools. Circular 10/65, requesting local authorities to submit plans for the reorganization of secondary schools on comprehensive lines, was introduced the year after Labour returned to power after 13 years of Conservative government. Yet, like so much else in welfare history, it is paradoxical that it was during Margaret Thatcher's time at the Department of Education and Science in the early 1970s that the largest number of comprehensive schools were approved.

The universalist–selective debate has never been entirely explicable on political party lines. Thus, Labour breached the principle of universalism in its espousal of NHS charges in 1950; while the Conservatives, in favour of selective secondary schooling, supported the comprehensive reorganization when they were in power in the early 1970s. In housing, because of the presence of a significant and growing trend towards owner occupation, universalism has always been fragile. In that sector, "the Conservatives have been the initiators of increases in selectivity, with Labour hostile but at least partly acquiescent" (Hill 1993). In social security, Conservatives were also more likely to initiate selectivist measures as, for example, in the early 1970s. This was in contrast to their Labour predecessors in the 1960s who "tried to move the system forward in a universalist direction" (Hill 1993).

The existence of broad bipartisan commitment to the features of the post-war settlement should not be allowed to obscure the dimensions of difference between them: differences that occurred not only between the parties but also within them.

Race and the consensus

As part of the Conservative party's rethink in the wake of its electoral defeat in 1945, Quintin Hogg (now Lord Hailsham) (1947) suggested that "the nation, not the class struggle, is . . . at the base of Conservative political thinking". In the period of so-called "consensus" both political parties were required to engage issues of nationality and nationhood in response to the predominantly "black" post-war immigration and the perceived threat to race relations in certain parts of the country. More recently, the "new racism" has emphasized the continuity of shared language, customs and institutions, "cultural codes of behaviour and expectations which are exclusionary towards the claims of black people" (Saggar 1992). By adding "nation" to the interconnected themes of work and family, it has been suggested, "we can be led towards a deeper understanding of the differential impact of welfare policies, to a more complex picture of the gains won and the losses suffered by the working class as a result of the ways in which the welfare state in Britain has developed" (Williams 1989).

It is generally agreed that one of the positive features of that development has been the strengthening of "claims based upon the equality of citizenship". But "not all those living within a given territory have counted equally as 'members of the nation' or as citizens, and not everybody has enjoyed the same rights of access to the Welfare State" (Pierson 1991). Such a conclusion goes beyond the identification of examples of racial discrimination practised by individual staff in welfare agencies. It suggests, rather, the existence of a structural dimension in "the hostility which immigrants and their British born descendants have had to endure." (Holmes 1991). In their study of Sparkbrook in Birmingham published in the 1960s, Rex & Moore (1967) drew attention to the way in which black people and Asians were discriminated against in the public housing sector, just as much or more than they were in the private market. "The working class through the Labour party had developed the council housing system to ensure housing rights for its own members. It now used . . . 'usurpatory closure' to deny the rights which it had won to newcomers" (Rex 1988). A more recent study (Amin with Oppenheim 1992) has indicated a variety of measures in the social security system, such as residence requirements, the "public funds" test and rules on sponsorship, all of which serve to "discriminate both directly and indirectly against people from ethnic minorities". The same report also highlights how Beveridge's contributory, insurance based system of income maintenance may work against the interests of people from ethnic minorities who tend disproportionately to be employed in lower paid jobs and subject to higher risks of unemployment. Because contributions are now earnings related, "people in lower paid jobs take longer to satisfy the contribution conditions", and because of their concentration in low paid work, and the likelihood that they will have interrupted work histories, it is women from ethnic minorities who are most likely to be excluded from the insurance sector of social security.

The employment issue transcends its relationship to the social security system, however, and has been central to the immigrant experience since the Second World War. Successive writers (Braham et al. 1992, Saggar 1992,

Skellington 1992) have addressed the interrelated themes of the pattern of employment (and unemployment) of particular migrant groups together with the fact that, during the 1950s especially, immigration was encouraged "specifically to resolve labour shortages in certain sectors of the economy" (Solomos 1993). But even in that period "migrants moved into public sector employment which was falling behind private industry in wage levels and into industrial jobs with longer hours, shiftwork or unpleasant conditions" (Brown 1992), often in sectors of the economy such as manufacturing which have subsequently steadily declined. At that time racial discrimination in employment was still lawful: it remained so until 1968. By the 1980s significant changes had taken place in both the migrant population and economic conditions. In contrast to the "full employment" of the 1950s, the 1980s experienced the highest levels of unemployment since the 1930s. Legal discrimination in employment had been unlawful for over a decade and, moreover, the black and Asian population had become a largely settled population of families for whom migration was mostly a memory. In relation to the experience of employment (and unemployment), however, a recent review of the evidence (Brown 1992) has suggested that while an increasing diversity has occurred in the pattern of ethnic minority employment "earlier injustices and imbalances continue to set the boundaries within which change can occur".

It has been suggested that such a pattern of employment disadvantage embodies longer established perceptions and experiences. In discussing employment within the NHS Williams (1989) points out

> . . . that the racist image of the Black woman as servant is as strong as that of carer in the acceptance of Black women in domestic, nursing and cleaning roles. To that stereotypical image from Britain's colonial past can be added the particular circumstances of immigration in the 1950s. That "migration" . . . was the consequence of a labour shortage, and did not put the minorities on an equal footing with whites – rather . . . it established the inequalities that have persisted since. (Brown 1992)

Nor can the existence of discrimination or disadvantage be separated from the politicization of immigration. Solomos (1993) has argued that in the post-war period, the state "far from simply responding to outside pressures played a central role in defining both the form and content of policies and the wider political agendas". In the specific context of the immigration from the "New Commonwealth" that developed in the 1950s, state activity then and subsequently has oscillated between controlling the numbers of those legally entitled to settle in the United Kingdom and attempts to create more harmonious relations between "host" society and minority ethnic groups. The first post-war imposition of immigrant controls occurred in the Commonwealth Immigrants Act 1962, although recent research has shown how the Conservative governments at various times in the 1950s sought to restrict entry into the United Kingdom, despite the labour shortages of the period. But in that decade "the terms of the political debate were by no means fixed purely by political party ideologies and there was opposition from both Conservative and Labour politicians to the call for controls and the abandonment of the free entry principle" (Solomos 1993). While sections of the Labour party "took an initial principled stand" (Holmes 1991) against the racism implicit in the legislation, when they returned to power in 1964 under the new leadership of Harold Wilson, they retained the Act and became increasingly committed to firm controls, an issue that continued into the Conservative legislation of 1971 that further redefined British citizen-ship. Public opinion and electoral expediency are usually cited as the reasons for Labour's move towards the longer tradition of immigration control that had characterized certain sections of the Conservative party since the late 1940s. It created in the process something of a bipartisan consensus.

From the 1960s, however, the immigration issue was constructed not only in terms of numbers but in relation to the potential strains for the infrastruc-ture of welfare services, in education, housing and employment; and much was made of the predisposition to criminal activity among certain sectors of the immigrant population. During its period in government in the 1960s Labour introduced a series of measures designed to reduce tension and improve race relations. Legislation was introduced designed to make racial discrimination illegal; organizations such as the Community Relations Com-mission, promoting racial harmony, were established; and extra resources were provided to local authorities in order to help meet the specific needs of ethnic minority groups. They may have represented "the liberal hour" (Deakin 1970) in race relations, "a unique period in which the civil and economic rights of black people were given some degree of priority by central government" (Saggar 1992). But other assessments are more critical. "Liberal" initiatives operated within the on-going framework of control, as the issue of the Kenyan Asians in the late 1960s made clear. For Rex, one of the consequences of the new initiatives was the redefinition of racial discrimination into "the more readily and easily understood problem of disadvantage" (Rex 1988), a dimension it has subsequently retained in the area of urban policy. Solomos (1993), in addition, sees in the liberal measures the primacy of political expediency rather than any commitment to justice and equality.

The period of so-called "consensus" was also a period of substantial bipartisan agreement on immigration issues and the way in which that debate was politically structured. But if there was substantial interparty agreement, there is also evidence of intraparty conflict.

Thatcherism and the welfare state

The debate

The values of Thatcherism appeared to challenge the principles implicit in the classic welfare state. Yet social expenditure continued to rise, the level of taxation increased and significant continuities with the past persisted. Nonetheless, especially after the Conservatives' third election victory in 1987, new policy initiatives were introduced that have created a more market orientated welfare system. Paradoxically, while they have espoused the consumer interest they have also increased central regulatory control.

A populist, pragmatic ideology, Thatcherism was composed of a variety of divergent strands: the fusion of neoliberal ideas concerning the supremacy of the market with the more "traditional" Conservative concerns such as law and order, patriotism, defence and security. This paradoxical alliance Gamble has termed "the free economy and the strong state" (Gamble 1988). This section aims to outline some of the central tenets of Thatcherism, its emergence in the 1970s and its impact on the welfare state.

Mrs Thatcher became leader of the Conservative party in 1975 and Prime Minister in 1979, a post she held until ousted by her own party in November 1990. She has frequently been described as more an instinctual than an intellectual politician. Nonetheless, despite the continuing disagreement about the coherence of the Thatcherite ideology, Wilding (1992) has identified several of its key facets. These encompass the challenge to collectivism, the promotion of markets, the new managerialism, cutting expenditure, the reduced role for local authorities, changes in aims, purposes and values, centralization, the mixed economy of welfare and the regulatory state.

Specific influences on this formidable programme have been varied: Enthoven's views about the internal market in the NHS, for example. But in

18

its early emerging configuration two main influences can be identified: Hayek and Friedman. There is a clear relationship between the Hayekian critique of socialist planning that negated individual freedom and restricted choice, and the Thatcherite commitment to roll back the frontiers of the state and set the people free. From the American economist Milton Friedman came another major challenge to the post-war settlement: the notion that inflation and not unemployment was the principal enemy. "Suddenly Keynes and Keynesianism had become dirty words" (Seldon 1991). Any policies involving the government in fine-tuning the economy in order to maintain employment levels were now perceived to lead only to inflation and inflationary expectations: a point made most forcefully by James Callaghan the Labour Prime Minister to his party conference in 1976. In this monetarist respect, Thatcherism predates Thatcher. Its implications were, however, to be worked out most fully during the 1980s. Since the "cure" for inflation lay in tight control of the money supply, there were implications for both the "corporatism" of the post-war settlement and the size and scale of the public sector.

Such a radical programme in economic and social policy was inevitably controversial. Three specific sources of opposition can be identified. In each case their influence was lessened or altered.

From its inception, professionals were an integral element in the wide range of services encompassing the welfare state. Increasingly, during the 1980s they were depicted as part of the non-productive public sector, a powerful constraint on change, acting more in their own interests than those of their clients and supporters of big government. For the Conservatives "the backlash against professionalism . . . had the advantage of appearing to offer a coherent alternative to the corporate high spending welfare state and to the Keynesian management of the economy which it claimed had failed" (Perkin 1990). The "corporatism" that had provided a place for professional providers in policy discussions was increasingly replaced by "conviction politics" and "transmission by think tank" (Self 1993). The Institute of Economic Affairs, the Centre for Policy Studies and the Adam Smith Institute "provided a vital arena for fusing academic theories with practical policies and for spreading the new gospel among politicians, officials, academics and the media" (Self 1993). But, furthermore, the environment of professional practice also changed. The emphasis on contract tendering, and quasi market competition in public services, as well as value for money and management practices imported from the private sector, fundamentally challenged the public service ethos as it was defined and practised in earlier decades (Hoggett 1991).

The civil service was also regarded sceptically. "Informed by experience and their liberal/conservative ideology, Mrs Thatcher and many of her Party colleagues mistrusted the civil service upon their election and regarded it as a parasitical organization" (Massey 1993). In fact the entrenched traditions of the civil service have been seen by both incoming Conservative and Labour governments since the war as a block to certain elements of their pro-gramme. But during the 1980s a significant change was introduced into its management. A report produced by the Efficiency Unit recommended the separation of executive operations from policy work. While the latter remains the responsibility of government departments, the executive opera-tions have been "hived off" to departmental agencies such as the Social Security Benefits Agency. Such agencies remain under arm's length minis-terial supervision but are free to manage their own day to day business within a framework negotiated between "agency, department and Treasury that sets targets and establishes performance indicators" (Gray & Jenkins 1993).

Local authorities, especially those controlled by Labour, represented the third locus of opposition to the Thatcherite programme. Pilloried publicly as "loony left" councils providing public funding for a whole variety of what were presented as "minority interests", the challenge between public services and market solutions was epitomized for much of the 1980s in the conflictual relationship between local authorities and central government. Central gov-ernment's answer was to abolish the metropolitan councils created only ten years before and transfer their powers to other bodies. But the 1980s also witnessed the progressive tightening of financial resources available from central government to local authorities to fund the services for which they were responsible, such as education and the personal social services. Its effect was to alter the balance of power between Whitehall and Town Hall in favour of the centre, a tendency that was also evident in measures such as the 1988 Education Act, the sale of council houses and the contracting out of local authority services.

As an alternative vision, elements of the Thatcherite agenda gained increasing legitimacy during the late 1970s as Britain became locked into the apparently intractable combination of rising unemployment and escalating inflation, low productivity, declining industrial investment and profitability and heightened industrial conflict. The impact of the oil price rise imposed by the oil producing countries in 1973 and the Labour government's shift in the direction of monetarism have already been noted. But the welfare state was also subject to other criticisms. The Oxford economists Bacon and Eltis (1976) argued that ever increasing public welfare expenditure had deflected resources from manufacturing industry on which, they argued, long-term economic prosperity and successful international competitiveness depended. There was also much contemporary discussion of government "overload". Paradoxically, democracy had both created increased demands on government and yet "severely restricted government's capacity – its authority and freedom – to act" (Mishra 1984). The fear was of ungovernability and the loss of legitimacy, exacerbated by the conditions of economic recession. "Slimming the state" looked a credible alternative.

Popular discussion of the welfare state in this period focused also on its beneficiaries. The tabloid press, in particular, highlighted the issue of welfare "scroungers" living a life of luxury on the dole (Golding & Middleton 1982). The issue is not whether the stories were accurate (in many cases they appeared not to be). It is that "scrounger phobia" dented the commitment of hard working, tax paying citizens (many lower income households were brought into the taxation system for the first time in the 1970s) to the principles as well as the practices of the welfare state and created the "Why work?" syndrome of that period. Another variant of the "popular experience" interpretation argued that

> The actual experience which working people have had of the corporatist state has not been a powerful incentive to further support for increases in its scope. Whether in the growing dole queues or in the waiting rooms of an overburdened National Health Service or suffering the indignities of Social Security, the corporatist state is increasingly experienced by them not as a benefice but as a powerful bureaucratic imposition on the people. (Hall 1985)

That perception, that public services were unhelpful and demeaning, became the springboard to a new perspective in which choice and freedom would be the hallmarks: at least for those able to afford them.

Whatever their relevance to the issues of the late 1970s, Thatcherite ideas have sustained electoral support for the Conservative party for a formidably long period of recent British history. That, of course, may owe more to a weak and divided opposition, as the Labour party was in the first half of the 1980s, as well as to "scare tactics" about tax rises during election campaigns, not to mention the "first past the post" system of electoral representation.

Yet during the 1980s, surveys about values showed that the Conservative party had failed to win the hearts and minds of most voters.

Polls suggested that on the whole the British wanted a society in which the state provided welfare rather than leaving individuals to look after themselves; they preferred a managed economy rather than a free market one. (Butler & Kavanagh 1992)

But in the future, it has been suggested, "elections will turn more than ever on the state of the economy", and increasingly that will depend "on international forces beyond the control of any British government" (Crewe 1993).

The issue that remains to be explored concerns the ways in which the varied ideological dimensions of Thatcherism impacted upon the welfare state. Was the result its destruction at the hands of expenditure cuts and progressive privatization or its restructuring?

There is an increasing consensus among social policy commentators that of the features of the post-war settlement "only the Welfare State survived largely intact into Mrs Thatcher's third term of office. But after 1987 even this last bastion of consensus came under attack" (Seldon 1991). This, of course, is not to deny the impact that the first two Thatcher administrations had on the welfare state: the sale of council houses, tax and social security changes, and reductions in public spending whose effects in the closure of wards of NHS hospitals and lengthening waiting lists, for example, attracted much media coverage. Sullivan (1992) suggests that popular opinion saved the welfare state from its potential destruction, although Deakin (1993) believes that this popularity has not saved it from the restructuring that began after the Conservative's third election victory in 1987. This "high noon of the government of Margaret Thatcher" (Morgan 1990) produced a more radical welfare state agenda, centring on competition, quasi or internal markets, opt-outs from local or district health authority control, the 1988 reform of education and the 1990 changes to the NHS, and the delivery of community care. The distinguishing features of the new managerialism that has accompanied this restructuring of state welfare services have included "the decentralization of day to day administration, the use of markets as the chief mechanism for resource allocation, greater responsiveness to the demands of consumers and an extended role for the private and voluntary sectors" (Taylor-Gooby & Lawson 1993). Several of these themes are treated in relation to individual service sectors in chapters later in this book. Their potential for future change is explored in Chapter 10 and critically assessed in Chapter 11.

There can be little doubt that Thatcherism represented a major transformation in British politics. "Both on the right and left the celebration of Thatcherism is a rejection of the social democratic consensus" (Taylor 1993).

Crewe suggests that John Major's replacement of Margaret Thatcher has "pushed both major parties back to the pragmatic centre ground of British politics". This, however, is not the centre ground of the post-war settlement of welfare Keynesianism "but a post-Thatcher settlement of the 'social market' within the European Community, in which the state's role is limited to the supply side of the economy and selective targeted welfare" (Crewe 1993). In interpreting the recent past the issue remains of the precipitants of change. An international assessment concludes that the changed political agenda of the 1980s "had more to do with the fundamental economic changes of the time than it did with the particular set of policy prescriptions that the radical right was advancing" (Glennerster & Midgley 1991). Similar changes to those introduced in Britain by the Thatcher Governments were also happening in many other countries. But if, for whatever reason, the post-war settlement is so extensively discredited, the issue for the future of welfare is about both values and management, market and state. Paradoxically, in that discussion a longer historical view that encompasses Britain before 1945 may not be inappropriate.

Gender and the welfare state

During the 1980s the gender analysis of welfare became the dominant perspective in the academic study of social policy. The Beveridge settlement was shown to discriminate against women in the social security system, while policies designed to promote community – rather than institutional – care posed additional burdens on women as carers in the home and called into question the political commitment to equal opportunities between men and women.

Since the end of the Second World War, there has been a paradox in women's experience. Employment opportunities have enormously expanded and their participation in the formal labour market has dramatically increased. This is not unrelated to the fact that the development of domestic appliances and their widespread availability has taken much of the time-consuming drudgery out of work in the home. "Full employment and higher living standards after the War together with the introduction of the National Health Service in 1948 brought incalculable gains for women's health" (Thane 1988).

On the other side of the equation, a different picture emerges: of women's greater income insecurity throughout the life cycle; a differential access to resources whether from the state or in terms of household resources; the persisting poverty of households headed by single women, whether of working age or in retirement; a health care system that has been criticized for trivialising women's problems of ill health (not least in relation to mental health); and a role that may have expanded to include work outside the home but in which women continue to bear a major share of domestic tasks and responsibilities, not least in relation to the home based work of tending and care. These are some of the elements encapsulated in the description of "the great majority of women . . . trapped in a vicious circle of domestic responsibilities and low paid, low status employment" (Lewis & Piauchaud 1987).

One of the contributions of the variety of analyses (Williams 1989) that comprise the feminist perspective concerns the relationship between women, work and welfare. This begins to explain the paradox that has just been discussed. But it also throws into relief the assumptions of gender relations and family structure on which the welfare state was created.

Since the end of the Second World War women have increasingly worked outside the home. Just over 70 per cent of all women of working age (between 16 and 59) in early 1993 were employed on some basis. Whereas at the end of the 1950s women accounted for less than one in three of all workers, they currently represent almost one in two of the labour force (Sly 1993). This increased female participation rate in the formal economy is the outcome of a variety of factors and their interrelationship. But it represents especially the shift of the British economy from its manufacturing base to the service sector. By 1992 only one fifth of all employees were in manufacturing; nearly three quarters were in the service sector (Social Trends 1993). But in that sector women predominate: 83 per cent of working women had jobs in the service sector in early 1993 compared with 56 per cent of men (Sly 1993).

In the process of increasing job opportunities for women, the expansion of welfare services has played an important role. "The welfare state is largely provided for, and by women" (Pierson 1991). The paradox is that welfare work often represents a transfer into the paid employment sector of the gender specific attributes, such as caring, traditionally associated with women in the home. "Women's labour is the key in the provision of welfare state services but women are still disproportionately concentrated in the least rewarded jobs" (Mayo & Weir 1993). Men disproportionately tend to be in managerial positions, while women are far more numerous in positions of direct service delivery such as health visitors, home care workers, nurses and social workers.

married women + emp⁵

Another emergent trend has been the increase in the proportion of married women in paid employment. Between 1951 and 1993 the proportion of the female workforce made up of married women rose from 38 per cent to 70 per cent (Lewis 1992, Social Trends 1993). Recent research (Dex 1988) however, suggests the pervasiveness of the view among both men and women that a married woman's primary responsibility is to home and family, with their wage-earning secondary to that of their husband's. Many of the terms, conditions and wages of the "flexible" part-time labour market are predicated on the assumption that they will be filled by "secondary workers".

But another feature, especially in the second half of the 1980s, was "the enormous and unprecedented increase in the numbers of mothers of young children who [became] waged workers": a phenomenon considerably at variance to the "strong appeals to the ideal of the traditional nuclear family" (Macdowell 1993) that characterized much of the political rhetoric on matters of social policy. Increasingly, "family members were left to work out their own solutions to the problems of combining paid and unpaid work . . . Issues of reproduction, including child care and the needs of other dependent relatives, were primarily regarded as matters of private concern rather than of collective responsibility" (Lewis 1993).

Women's increased entry into paid employment since the Second World War has "masked significant changes between women as well as between women and men" (Mayo & Weir 1993). The contrast is between the "career woman" and the casual, part-time worker. Women in the former category are

> . . . more likely to be in a position to afford full-time child care which, in turn, enables them to avoid career breaks and part-time work. Conversely . . . women in routine clerical and unskilled manual work, the more typical occupations for women, are precisely those . . . most likely to become trapped in low paid and casualised part-time work to fit in with their caring responsibilities and most likely to be adversely affected by reductions in public services such as local authority nurseries and holiday play schemes. (Mayo & Weir 1993)

In addition, part-time work, which represents an increasing share of women's paid employment (Employment Department Group 1993), may entail lower rates of pay (potentially, therefore reinforcing women's dependency in marriage) and the need to work antisocial hours. It offers less job security and fewer employment and social security rights, not least in relation to pensions. The insurance sector of the income maintenance scheme is

P/time work

25

"not well organised to deal with intermittent workers or those in-part time jobs – just the type of employment which is . . . very much on the increase particularly among women" (Millar 1989).

The notion that women's work is secondary employment has an especial significance for women who live alone: both single women and the increasing number of lone mothers. A number of elements flow into the recent (early 1990s) political construction of "lone parenthood". The increase in the number of marriages ending in divorce – from 28,000 in 1951 to 152,000 in 1988; the Conservative government's rhetoric about "traditional" family values; the rising proportion of dependent children living in lone parent families; the rising costs of the social security budget and the American debate on "the underclass" which, in Murray's (1990) formulation gives a central place to illegitimacy as "the best indicator of an underclass in the making". The issue of lone parenthood is in practice overwhelmingly that of lone mother families. Such families have presented governments with a long-standing ambiguity: "whether to treat these women as mothers or as workers, in other words whether to promote dependence on the state or the labour market" (Lewis 1992). In theory, modern welfare states may have tended towards the view that "women's primary duty is motherhood", yet in practice "their access to social welfare programmes has been, as per Beveridge's proposals, determined by marriage rather than motherhood" (Lewis 1992). Beveridge himself discussed the issue of marital breakdown and favoured the introduction of a separation benefit as a means of replacement income. His proposal for such a benefit, however, "floundered over the issue of fault". As a result, lone mothers are excluded from the national insurance benefits system and have to resort to second class social assistance programmes. But women also find the cost of child care arrangements or its availability a barrier to paid employment. Financial assistance introduced in the 1993 budget to help with such costs may extend the choices available to lone mothers and offer the beginnings of a route out of the poverty of lone parenthood. A similar objective was implicit in the establishment of the Child Support Agency designed to transfer responsibility from publicly financed services to absent fathers. In attempting to do so, however, it has produced significant levels of opposition from both women and men.

There are elements of both continuity and change in women's experience in the welfare state. But there can be little doubt that patterns of difference between women have become of greater significance. Such differences are related primarily to their differential positions within or outside the paid employment sector and the opportunities or restrictions on choice that

26

welfare states creates dependency

ensue. Such an increasing diversity of experience may carry not inconsiderable implications for the support among women for the principles and practices of a universal and solidaristic welfare state. That same welfare state since the Second World War has expressed a continuing set of assumptions about women as wives, mothers and workers. But in the intervening 50 years change and diversification have increasingly been the world of women's experience at home, in employment and in family and household structures.

In this chapter, each of the sections analyzing the welfare state in relation to class, race and gender have treated those dimensions separately. But, as other writers have pointed out, in many respects they are interrelated structural dimensions of disadvantage and inequality that have persisted despite the promised universalism and social citizenship implicit in the welfare state. The debate about the future of welfare is inevitably structured by the varying assessments of its past performance: with what it has accomplished, as well as the objectives and aspirations it has failed to achieve. "One of the tensions that still remains unresolved is how to develop universal welfare policies which are neither monolithic nor uniform but which are able to meet the diversity and difference of people's welfare needs in forms which do not reproduce difference in unequal ways" (Williams 1993)

The debate about the future of welfare is also set within a framework of change: in employment patterns, family structure and population profile; in electoral support and political legitimacy; in values and purposes as well as the changing context of national and international economic decisions. "Even if the structure of welfare services had been ideal for the 1950s or 1960s, these changes raise questions about whether they now need to be adapted to deal with a different world from that envisaged by Beveridge and others fifty years ago" (Hills 1993).

Suggested reading

The studies by Hill (1993) and Lowe (1993) are indispensable. The general history of the post-war period is well covered by Kenneth O. Morgan (1984, 1990). Cronin (1991) is especially strong on economic policies, but aspects of social policy are also discussed. An authoritative review of the British welfare state since 1974 is provided by the contributors to Hills (1990). The same author has also discussed *The future of welfare* (1993). For the analysis of the welfare state in terms of class, gender and race see Cochrane & Clarke (1993), Pierson (1991) and Williams (1989).

CHAPTER 2
Education:
the changing balance of power

John Barnes

In the last five years, "educational issues have acquired an almost un-precedented prominence on the British political agenda" (Broadfoot 1991). Although the 1988 Act is unquestionably the most important, not a parliamentary session has passed since it was enacted without a new law being added to the statute book. The local education authorities (LEAs) have lost control of their polytechnics, further education and a sizeable number of schools and they have been forced to contract out many of their services. A new type of school, the City Technology College, has been created and more recently the concept of bringing failing schools under new management further varies the pattern of school provision. The polytechnics have been rechristened and brought together with the older universities under the aegis of a new funding council (HEFC), replacing the separate funding councils established by the 1988 Act. Funding councils have also been created to deal with the further education sector and grant maintained schools. A National Curriculum Council and a Schools Examination and Assessment Authority were created to develop in detail a national curriculum and new methods of assessing it, and have since been abolished in favour of a single Schools Curriculum and Assessment Authority (SCAA). The National Council for Vocational Qualifications (NCVQ), created in 1986 to provide a single framework for all vocational qualifications, whether obtained at work or in an FE college, has been given the task of creating a new set of General National Vocational Qualifications (GNVQs) to parallel GCSE and GCE A level examinations. No alternative qualifications can now be offered without the sanction of either SCAA or NCVQ. The independent examination boards have been made subject to a mandatory code of practice and both SCAA and NCVQ operate in a quality assurance role. Her Majesty's Inspectorate (HMI), once an important part of the Department for Education, has been hived off as an independent agency (OFSTED) to preside over the process of school inspection. This is now to be carried out more extensively and regularly than at any time since the nineteenth century. New methods of funding education at every level have been set in place and they have in common some, though not total, adherence to quasi market principles.

This is a formidable body of legislation, and it is little wonder that students, faced with it and a rapidly changing educational scene, are inclined to minimize the earlier pace of change, to emphasize the way in which consensus has given place to conflict, and to ignore the fact that education, at least since the Second World War, has always been an important part of the political scene and has been shaped to a very considerable extent by political considerations. The 1944 Act, which largely created the framework within which the educational world operates and that dominated the scene for the next 40 years, was itself a compromise, put on the statute book by the wartime coalition government, but significantly modified in its operation by the need to rely on the LEAs and on the teaching profession to translate the legislation into practice. Secretaries of State who neglect the question of implementation are liable to find out the hard way, as John Patten did over testing in the summer of 1993, that they are very dependent upon the consent or at least the acquiescence of teachers, heads and school governing bodies.

Policy networks

Policy in the educational field is made at different levels, in Cabinet Committee, by the Department, in the funding councils, in statutory bodies like the Schools Curriculum and Assessment Authority, the National Council for Vocational Qualifications and the Office of Standards in Education, in LEAs and at the level of the individual institution and its component departments. To complete the picture of those involved in the educational field, one would have to list other providers like the diocesan authorities of the Church of England and the Roman Catholic Church and the Pre-School Playgroups Association, the Independent Schools Information Service and Headmasters' Conference (HMC), which speak for the private sector, the various teachers' associations, the national bodies speaking for parents and governors, the examination boards and other awarding bodies, pressure groups like the Campaign for the Advancement of State Education, the education correspondents and the specialist education press. These bodies are linked in what may be described as a policy network or, more accurately, a whole series of them. What links these organizations is their dependence on one another for resources, whether financial, organizational, expertise or communication.

In education, policy networks differ in terms of their relative integration, stability and exclusiveness and a number operate in parallel. The linkages between the Department, local authority associations and teaching unions for example, operate alongside both a professional and a party political network. Nor is the assumption justified that central government (to be more precise the lead department in each policy area) is the focus and dominant element in each network (Rhodes 1988, Rhodes & Marsh 1992). Policy decisions can be the end product of local decision-making, while professional interests or producers can also dominate a network. Curriculum development, for example, was very much a professional matter until the mid 1970s, led by the teacher dominated Schools Council.

In the immediate post-war years, a near classic example of a policy community was in operation, characterized by a process of elite accommodation in which three men met regularly, the consensus reached determining the course of policy. Other interests were either excluded wholly from what was going on or marginalized. The outcome clearly suited the three parties involved. They were the Permanent Secretary of the DES, the secretary of the Association of Education Committees (AEC), and the General Secretary of the National Union of Teachers (NUT). The balance of power survived even a major change imposed by the Treasury and the Ministry of Housing and Local Government: the shift from percentage grants in aid of educational spending to the block grant system in 1958, which all three resisted. It also proved resistant to changes in the terms of trade sought by the Department.

Two factors especially operated to break up this tight knit community. First was the end of the AEC's role. Local authorities saw the need to speak jointly to central government on a whole range of issues, but counties, municipalities and districts had never seen eye to eye, hence the existence of three separate associations, each with a different point of view and a different financial case to put. Although the AEC was a powerful counsellor in regard to government, it was widely regarded in the local authority associations as a "cuckoo in the nest", the more dangerous since education was the largest spender. Other services competing for their share of block grant resented the semi-autonomous role Education Committees appeared to claim. After local government reorganization in 1974, the Association of County Councils (ACC) and the Association of Metropolitan Authorities (AMA) created their own education committees at the expense of the AEC. The Council of Local Education Authorities, drawn from these committees and speaking for them where there was a common interest, retained something of the AEC's role for the next decade. With party politics increasingly dominant, it became irrelevant, and the intergovernmental network (in so far as it operated), comprising the rival ACC and AMA, offered the Department for Education (DfE) considerable opportunities to divide and rule.

The second factor was the changed balance of power between the NUT and rival unions. As the largest body of teachers, the NUT exercised very considerable influence for almost three decades after the war. By the 1970s, however, the National Association of Schoolmasters, under the leadership of Terry Casey, began to challenge the NUT's dominant position. Their rivalry led to a more abrasive trade unionism and precipitated the creation of the Professional Association of Teachers that gained from abjuring strike action. Clearly, this fragmentation of teacher representation has been a major factor weakening their overall influence. Head teachers, meanwhile, also have their own associations: the National Association of Head Teachers and the Secondary Heads Association.

Although the NUT was a powerful advocate for the profession, teachers have always been part also of a series of overlapping professional networks linking them, for example, through their subject associations, their role as examiners, and their participation on the subject advisory committees of the various quangos set up by the Secretary of State, linking also HMI with local inspectorates and advisory services, and with senior education officers (almost all former teachers). These networks were more powerful when the curriculum was regarded as their own "secret garden" and teachers dominated the Schools Council and its thinking, but the influence of these professional networks remains greater than most commentators are prepared to recognize. Much of the detail of the National Curriculum, for example, has been filled in by members of these professional networks, while the way in which it is translated into effective practice is almost entirely in the hands of the teaching force.

What to many educationists are purely professional networks have taken on, so far as the "new right" are concerned, the stigma of a producer lobby (Henney 1984). Public choice theorists, whether of the left or the right, offer good grounds for believing that the ways in which professionals model the education process articulate, particularly, the self-interest of those concerned. Slowly, but gaining pace since the 1970s, associations of governors

31

and of parent/teacher associations have emerged to reflect other interests in the process. Their links with their constituents seem as yet relatively weak and their influence diminished as a result. Nevertheless, with current political argument running in the direction of "consumerism", their potential for acquiring legitimacy and influence is clear. To some extent the battle that the government lost in the summer of 1993 was one for their hearts and minds. Arguably, therefore, what was once a policy community has become an issue network, relatively accessible, offering the government more chance to manoeuvre, but with outcomes more variable and uncertain.

These observations suggest that the classic model of the policy process in education persists (Kogan 1978), although it derived from experience of the years 1955–75, and its emphasis therefore was on the partnership between the Department of Education (DE), local education authorities (LEAs) and the professionals in the field. Given that these are not all the groups that might have been involved, the model is best characterized as one of skewed pluralism.

Pluralism

Pluralists argue that it is possible to assess the concentration of power in any community by looking to see who wins in decision-making conflicts and they conclude that power is diffused among many different groups, and that it is arranged non-hierarchically and competitively. In the classic pluralist model, political outcomes are the result of government trying to resolve the competing demands of the various groups: in this process the "state" becomes almost indistinguishable from the interplay between the various organized interests.

Kogan rightly suggested three significant reinforcements to pluralism within the education system as he knew it. First, the partners recognized themselves to be in partnership and that their roles were complementary. This coloured their thinking and meant that DE was reluctant to move too readily into prescriptive mode. Secondly, the system enjoyed a very considerable degree of indeterminacy and it was therefore difficult for anyone to grasp, let alone plan, what might be involved in a change of policy. Finally, since the heart of the education process is to be found in the schools and in their classrooms, it is not that easy for the DE to make effective general policy, let alone implement it in any controllable way, should they wish to do so. Only the first of these points looks outmoded today.

Ministers and civil servants continue to find that the Department neither possesses nor controls all the resources necessary to accomplish its goals. To the extent that funds, facilities, information, personnel or other resources are deficient, it must enter into a relationship with other bodies to supply what is required. But that relationship is one of interdependence. At the centre the department fights for increased resources from the Treasury, although these are then channelled to the LEAs as part of a block grant in support of all local authority functions. That means a further struggle for the allocation of resources at local level, with distribution of the total allocated, once solely the function of the Education Committee, now subject to both regulations and guidance from the Department. The specific local formula, however, is a matter for local initiative and central ratification. The way in which those resources are further distributed within the school, the employment of heads and teachers, and the purchase of relevant books and equipment are matters for school governors, advised by the Head. The curriculum offered within the school, however, since 1988 has been heavily constrained, although not totally dominated, by the introduction of a nationally prescribed curriculum and the accompanying assessment regime.

This very considerable degree of interdependence does not preclude the possibility of conflict. The government's National Curriculum role is a powerful reminder, however, that the Department controls the legislative framework into which the system is set, as well as the process by which it is modified. It is therefore in a good position to shape the outcome, but is it determinate, as Kogan supposed? The radical reshaping of education law by Kenneth Baker and his successors was the culmination of considerable debate lasting two decades, but Julian Haviland's compilation of the results of the consultation done prior to the 1988 Act makes clear the extent to which the reforms were carried through without support from those making up the policy network, in some instances even without support from those whose party allegiance predisposed them to favour the government (Haviland 1988).

Given continued electoral support, the government can evidently determine most of the ground rules, but that does not render it immune from pressures, both direct and indirect, particularly from members of the governing party, the mood of the electorate, and demands from industry for the right kind of manpower. Since business is the principal vehicle not only for the provision of jobs but the economic growth upon which the expansion of public services exists and governments are judged, it requires no special insight to see why its influence is so considerable. The decision to shift

British education towards the "new vocationalism" in the late 1970s was the result of businessmen's dissatisfaction with the output from the schools and government consciousness that Britain was in increasingly rapid, if relative, economic decline and that most of its workforce lacked the skills necessary to economic regeneration. However, pluralism can be skewed in favour of other groups. The teachers themselves benefited when the curriculum from 1945 until well into the 1970s was characterized as being for professional judgement alone.

Valuable though the insights into policy-making afforded by neopluralism are, the importance of factors other than interests should not be discounted. The "party government model" of policy generation is illuminating, particularly in relation to areas seen as central in terms either of values or the logic of party competition. Powerful policy networks operate within parties also. The Conservative local government committee and conference, its policy liaison group, and the Conservative National Advisory Committee on Education have proved influential bodies (Knight 1992, Gyford & James 1983). There are parallel organizations in the Labour party.

The process by which the pursuit of comprehensive reorganization became a flowing tide that the Department was powerless to resist, but which it took a Labour government to make the norm, provides a good illustration of how the changing climate of ideas, local initiative and pressures, party ideology and party competition contributed to policy change. The comprehensive school became the dominant form of secondary school organization, but the type of comprehensive school that emerged was seldom that willed by the idealists who had first put the idea on the policy agenda. Policy outcomes rarely conform to those sought by particular actors in the process.

The last half century has been characterized by major shifts in policy, and radical changes also in the ways in which policy is developed. As a result, the initiative has shifted, first from the Ministry of Education to the local education authorities, and then, from the mid 1970s, back increasingly to the Department of Education. A distinction can be made between the first 25 years when a relatively tight knit policy community operated, at least so far as schools and further education were concerned, and the more recent period when a great many more actors impinge on the process and the Department's aspirations have grown.

Against that background, the rest of this chapter examines a number of themes in the past 50 years of educational history. These include the settlement introduced by the 1944 Education Act, the shift towards comprehensive schooling, the new vocationalism and the changes of the 1980s with their emphasis on school choice, parent power, local management and national curriculum.

The first phase: a tripartite system

The 1944 legislation that governed the system for almost fifty years was produced by the wartime coalition. It was designed to go through a Conservative dominated House of Commons and to meet a Prime Ministerial requirement that nothing controversial should disrupt the unity essential to winning the war. Apart from the exclusion of the independent sector from reform (its future was to be considered by a government-appointed commission, whose conclusions were never implemented), the Act nevertheless satisfied the widespread desire for educational reconstruction and went far enough to marginalize those, principally members of the Labour party, who wished for a much more radical shift in the direction of multilateral or comprehensive schools. Even the agreement reached with the providers of church schools, unpopular though it was with LEA officials, proved a durable compromise. Not until the 1970s were any serious misgivings voiced within the Labour party about the existence of "voluntary aided" schools, and in general church schools are attractive to parents.

The Act extended the principle of free secondary education, initially to the age of 15, to all pupils and established the modern distinction between primary and secondary schools. Both at the time and subsequently left-wing critics argued that it was the product of departmental thinking and was strongly coloured by the desire to maintain the existing social structure. They identify an implicit hierarchy of schools with the independent schools at the top, grant aided grammar schools under independent governors (direct grant schools) next, and then in the "maintained" (state) sector, grammar, technical and modern schools. The working class, they argue, was destined for the modern school where they would be prepared for the kind of jobs that would keep them in their place. Both the conclusions of the Norwood Committee, appointed to consider curriculum and examinations, and the design of the new GCE examination, which was taken at 16, one year after most children had left school, were seen to reinforce this hierarchical system. There were civil servants who thought that children naturally fell into the Platonic categories of gold, silver and lead, but in general neither their patterns of thought nor the issue on which they focused were those ascribed to them.

Radical critics believe that the process of differentiation is the cause of differences between children and that only by its elimination can equality of opportunity be achieved. They look not only to the comprehensive school but to an undifferentiated curriculum taught in mixed ability classes as the only acceptable pattern of reform (Simon 1991). Even within the Labour party this was never the majority view, nor has it ever prevailed among teachers. Initially the Labour party saw the multilateral school, which contained separate grammar, technical and modern streams within a common social grouping, as the way to maximize educational opportunity and deal with the distorting effects of social snobbery. Others, including R. A. Butler, agreed that it would be worth experimenting with an institution that allowed differentiation on grounds of ability and aptitude without forcing children to attend separate schools and wear different uniforms. But it is anachronistic to assert the virtual identity of multilateral and comprehensive schools at that time, and wrong to suggest that the Labour party were committed already to the comprehensive school.

The emergence of a tripartite system of grammar, technical and modern schools was not the product of Whitehall dominance over weak Labour ministers, nor was it the result of social prejudice. The principal objections to the multilateral school were threefold. Not the least important at a time when demographic pressures on the building programme were acute, was that it did not make the best use of existing buildings. But there were major doubts because such schools were untried and would inevitably be very large. The same objections were deployed against the comprehensive school when LEAs like the London County Council and Coventry made them part of their post-war plans. Significantly, the Department argued that selection would in any case continue within these schools. They also thought that schools worked best when they had a single specific aim or function.

If the absence of any change in policy when the Labour government took office in 1945 raises questions about the potency of the departmental view, or, more accurately perhaps, professional influence, the evidence contradicts any suggestion that Ellen Wilkinson was a weak minister, although her successor, George Tomlinson, can be seen as more ambassador for the Department than master of it. The man she chose as her Permanent Secretary saw no reason to interfere with the only successful model of state secondary education: "It would have been mad as well as impractical to scrap [it] in favour of any one alternative. It was right to expand it on a grand scale and make it available to all children who had the ability and aptitude to profit from it" (Redcliffe-Maud 1981). Most Labour-controlled LEAs also saw grammar schools as the best available route to social equality for the bright working class child. Ellen Wilkinson was therefore far from alone in resisting those in her party who wished to rush into change, but her vision of the future was the modern school, which would provide a liberal education free from the tyranny of examinations. If successful, they would evolve into the only mode of secondary education.

Crucial to understanding the possibilities as Ellen Wilkinson saw them was the Norwood Committee's recommendation that, with the exception of an examination at 18 for the purposes of university entrance, there should be no external examinations. However, parity of esteem between grammar and modern schools was destroyed by the decision in 1948 to include an ordinary level in the new GCE examination, initially to be taken by 16 year olds, but which rapidly became a school leaving examination, confined mainly to grammar schools. Parents saw examination success as the way to a secure job, and employers' attitude to the GCE examination confirms their realism.

Comprehensives become a party issue

Once in opposition, the Labour party made advocacy of the comprehensive school a central feature of their education policy (Barker 1972). Conservative ministers proved increasingly hostile to comprehensive schemes and the ability of the grammar schools to produce a genuine meritocracy appears to have strengthened official resistance to their destruction. However, little was done to tackle the increasingly low esteem in which modern schools were held. Instead the Department turned their minds to the further education system. In this they were at one with their minister, "the first . . . to assume that education was an economic investment" (Kogan 1971). David Eccles was keen to respond both to industrial pressure for more skilled manpower and parental disappointment with modern schools by developing "an alternative route to high qualifications and well paid jobs via secondary modern and technical schools and technical colleges" and by expanding technological education. Despite the financial problems of the government, Eccles, with Prime Ministerial backing, was able to make further education a priority, establish Colleges of Advanced Technology, and create new technological qualifications. His success may be measured in terms of the direct comparability between Britain and the United States so far as social mobility is concerned (Kerckhoff 1990), but the technical school fell victim to his desire to spread technical courses through all types of secondary school. Although educating only one pupil in 25, scarcely "appropriate to the needs of a commercial and industrial nation" (Venables 1955), they were appropriately orientated towards industry. This could irritate purists: schools were not "sub-assembly lines", Boyle said, and did not need to ape the technical colleges (Sanderson 1991).

Party conflict over secondary education set a term to consensus, although not until the Labour party, aiming to still persistent doubts about the concept among the leadership and in many LEAs, redefined comprehensive reorganization as the extension of "grammar school education" to all. Eccles and his successors were slow to react and ineffective when they did so. Their reluctance in the late 1950s to expand the number of grammar school places, the consequent extension of the GCE examination into modern schools, the disparities of grammar school provision from one LEA to another, and the inaccuracy of the selection system made the modern school the target of a middle class revolt. Academic research played a key part in changing the intellectual climate and legitimized their resentment. Sociologists, principally but not exclusively at the London School of Economics (LSE), identified apparent biases in the system against the working class while the errors in the testing process were highlighted by influential social psychologists. Boyle, when he became Minister in 1962, found plausible the academic contention that intelligence could be acquired; and his principal legislative legacy was provision for the middle school system, which was designed to minimize the size of comprehensive schools and make them more acceptable to his own party.

The education system was now operating in a very different way from that envisaged in the 1944 Act. Development plans were a dead letter: ministerial powers of approval and disapproval operated in regard to particular schools only. More important still, Maud's view that the curriculum was a matter for those who taught in the schools had become the prevailing wisdom. While the DE retained a tight hold on capital spending, its ministers lost an important battle over local government finance. They had wished to retain their ability to influence education spending through the percentage grant, but the Treasury in alliance with the Ministry of Housing and Local Government imposed the block grant system in 1958. While central initiatives were still possible, as the five year building programme to expand technical education shows, power had shifted towards the LEAs.

The forward planning of building programmes became the most obvious way in which the DE could influence the educational system, and *Technical education* (1956) (Cmd 9703) was followed by a further White Paper on school building in 1958, setting out a five year programme to complete the elimination of all-age schools and to improve science facilities. A further three year programme to cover the years 1965–8 followed in 1963, again with indications of the criteria that would govern successful LEA bids. By 1968 this device had taken on the shape of a three phase programme, a preliminary list approved against specific criteria seven to five years ahead of actual building, a design list a year in advance and a starts list. Given this degree of control, it is not surprising that, when Anthony Crosland decided in 1965 to promote comprehensive education, he relied on his control of the capital programme to achieve his aim.

The other mechanism used to promote policies was more traditional: the use of advisory committees appointed by the Minister and serviced by Departmental officials. The Central Advisory Councils for England and Wales were given a three year term and a specific remit after 1951. All but one of their subsequent reports, *Early leaving, 15 to 18, Half our future, Children and their primary schools* (Central Advisory Council for Education [England] 1954, 1959, 1963, 1967) were important planning documents, influencing the planned expansion of higher education, the decision by Edward Boyle to raise the school leaving age to 16, the setting up of educational priority areas by Tony Crosland and the commitment to universal nursery education made by Margaret Thatcher in 1972. They became a focus for debate, helped change the appreciative system of all those concerned, and induced consensus around their conclusions. They helped to build a policy community on which the DE could rely to deliver agreed policies.

The comprehensive revolution: from consensus to scepticism

In its early stages the comprehensive revolution was less a party product than the outcome of local pressure and LEA initiatives. Even before the Labour party came to power in 1964, the comprehensive tide was running strongly and the return of a Conservative government six years later could not halt, let alone reverse, what was happening. In the circumstances it might have been wiser for the Labour government not to have made comprehension a national political issue: as it was Crosland acted wisely in avoiding legislation and leaving considerable room for LEAs to decide on the scheme they wanted. The initial response from the Conservative opposition was to endorse the view that it was an issue for local decision.

By the end of the decade, however, attitudes were hardening, in part because of a growing conviction that progressive methods were lowering standards in both primary and secondary schools, but also from fears that the adoption of the comprehensive system would be followed by a shift to mixed ability teaching. A relatively small group of critics, some of them Labour supporters of working class origin, developed their critique in an increasingly sophisticated series of Black Papers (Cox 1992). They had few allies in the specialist educational press, but they strongly influenced the Conservative backbench education committee and many on the Conservative National Advisory Committee on Education (Knight 1992).

Three key developments accentuated the politicization of education and helped shift the balance of power within the system towards politicians and parents. First, the decision of Edward Short in 1969 to introduce legislation to make comprehensive education mandatory: this contributed to an atmosphere within the Conservative party that saw the increased politicization of local government as welcome. Local government reorganization and the reselection of County Councillors accelerated the process in shire counties, and foot-dragging over comprehensive reorganization turned into active resistance, coordinated by informal meetings of those concerned and encouraged by a marked shift in public opinion in favour of the grammar school, and, to a lesser extent, the selective system.

Secondly, the sheer size of the 11–18 comprehensives – many had 10 to 12 forms of entry – worried parents and created problems with their management and leadership. It took remarkable personalities to give such schools an effective lead. Judged on academic results the new system appeared successful. There was a steady rise in standards as measured by GCE results, and when the Certificate of Secondary Education was devised to provide a summation for pupils of lesser academic ability, that too showed a gratifying improvement in measured standards. The public remained sceptical, rightly perhaps, since comparisons with the tripartite system, more particularly as it evolved in those authorities that retained it, cannot be made with any confidence (Marks et al. 1983, Glennerster 1990b). The best comprehensives were excellent, but the press and public chose to focus on the failures, more particularly in the inner cities. It was soon to be clear from academic research that comprehensive schools varied greatly in effectiveness (Rutter et al. 1979, Smith & Tomlinson 1989).

For all its faults, selection had extracted able working class children from their locality and had educated them alongside their intellectual peers. The grammar school ethos involved setting a high value on education, expecting effort and rewarding achievement, and this too was helpful. Compelled to select their pupils on the basis of where they lived, comprehensive schools tended to become neighbourhood schools. Some flourished: with social trends set firmly towards home ownership, all too often house prices within catchment areas reflected their success. In many parts of the country middle class children attended predominantly middle class comprehensives. Since council houses tended to be grouped in large estates, the converse happened in working class areas. It could be said therefore that, except in predominantly rural areas, selection by class had replaced selection by merit. If the schools were good, this did not worry parents; but, where they were poor, choice seemed the only alternative to wealth as a means of escaping the prison of the geographical catchment.

The shift in attitudes towards comprehensive schools was fuelled thirdly by distrust of the progressive methods favoured by the idealist teachers, who, all too often, were the only teachers prepared to go to difficult areas, and it was accompanied by suspicions that the major shift in primary practice, inspired by the Plowden Committee, had some undesirable side effects. Stress on the uniqueness of the individual child and the ability of children to engage in an active process of learning meant that classes were treated "as a body of children needing individual and different attention". Theoretically teachers took into account each child's intellectual, emotional and physical development. Increasingly mixed ability classes and project work became the norm, although there were doubts already about the underpinning theory (Peters 1969). The ideology (for such it was) took deep root in the education departments of the teacher training colleges and attracted immediate hostility from the "Black Paperites", who called for more school based teacher training and rigorous testing at the ages of 7, 11 and 14 (Cox & Boyson 1975).

Enriching though it was, in the hands of too many primary teachers, active learning and discovery were accompanied by a lack of focus, structure and direction. Teachers found it impossible to give the individual attention to which they had been taught to aspire: and, when they did so, it was inevitably spread very thin. It was less than reassuring that the Assessment of Performance Unit found that large classes, where more formal teaching was essential, often performed best. As "the spotlight shifted to the curriculum as a whole, to its scope and balance, to consistency, continuity and progression, and to the place of subjects like science, the efficacy of the class-teacher system was open to question" (Alexander 1992). But HMI's attempt in 1978 to nudge the system into better structured and less circular topic work, properly conceived science teaching and consultant-led whole school curriculum planning proved ineffective in the face of LEA reluctance to abandon such an inexpensive system and the bias towards it in the primary school culture (Alexander 1984).

If Bennett's research into teaching styles, vulgarized by the press, focused doubts about the effectiveness of informal teaching (Bennett 1975), it was the William Tyndale affair in 1976 that showed how far some teachers were ready to take their progressive ideology. Press reports of their activities, and of the subsequent Inner London Education Authority (ILEA) inquiry, account for a marked shift in the political climate, which put teachers on the defensive and ensured that the Conservative party's emphasis on the need to maintain standards became the common currency of public debate.

The new vocationalism

In Downing Street the recognition that the Labour government needed to find a way of outflanking the Opposition on this question was reinforced by growing complaints from industry about the absence of basic skills in their young recruits (Donoughue 1987). The economic climate contributed greatly to what its proponents would describe as an onset of realism. The 1972 White Paper with its promise of improved pupil/teacher ratios, universal nursery education and the replacement of outdated primary schools was a victim of the "oil shock" in 1973–4. In the aftermath of the 1976 sterling crisis, five per cent was cut from education spending in a year and inflation imposed its own form of cut. But the system also faced devastating criticisms of its performance. Weinstock's savage attack, "I blame the teachers", in the *Times Educational Supplement* (1976) was followed by more measured criticism from the CBI and others, neatly summarized by Chitty – "unaccountable teachers, teaching an irrelevant curriculum to young workers who were poorly motivated, illiterate and innumerate" (Chitty 1988, Jamieson & Lightfoot 1982).

Callaghan's Ruskin College speech addressed these concerns and was largely responsible for the "new vocationalism" that dominated education and training for a decade and is still influential. The Department had a separate agenda. They had begun to revive their interest in the curriculum before James Hamilton became Permanent Secretary in 1976, but his belief that "the key to the secret garden of the curriculum must be found and turned" and that greater centralization was desirable drove them on (Fenwick & McBride 1981, Maclure 1983). The "Yellow Book", prepared as a brief for the Prime Minister and leaked in October 1976, signalled their concerns. In primary education a "corrective shift of emphasis" and a more systematic approach were needed. Secondary schools were undemanding and set inadequate standards, particularly in the formal subjects. Employers' complaints about the lack of basic mathematical skills as the basis for technical training were thought to be right and there was concern that too few pupils were opting for the scientific and technical subjects, essential to Britain's future. Teachers were inadequately qualified and had concerned themselves too much with preparing children for their place in society and not enough with preparation for the world of work. Was the time ripe therefore for the establishment of a core curriculum, the document asked, which would include vocational elements?

Although the "new vocationalism" owed much to the thinking of the Manpower Services Commission, the extent to which it was infused by a professional agenda, which "had been suppressed by the inertia of formal, academic traditions and the vested interests they had accreted" (Tomlinson 1989), further emphasizes the complexity of policy-making in a plural society. The explosion of knowledge, demands for new skills and knowledge in a changed social and economic structure, rapidly changing mores, and the inability of the "bottom 40 per cent" to respond effectively to what they were being taught made the curriculum problematic. A month before Callaghan's speech, a start was made on a joint HMI/LEA curriculum project to cover the ages 11–16 and this produced a series of influential reports, beginning with working papers, moving to a review of progress in 1981, and culminating in *Curriculum 11–16: towards a statement of entitlement* published in 1983 (DES 1983). As Tomlinson notes, "the notion of a broad and balanced curriculum, diversified according to individual pupil need, coherent as received by the pupil, and progressing in a planned way through time" is taken forward in the White Paper, *Better schools* in 1985 and in the opening section of the 1988 Act (Tomlinson 1989).

Capability became the new watchword, emphasizing that in addition to analysis and the acquisition of knowledge, a well-balanced education must include "the exercise of creative skills, the competence to undertake and complete tasks and the ability to cope with everyday life; and also doing these things in cooperation with others" (*Education for capability* 1978). There were overlaps with the idea of competency based education that found favour with the Employment Department (Cmnd 8455) and the development of programmes to give all under 18s some kind of education or training if they could not get a job were bedevilled by "turf fights" between the Department of Education and Science (DES) and the Manpower Services Commission

(MSC). Shirley Williams, then Secretary of State for Education, had envisaged that the education service and youth agencies would run such a programme, with the participation of employers. But the MSC argued successfully that the DES lacked the experience and ability to run such a scheme effectively, let alone introduce it with the necessary degree of urgency, and had no mechanism to ensure that money given to LEAs for the purpose would be spent on the scheme.

The final shape of the Technical and Vocational Education Initiative (TVEI) was, DES officials believed, a successful rearguard action to regain control of a programme approved by the Prime Minister, the head of the MSC, and their own minister, without their knowledge. It remains unclear whether Secretary of State for Employment David Young's threat to reintroduce technical schools under the MSC's aegis was simply intended to get the DES to act, or a genuine attempt to use the MSC as a vehicle to transform education. In the end, the planning and supervision of the scheme was done by a group dominated by educationists, but its funding remained with the MSC and schools were in effect contracted to deliver a programme against specific criteria. Despite criticisms that thought work experience, the teaching of technology and new forms of active learning were narrowing and threatened the whole comprehensive ethos (Golby 1985, Chitty 1986), teachers found in practice that the scheme gave them room to further their own agenda. Indeed, it proved so successful that the government resolved to extend it to all 14–18 year old students between 1985 and 1995.

Despite the approval for TVEI in *Better schools* (Cmnd 9469), there were obvious tensions between its approach, which emphasized active and collaborative learning and technology across the curriculum, and the subject based national curriculum introduced by the 1988 Act. These were accentuated by persisting problems in deciding what technology amounted to as a subject in its own right (Graham 1994). The compromise eventually agreed between the departments of state, with strong support from the National Curriculum Council (NCC), centred on the notion of cross curricular themes, but little has been done to develop them. However, it is likely that one outcome of the Dearing (1993) review will be further thought and debate about the needs of the 14–19 age group, both in schools and in further education.

Further education in the 1980s was heavily influenced by its dependence on the MSC for a substantial part of its funding, but its courses and clientele remained diverse and its shape was dependent also on local and institutional aspirations (Reeder 1979). The creation of the Business and Technician Education Council (BTEC) in 1976 had been intended to bring some order into the field on a national basis, with skill training central to TEC, and occupational socialization arguably the concern of BEC courses (Avis 1981). However, BEC courses, while basically vocational, were intended also to offer a broad education and, as such, made some headway in the schools. The result of a joint MSC/DES review of vocational qualifications in 1986 was the creation of a new body, the National Council for Vocational Qualifications (NCVQ) whose task was both to incorporate existing qualifications, wherever appropriate, into a national framework, operating at four distinct levels (five from 1989), and to work closely with the MSC and industry to foster the development of employment related standards for incorporation into that framework. The development of these competence based standards had obvious consequences for the curriculum, teaching styles and organization of FE Colleges (Burke 1989), but they were not really appropriate for schools.

The question of what was appropriate, particularly for the bottom 40 per cent, became the subject of debate in the early 1980s. The DES asserted their minister's "inescapable duty" to satisfy himself that "the work of the schools matched national needs" (Cmnd 6869), but they had to win a struggle with HMI and the Schools Council before translating their concept of the curriculum into legislation. The Schools Council was handicapped by the fact that it had been the main source of advice since 1964 on curriculum and examinations, and it was abolished in 1982. The DES's own *Framework for the curriculum* (1980) and still more *The school curriculum* (1981) were subject to so much adverse criticism, however, that ministers would not consent to legislation.

School choice

As a member of the market right, Keith Joseph as Secretary of State for Education was hesitant in any case about prescription. His own sympathies lay with those who wished to leave responsibility for curriculum content and standards with parents, arming them with an educational voucher, which they could "cash" at the school of their choice. Their aim was to transfer power from providers to consumers, the parent being the best available surrogate for the child, and to induce their active involvement with their child's education (Barnes 1991). Vouchers could be weighted for age and educational need; confined to the public sector or allowed to offset the costs of an independent school; taxed or topped up; additions might be made for those who did not obtain the school of their choice. But some things were constant: there was direct accountability from school to parent and there was a right of exit, leaving unsatisfactory teachers to their empty classrooms and pushing Heads into remedial measures. Against arguments that education was not a supermarket good and too important to leave to those whose own information and education might be deficient, voucher advocates suggested that officialdom would pursue its own interests, and that appeals systems benefited only the articulate middle class.

They were not able to persuade Joseph's predecessor, Mark Carlisle, but had high hopes of Joseph when he became Secretary of State in 1981. They were correspondingly disappointed when he backed away from the idea two years later. The real objection was not, as claimed, departmental advice that the scheme was administratively impractical but the impossibility of establishing a sufficient consensus among parents in favour of the reform to ensure its survival if there were a change of government. The Prime Minister continued to find the idea attractive, but lacked the time to give it a sustained push.

What this episode reveals is the importance of the party channels in getting ideas on to the policy agenda. Education vouchers had been canvassed by the Institute of Economic Affairs since 1964. It was not until 1975 that they began to attract the attention of a substantial number of influential Conservative educationists with good access to party leaders. To succeed, however, the idea needed a more specific commitment from the party and/or a determined minister who would push it through.

Vouchers squared with the emphasis the party put on parental choice in *The Parent's Charter* (1974), but it proved possible to meet that commitment with measures that were more acceptable to paternalists within the party. Clear obligations were imposed on LEAs to take account of the wishes of parents in Carlisle's 1980 legislation, and an appeals system established for parents dissatisfied with the allocation of schools. Catchment areas and local authority boundaries were outlawed. However, the reform that might have made a reality of parental choice, provision for a flat rate charge on all school transport whether to the nearest appropriate school or not, failed to get through the House of Lords. A second set of measures to strengthen parental power may have originated in the decision by some Conservative LEAs to include parents on school governing bodies. Well before the Taylor Commission was appointed to consider school government, the *Parent's Charter* committed the party to elected parent governors; and the 1986 Act modified the Taylor recommendations in such a way that elected parents and, to a lesser extent, teachers dominated new style governing bodies. Accountability too was pursued, with schools compelled to publish details of their record, specialities and objectives and governors having to account for themselves to an annual meeting of parents.

Parental power, increased accountability and choice were one strand only, however, in a complex debate within the Conservative party. There were marked differences, as commentators have noted, between those "who believe in enterprise (the Lord Young Group) and those who believe in standards (the Hillgate Group)" (Gleeson 1989). The latter not only saw TVEI as a threat to subjects and externally assessed standards, but were increasingly involved in a debate also with the market right about the extent to which parents could be relied on to safeguard standards. Rather than accept the case for vouchers, they took up the case already pressed by the Selsdon and No Turning Back groups for the reintroduction of grant maintained schools. They also wanted to create a national curriculum, to introduce testing at the end of each key stage in a child's development, and to shift the balance within the new GCSE examination against coursework.

The 1988 Act

When he became Secretary of State in 1986, Kenneth Baker was aware of the complex debate taking place within the party and of the solutions on offer. He had to find a way of bringing these ideas together so that they would satisfy the Prime Minister and all groups within the party. Baker's own account makes clear his distrust of LEAs, the educational establishment in general and the teacher unions in particular, and his wish to make parental responsibility for their childrens' education more of a reality.

Three key features of the legislation, open enrolment, formula funding and local financial management, together come close to being a voucher system. The subject based national curriculum and the provisions to test it by written tests at each key stage as well as by teacher assessment met the demands of the traditionalists and provided Baker with the overall framework that he believed essential both to ensure that national needs were met and that pupil entitlement was safeguarded in what was bound to become a highly decentralized schools system. The traditionalists were less happy with the emphasis on criterion based assessment, already applied to GCSE, and arguably one of the DES's main contributions to the Act. They were openly sceptical about the ten level scale devised to monitor pupil progression, perhaps not surprisingly since this was devised by a professional team dedicated to building on good classroom practice (Maclure 1992). The restoration of

47

the direct grant system, first promised by Boyle, was finally accomplished. However, Baker probably realized that, if the experiment was successful, not only would it need a funding agency to operate the system but it would be hard to resist the arguments for a common funding formula. Vouchers might then return to the agenda. Credits for students in further education, and a boost both for the inner cities and for technical education in the form of City Technology Colleges completed the package. Reforms to teacher training were left aside, but continuing suspicion of the progressive ideology that Conservatives see as dominant in that field has led to the view that a larger share should be done by professional mentors in schools, a reform that Kenneth Clarke set in train.

The final part of the 1988 Act dealt with higher education. Policy towards the universities until the late 1970s largely took the form of benign neglect. The expansion in the number of university students, which resulted from the Barlow Report in 1945, was accelerated in the wake of the Robbins Committee's recommendation in 1963 (Cmnd 2154) that a place should be available for all qualified applicants. The major government initiatives, however, were in the local authority sector: the creation of the College of Advanced Technology (CATs), which became new universities in the wake of the Robbins Report, the designation in 1965 of polytechnics and the creation of the Council for National Academic Awards (CNAA) to supervise their quality and award degrees to their students. Against Robbins's advice, they were deliberately left under LEA control, and, in terms of preventing academic drift, this made sense. Not all local authorities, however, were helpful, and pressures from the polytechnics for their incorporation grew. By 1978 their standing was such that the Lindop Committee recommended a substantial relaxation of the CNAA regime, and moves to accreditation were set in train. In the university sector the effort to drive down costs was followed by savage cuts in the early 1980s (Kogan & Kogan 1983). When, contrary to expectation, the demand for higher education actually grew, it was the polytechnics that responded. The government not only took credit for their figures, but set in train an expansion to ensure that one in three young people would enjoy a higher education by the year 2000. The polytechnics were rewarded for their efforts with incorporation under the 1988 legislation, but the question of how the continued expansion was to be funded has yet to be addressed properly. Kenneth Clarke legislated to end the "binary divide" and to establish a single funding agency for higher education in 1992, and an expensive loans scheme was set in place to make long-term savings on the cost of maintenance. However, these sums will not be available to boost expansion, and in the meantime demand has been constrained and grants to universities have been cut.

The 1988 Act in retrospect looks a surprisingly coherent package, but major problems have arisen over the demands made by the national curriculum and, still more, the elaborate and cumbersome assessment scheme devised by the Task Group on Assessment and Testing working party. It is possible to argue that the latter derives from the ten level scale that Black and his colleagues devised to emphasize progression, but the Dearing review, set up in response to teacher action in 1993, while suggesting some radical modifications to the scale, is unwilling to abandon it without further reflection and research. Instead it has drastically lightened what has to be taught at both Key Stages 1 and 4. A pupil's entitlement to a broad based curriculum will now end at the age of 14, and it is evident that Sir Ron Dearing believes that this will contribute to the enhancement of standards at that age. Beyond the age of 14 he has deliberately created room for the inclusion of a vocational element, and it is clear that he envisages an other than traditional approach to this.

The need for General National Vocational Qualifications was first identified in the White Paper, *Education and training in the 21st century* (1991) and five were rapidly developed in the course of a few months to the point where they could be piloted. Inevitably there were pitfalls in such rapid progress, identified in evaluations and taken into account when NCVQ and the three awarding bodies, BTEC, City and Guilds, and RSA, revised the existing GNVQs and produced second-wave qualifications. Despite criticisms that GNVQs sacrifice knowledge and understanding to the pursuit of competence related measures (Smithers 1993), the evaluations that have been carried out are largely favourable, and the OFSTED report (which critics misrepresent) makes it clear that at the advanced level, the new qualifications are well on the way to equivalence with GCE A level. There are more problems at the intermediate level, however, that will have to be resolved if Dearing's concept of what is to be available to 14–16 year olds is to be achieved.

The principal beneficiaries of the government's reforms look to have been the secondary schools, which are in general enjoying the ability to manage their own affairs and have weathered the change to formula funding. The burden falling on governors, however, may make recruitment difficult, particularly at primary school level, and there is evidence that some primary school Heads are failing to cope. The principal casualties have been the LEAs. In quick succession they lost first polytechnics and then the whole of further education. Some have also lost large numbers of secondary schools to the grant maintained sector. They looked to have discovered a new role in quality assurance, as enablers, and as suppliers of services. But the decision that inspection would become a semi-privatized service regulated by OFSTED, when coupled with stringent regulations about the amounts they should disburse to schools, has induced thoughts of their demise. The creation of a funding agency to deal with the Grant Maintained (GM) schools will not only lead to an expensive duplication of services but, given-over provision of secondary school places, to clashes with LEAs over whose schools to close, with the Secretary of State drawn in to arbitrate. Further change therefore looks inevitable, even though the outcome of local government reform has been limited.

Conclusion

Policy is an outcome, the product not of any single conscious intention, but of forces in interaction, whether the mode be discussion, argument or conflict. Potentially the Education Department is the most important actor, and a shift in its thinking from self-conscious partnership towards a desire to dominate, not least in terms of the curriculum, is discernible from the mid 1970s. However, Britain has party government, and the role played by party in disrupting the post-war consensus and later in bringing fresh modes of thinking and new actors into play is key. One cannot understand the 1980s without consideration of currents in Conservative thinking. Nevertheless, paradoxes remain. A broad consensus existed not only in the earlier period, but about the policy agenda and many of the solutions proffered since 1976. The latest consensus is more dynamic, however, and less complete. Finally, the system remains "bottom heavy" with institutions and teachers key actors in the educational process. Intermediary institutions have proved vulnerable to government action, but, as the translation of the Dearing (1994) review into practice shows, both the detail and the execution of policy remain with those in the system, and not at its top: and the devil as always is in the detail.

Suggested reading

Brian Simon (1991) offers a comprehensive, scholarly account written from an avowedly left wing standpoint. There is much useful material in Gordon et al. (1991). Ball (1990) provides an account of the origins of the 1988

Act and Maclure (1992) provides a commentary on it. Richardson (1993), Knight (1992) and Lawton (1980) help illuminate factors in the policy process as well as offering valuable subject matter.

CHAPTER 3
Employment policy: a chronicle of decline?

Noel Whiteside

Introduction

One of the largest changes in economic policy since the war has been the virtual disappearance of full employment as a policy objective and its replacement by the control of inflation. Inflation, we are led to believe, is caused by governments expanding the amount of money in the economy in order to create jobs. While unemployment afflicts an unfortunate minority of the working population, inflation presents a more general and potent threat: corroding savings, damaging the lives of those on fixed incomes (especially pensioners), undermining long-term investment, fostering industrial militancy, while reducing confidence in sterling and destroying its trading value on the world's money markets. Inflation threatens those traditional social values – hard work, self-reliance, personal enterprise and thrift – that are commonly regarded as the bedrock of a prosperous, stable society. Containing inflation will encourage investment, thereby restoring economic prosperity and social wellbeing. Seen from this angle, we might well conclude (in ex-Chancellor Norman Lamont's phrase) that unemployment is a "price well worth paying" for the restoration of financial stability.

Viewed historically, this was not always so. For a quarter of a century after the war, both the main political parties endorsed the view that it was government's role to maintain full employment as a principal object of economic policy. Less general agreement existed about how this might be achieved: the Labour party being more convinced of the merits of central planning and direct state intervention than their Conservative counterparts. In the 1950s and 1960s, Britain enjoyed high levels of employment and relatively low levels of inflation. Unemployment, much like cholera and typhoid in the previous century, was viewed as a problem of the past that had fallen victim to the march of human progress. By the early 1970s, governments of both political persuasions were intervening in the labour market more than ever before; there was strong political consensus about how manpower policies might be improved. From the middle of the 1970s, all this changed. The election of the first Thatcher administration in 1979 witnessed the virtual disappearance of the unemployment issue from the political agenda. The reasons for this change of heart – and some comments on its consequences – will be made in the course of this chapter.

Over the last 20 years, governments have tended to judge employment and manpower policies solely in terms of their impact on the economy, presumably on the assumption that economic growth automatically cures all social ills. It is a mistake, however, to ignore the wider consequences of high unemployment. Waged work is endowed with enormous social value in our society. To be deprived of access to it is to subject the individual to grave social disadvantage. Aside from the humanitarian aspect, we must recognize that joblessness entails high economic – as well as social – costs. Unemployment is associated with some pretty unpleasant social consequences and, one way and another, these translate into higher rates of social expenditure. The unemployed show a greater propensity for alcohol and drugs. Their marriages are more likely to fail; their children are more liable to suffer from low birth weight, poor health, low educational achievement. High levels of unemployment are associated with rising rates of physical and mental sickness, and areas of high unemployment (particularly inner cities) also suffer from higher rates of crime. In these ways, unemployment (when twinned with a criminal conviction or a poor health record) converts itself into unemployability – and thus permanent social dependency. Although it is hard to prove that unemployment alone causes these social problems, the fact that their incidence is worst in areas where joblessness is greatest indicates, at the very least, that a community living with high unemployment is liable to experience a growing reliance on the police, social security and the social services. It is no coincidence that Conservative governments in the 1930s and in the 1980s and 1990s have had great difficulty in keeping public expenditure under control.

This chapter is divided into four main sections. The first two outline the changing economic framework within which employment policy has been located since the war. The third looks at the objects of manpower policy: that is to say policies dedicated to training and re-deployment – an area in which Britain is extraordinarily weak, when compared to countries like Germany and France. The fourth traces manpower policy development in Britain. The concluding section will place policy developments in a broader context and will explain why the problem of unemployment has been so peculiarly persistent in recent years.

Employment policy and economic policy: Keynes and after

Employment policies in the 1940s grew from the experience of the slump years. The 1930s – the "devil's decade" in the words of the journalist Claud Cockburn – had been disastrous: widespread unemployment and poverty at home and chronic political instability abroad, culminating in the triumph of Nazism and the outbreak of the Second World War. By the end of hostilities, common political consensus existed that such conditions must never recur. Hence the wave of policy statements, committing each government to the maintenance of full employment, issued by the Allies after the war. As soon as the war was over, the Western powers turned their attention to destroying the conditions that had made the 1930s possible. The 1946 agreement at Bretton Woods involved the signatories in new commitments to facilitate trade and underwrite economic growth on a worldwide scale. The interdependence of Western industrial economies was recognized. The outbreak of the Cold War in the late 1940s reinforced this commitment, as the United States moved to guarantee European security against the Russian threat by rebuilding the economies of Western democracies under the Marshall Aid programme.

In Britain, fears abounded that a short boom, followed by a longer economic depression – the pattern that had followed the Armistice of 1918 – would be repeated. However, the war itself had transformed the relationship between state and society. J. M. Keynes, the best-known critic of inter-war economic policies, had been appointed Economic Adviser to the Cabinet under the coalition government: a position that allowed his ideas on official economic management to infiltrate Westminster and Whitehall. In 1936, Keynes had published an influential treatise on mass unemployment and the means that governments could employ to eliminate it (Keynes 1936). Neo-classical economic theory, which dominated the Treasury at that time, dictated that recession should be met by reductions in wages and public expenditure, to enable British industry to reduce its costs, allowing exports to compete more effectively in overseas markets. In this at least, it endorsed an approach remarkably similar to monetarist policies pursued in the 1980s.

Keynes argued that such strategies were mistaken: that, left to its own devices, a free market economy did not automatically stabilize at the level of full employment (as the neoclassical school claimed). Wage cuts and redundancies reduced domestic demand for consumer goods which depressed those industries supplying the domestic market, leading to more lay-offs and wage reductions. This "downward spiral" discouraged investment and undermined growth. Jobs for all, Keynes argued, could only be guaranteed by government accepting responsibility for the maintenance of domestic demand: either indirectly (the preferred route) through redistributive taxation and lower interest rates to stimulate investment, or directly — through public expenditure on capital projects, industrial investment, even welfare benefits — which would raise working class consumption. As the poorest spent a higher proportion of their income, redistributive taxation would foster higher rates of economic activity. The wealthy allowed money to languish as "idle savings" (in property, jewellery, *objets d'art*) and this did not stimulate enterprise. Albeit that Keynes was a Liberal, some of his recommendations thus harmonized well with the aims of the incoming Labour government in 1945.

During the war itself, the chief problem had been a shortage (not a surplus) of labour and Keynes's main energies had been directed towards inflation. Wartime manpower questions were subject to direct government controls. Conscription was introduced for men (and many women). Manpower budgets facilitated the direction of man- (and woman-) power to where it was needed; rationing and price controls reduced the direct inflationary threat and provided the foundation for wartime voluntary wage restraint agreements with the trade unions. The unions were promised a return to pre-war practices, which meant the restoration of free collective bargaining and the free movement of labour, when hostilities ceased. Full employment became a central issue in reconstruction planning. Without full employment, or something very like it, Beveridge's plan for comprehensive social insurance would collapse, for the Beveridge Report (Cmd 6404) made claimants' rights to social security dependent on their contributory record; without employment, contributions would not be made. Hence Beveridge followed up *Social insurance and allied services* with proposals detailing how full employment was to be achieved (Beveridge 1944). Rumours of this publication pushed the War Cabinet into issuing a White Paper, *Employment policy* (Cmd 6527), in 1944, largely to prevent Beveridge stealing a march on the government's reconstruction proposals for a second time.

Although both publications aimed at a common objective, their content differed quite substantially. Beveridge wanted a labour market where there were always more job vacancies than job seekers; to secure this state of affairs, he was willing to endow central government with powers over investment and even industrial ownership, should the market mechanism fail to respond to indirect incentives. The White Paper, on the other hand, was far more conservative and, in some respects, a jumble of internal contradictions: reflecting the battle within Whitehall between the more radical economists in the Economic Advisory Section and the Treasury mandarins, who remained sceptical of any state intervention in the management of the economy. Hence, although the White Paper acknowledged the possible need for some Keynesian measures, such as deficit budgeting, regional policy and alterations in the rate of National Insurance Contributions (NICs) to accommodate booms and slumps, it also retained traditional methods of tackling unemployment. Beveridge dismissed it as a public works White Paper, not a plan for full employment. Both publications, however, effectively transferred power over employment policy into the hands of professional economists. There it has rested ever since. As in other areas of welfare, this proved to be a lasting legacy of the war: the removal of policy from popular control and its relocation firmly in the hands of professional experts operating within central government.

Employment policy demonstrated that, in some parts of Whitehall, traditional economic concepts were being abandoned. In itself, however, it had little influence on policy. The post-war Labour government's plans for economic regulation relied more on central state controls than on the use of fiscal and monetary incentives to create jobs. To the development of regional policies (mentioned in the White Paper), it added a programme for extending public ownership through nationalization and the creation of a welfare state. All provided, through state management, avenues for job creation over and above Keynesian strategies. Moreover, Keynesian policies proved unnecessary. As during the war, the post-war problem was one of continuing shortages of manpower and materials: both of which were needed not only for necessary capital works, to build or repair factories, schools, hospitals, houses, but also for the export drive vital to meet Britain's many and urgent external financial obligations. In the late 1940s, appeals were being made to women to stay at work and the first inflow of immigrants from the "New Commonwealth" were being recruited by employers, with official encouragement, to staff those jobs (commonly located in the public service sector) too low paid and unappealing to attract British recruits. The threat of inflation was also contained, as during the war, by direct controls on consumption, less through the use of Keynesian strategies. Rationing persisted and price controls were used to counteract the growing cost of imports. The Labour government's view of a planned socialist economy differed considerably from the managed capitalism envisaged by Keynes. To talk, therefore, either of a "Keynesian revolution" in the 1940s, or of consensus between Labour and Conservative forms of economic and social policy in the immediate post-war period, is somewhat misleading (Jones 1992, Rollings 1988, Tomlinson 1993).

While not denying the mutual commitment to full employment, the post-war Labour government, working on the principle of "fair shares for all", had fewer reservations about the use of state controls than had its Conservative successors. Using central powers, Labour aimed to modernize the public and private sectors, raising productivity and enhancing training: promoting regular contracts of employment that included weekly wages (and overtime rates), holidays with pay and other benefits that had been far from universal in pre-war days. Modernization initiatives were largely stifled by opposition from industrial employers, who saw such official regulation as a thinly disguised move towards nationalization (Tiratsoo & Tomlinson 1993). The other major problem was inflation. Price subsidies rose alarmingly in the late 1940s and, to control wages, the government was forced to go cap-in-hand to the TUC to negotiate a wage freeze in 1948. This was, however, only a temporary solution to what proved to be a continuing problem. In the winter of 1950–51, the Cabinet discussed a new Full Employment Bill, never presented to Parliament, which, while reiterating the measures the government would adopt to counteract a slump, extended official economic regulation to contain inflation. The Chancellor (Hugh Gaitskell) was exploring mechanisms to allow state guidelines to form a framework for determining wage rates and incomes. Labour's faith in the ability of Keynesian economic management to secure full employment without inflation remained limited (Rollings 1993).

Differences in strategy between the parties signalled important ideological divisions. For the Labour party, long-term security of employment required central planning to raise industrial efficiency and to regulate the economy on a scientific basis, for the good of all. In many ways similar to the ideology underpinning the Liberal welfare reforms of the early twentieth century, such policies assumed the efficacy of the state as an agency of social and economic amelioration: a faith rooted in a belief in scientific method and national regulation. This socialist vision was not supported by all in the Labour movement, still less within a Conservative party which, while acutely aware of its electoral image as the party of mass unemployment, still retained a basic faith in the merits of free market economics and the sanctity of private property. The Conservative governments of the 1950s unpicked Labour's state controls and Conservative Chancellors of the Exchequer adapted Keynesian strategies to sustain full employment and economic growth. They also revived other traditional economic objectives: the balanced budget, the promotion of free trade, the restored convertibility of sterling and the general integration of Britain into the international economy. The overwhelming priority given to the maintenance of full employment by Labour ceased to dominate and became one of several policy objectives. The Conservatives in the 1950s eschewed the prospect of raising unemployment in order to contain industrial unrest and rising wages. The problem of inflation, although present, was nowhere near as severe as it later became, the economy was growing (although not as fast as that of its competitors) and the party, thanks to its association with the policies of the slump years, was peculiarly sensitive to the unemployment issue.

In the event, the commitment of the Conservatives to full employment was never put to the test. The 1950s proved unprecedented in terms of general prosperity. When Macmillan took the Conservatives into the general election of 1959 under the slogan "You've never had it so good", the electoral response indicated that he was only too right. Appearances, however, proved deceptive. Behind the façade of full employment and rising living standards, problems were brewing. First, the "hands off" approach adopted by the Conservatives allowed traditional managerial and union practices to reassert themselves: practices that were sadly out of keeping with the new competitive international environment of the 1960s, as the economies of Germany and Japan recovered. Secondly, the use of budgetary devices to "fine tune" the economy (or "stop-go" as the practice was commonly termed) was adapted more to political needs than to economic ones: economic expansion being stimulated for electoral purposes, with subsequent retrenchment to prevent inflationary overheating. Such practices undermined investment; businessmen could not count on any period of sustained growth. Hence British industry continued to be characterized by low investment, antiquated plant, an underskilled workforce, overmanning and low levels of productivity. Consequently, demand management techniques to stimulate economic growth began to come unstuck; instead of stimulating further investment (and more jobs) at home, they tended to suck in cheaper imports manufactured elsewhere, damaging Britain's balance of payments and, with this, confidence in sterling. The international money markets did not wait for such effects to work themselves through. Rather, signs of state-funded economic expansion provoked a sterling crisis, forcing governments to rein back on programmes of expansion. The alternative was to devalue the pound: a less attractive option requiring a formal political decision (in the era of fixed exchange rates), and one which damaged the reputation of currency and government, at home and abroad.

These factors explain why Keynesian strategies ultimately failed to maintain full employment. An increasingly competitive international environment exposed the weaknesses of Britain's economy. Government aid designed to expand new industries was used to shore up old ones; the stimulation of domestic demand did less and less for home based growth and more and more damage to the currency. Even though union leaders were sympathetic to the Labour governments of 1964–70 and 1974–9, the influence of more radical shop stewards and the power they had acquired in the period of full employment made such endorsement nearly worthless. Neither the TUC nor the union leaders could control the behaviour of their rank and file. Ordinary workers, frightened by a rising rate of inflation and government's efforts to impose statutory controls over wages, imposed ever-higher wage demands – which made a bad situation worse. Industrial conflict escalated as workers placed increasing faith in their industrial muscle to protect themselves against the rising cost of living. Strikes (or the threat of them) worked; state planning apparently did not. This breakdown in political consensus on the purposes and form of official economic strategies caused both parties to search for a more workable solution.

Employment policy and economic policy: the monetarist alternative

There is insufficient space here to trace a detailed course of British economic policy in the 1960s and early 1970s, which eventually resulted in the disappearance of full employment as a primary policy objective. Denis Healey's budget of 1975 is commonly understood to be the first to abandon full employment: a position reinforced by the terms of the IMF loan the following year, which required extensive public expenditure cuts, involving a necessary loss of jobs. Further, by the mid 1970s, civil servants and politicians who recalled the slump years were passing into retirement. Their place was being taken by younger men and women who had little knowledge of (and less interest in) historical precedent, who argued that inflation threatened the livelihoods of a larger section of the electorate than unemployment ever did and should be given the higher priority. The election of Mrs Thatcher in

1979 allowed policy rationalization to come into line with policy practice. The Conservative governments of the 1980s made no secret of their objectives: to restore economic competitiveness through a programme of cutting costs (both private and public). Monetarist doctrines, adopted to justify these strategies, dictated that increases in the money supply, the inevitable consequence of official economic expansion, raised the rate of inflation while failing to affect unemployment. Only by eliminating inflation, the Conservatives argued, could investment be encouraged and "real jobs" sustained. The reduction of state intervention in the economy would stimulate the free market, foster more competitive enterprise and reverse Britain's economic decline. The role of government was to make the labour market work as monetarist doctrine suggested it should, by removing impediments to wage reductions and greater labour mobility. The Non-Accelerating Inflation Rate of Unemployment (NAIRU) – an irreducible minimum – was basically determined by the state of the market and could not be affected (except adversely) by state intervention. If unemployment remained above NAIRU, this was because unions were "pricing their members out of work". We thus return to an ideology that blames the incidence of a problem on the victims themselves.

This perspective underpinned the employment policies of the Thatcher years. In economic terms, this represented a complete reversal of what had gone before and a return to supply-side principles. Impediments to reductions in industrial costs (which meant wages), like trade unions and wages councils, were attacked. More stringent regulations were placed on access to unemployment benefits – particularly for women; official efforts were made to promote job sharing and tax cuts were promised to raise work incentives (although, thanks to the rising social security budget, these proved unviable before the mid 1980s). Agencies for channelling public investment in the private sector (like the National Economic Development Council) were wound up and grants in aid to both public and private sectors became much more stringently controlled. "Privatization", the return of public services to the private sector, became a hallmark of economic policy: a process that not only involved the transfer of ownership of gas, electricity and other public utilities, but also the "contracting out" of cleaning, catering and general maintenance services by schools, local authorities and the NHS.

Manufacturing industry contracted rapidly: a collapse exacerbated by contractions in the international economy (caused by the second oil price shock in 1979) and by the government's insistence that industry should stand on its own two feet. Unemployment, which had stood at 1.25 million on the eve of the 1979 general election, more than doubled in the first 18 months of the new Conservative government and went over three million by 1985. In spite of frenetic efforts to massage the figures back to a respectable level (which meant tightening rules on "availability for work", promoting early retirement for the over-50s and pushing large numbers onto government training schemes), the official figure dropped below three million only in 1986–7 and has stayed stubbornly over two million more or less ever since. At the same time, the number of long-term unemployed (those out of work for more than a year) reached 1.5 million by the mid 1980s – a figure three times higher than that reached in the 1930s. And the number of long-term sick (invalidity benefit claimants) rose by a factor of five between 1979 and 1993, reflecting the problems experienced in a tight labour market by those in less than perfect health. The results of Thatcher's employment strategies led to a permanent rise in social dependency (which John Major has inherited and which explains the large 1992–3 public sector deficit). The contraction in the public sector and the spread of subcontracting removed security of employment: many more are now in part-time work or on short-term contracts, often under the label "self-employed". These now make up over one in three of the workforce and the figure is rising. Subcontracted employees have no right to statutory job protection, sick pay, superannuation or any of the other benefits taken for granted by their colleagues in conventional full-time work. This allows employers to save on employment overheads, while fostering, so the Conservatives claim, a "flexible", more competitive labour market. The costs of business fluctuation are borne by the employee alone; untold and inestimable amounts of work have been lost by the "self-employed", who have little choice but to struggle on, working ever longer hours at ever lower rates, trying to make ends meet.

In response to the question, has Conservative economic policy made a difference to employment, the answer is an unqualified "yes". Unemployment has all but disappeared from the social policy agenda. In the 1980s and 1990s, official efforts to cut public expenditure have pushed more and more people onto the labour market, without any reflection on the consequences for the large numbers already there. The object has been to allow new labour market entrants – single mothers, school leavers and the rest – to offer their services at "competitive" (meaning lower) rates of pay. Without any expansion in the job market, however, the successful insertion of one applicant must result in the expulsion of another – who in turn becomes a dependent of the state. The assumption underpinning supply-side strategies, that economic growth will generate jobs, is unfounded; "jobless" growth is a well known phenomenon. Unemployment is now higher and more persistent than it has ever been at any point in British history, including the 1930s. This goes a long way towards explaining the rising rates of poverty that have characterized the last 15 years.

Manpower policies: the problem

Employment policy is not only about the provision of jobs. Aside from stimulating demand for labour, post-war governments have taken an active interest in the quality of its supply: providing official programmes to facilitate recruitment, training, placement, redeployment and so on. In this field, Britain's performance has lagged well behind France, Sweden and Germany and repeated efforts to improve matters have generally had little impact. It is as well that we understand why. The answer is to be found in an area generally ignored by students of social policy: namely industrial management and industrial relations. In trying to develop manpower policies, governments have been invading a territory already colonized by industry itself. Both employers and unions have sought to exclude the state from areas regarded as the proper provenance of managerial prerogative and free collective bargaining. Research into the post-war Labour governments has stressed the general opposition from private employers to official policies to reform managerial practices. Equally, manufacturing trade unions, operating within a framework of wage differentials based on skill, have looked askance at official initiatives that would disrupt traditional practices and flood the market with state trained labour: even from a government ostensibly committed to their interests (Whiteside forthcoming 1995). Trade unions have tended not to take kindly to measures that will undermine bargaining power and, with this, wages. Every attempt by any government since the war to interfere with manning levels, impose wage controls or promote industrial restructuring has met with strong opposition. Preference has been given to traditional systems of apprenticeship. Yet such systems only permit training for present – not future – needs and may not endow the recipient with skills transferable between firms. Further, British industry has an appalling record of industrial training and, in periods of recession, has cut back on such training programmes as exist. All these factors have proved continuing problems for governments determined to raise productivity and promote growth in the post-war period.

The objects of state action have remained, however, unclear. Most obviously, positive manpower policies are designed to promote economic prosperity by ensuring the effective deployment of manpower and by raising levels of skill and adaptability in the labour force. This "investment in human capital" requires a total manpower policy, not simply programmes for the unemployed. Alternatively, focusing training on the jobless allows labour surplus to one sector to transfer to another, preventing the "deterioration" of the unemployed. Finally, and developing from this strategy, training need not require the acquisition of skills at all. "Training" can simply refer to the imposition of work discipline on the idle. Government schemes serve to allay the irritation commonly provoked by the thought that some people are able to live at public expense without having to stir a finger to earn their keep. The idea that the unemployed be required to accept a place on a training scheme as a condition for receiving benefit has been revived sporadically since the 1970s. "Workfare" is often presented as a new idea, originating in the United States. However, identical principles underpinned the English poor laws since the days of Queen Elizabeth I – with the able-bodied poor being set to work in return for the receipt of public relief. It is the expense of such measures, as well as their unpopularity, that has prevented their reintroduction.

Training policies have thus been required to serve a variety of ends. For this reason, there has been a tendency for official programmes to fall heavily between two stools. A complete manpower policy being both expensive and industrially unacceptable, official initiatives have tended to focus on the unemployed. If they promote "real" training in marketable skills, they are damned for trying to make a silk purse out of a sow's ear, the unemployed being the rejects of the labour market and therefore the least likely to give the nation a good return on its investment. Further, government trainees compete for jobs with those trained elsewhere and are regarded as second rate by comparison. If, on the other hand, government programmes are little more than "setting the able-bodied poor to work", then a different, but related, set of problems emerges. Extensive state activity will end up exacerbating the unemployment problem, not alleviating it. If state-sponsored trainees work in areas where commercial interests are already active, the agency operating with a public subsidy will offer a cheaper service than its commercial rival and will drive the latter out of business. Similarly, if employers are offered money to take on government "trainees", then they will see this labour as a cheaper alternative to taking on their own and will cut their recruitment accordingly. If, on the other hand, the government funds projects that no commercial undertaking would touch, because of their inherent unprofitability – then the unemployed working on them are not being prepared for "real" jobs in the "real" market economy. State policy is thus failing in one of its primary aims: to restore the jobless to financial independence.

Manpower policies in practice

The final, and most fundamental, difficulty that has dogged manpower policy is the low esteem afforded technical training in this country. The post-war Labour government ran up against the difficulty when instructing the education establishment – and the Treasury – to promote technical educa-tion in the tertiary sector. In this instance, the universities seized the lion's share of public funds put aside for the expansion of adult education and training. While some of this helped expand medical schools and up-grade engineering faculties, it generally served to reinforce the Oxbridge tradition of higher education in the classics and the liberal arts: an education similar to that received by the politicians and senior civil servants themselves. Simi-larly, when Labour expanded higher education in the mid 1960s (including the creation of the Open University), the new courses in the new universities and polytechnics rapidly became very similar to those already provided in traditional universities. Technical courses of the City and Guilds variety were left to the smaller, and less well endowed, colleges of further education, which only trained those who failed to achieve higher academic standards. The pre-eminence of the academic was reflected at school level, where tech-nical subjects were equally neglected. "Technical" schools found their way into Butler's 1944 Education Act but never appeared in the flesh – so to speak. In the mid 1980s, the idea was taken off the shelf and presented (as a "new" policy) to the public in the shape of the Technical and Vocational Education Initiative (TVEI), a training programme to be run within existing secondary schools and supplemented by the introduction of 20 City Tech-nology Colleges. As the latter were to be funded by industry, and as govern-ment refused to fund this policy in anything like an adequate manner, this initiative has not overcome the bias in British education. Technical subjects are still the purview of academic failures.

During the 1950s, governments slowly became aware of the threat to the country's future imposed by Britain's failure to train. Efforts to improve matters were confined at this point to private exhortations to industrial employers – exhortations that were generally ignored. Employers covered their training requirements through the traditional mechanism of poaching skilled manpower from rival concerns with the promise of higher wages. In the 1960s, both Conservative and Labour governments moved to remedy this state of affairs. In 1964, legislation was passed allowing the Ministry of Labour to create Industrial Training Boards (ITBs) for specific industries. The ITBs were to be representative of both sides of industry and a levy on all employers in the specific industrial sector would fund common training programmes to replace, or at least augment, traditional apprenticeship systems and to ensure common standards of attainment. These failed to win much support. By the mid 1980s, all but seven of the original 27 created under the Wilson Government were scrapped. Small employers found the levy burdensome and argued that they gained no benefit from the training programmes; trade unionists opposed measures that diluted union control over recruitment. There were other reasons why the ITBs fell well short of Britain's training requirements. First, they only trained a proportion of recruits coming into the industry – doing nothing to retrain manpower already there and very little to raise technical awareness within schools and colleges. Secondly, their creation was patchy: less well organized sectors of the economy did not possess the means, let alone the will, to create ITBs. Thirdly, the rate of training was uneven. Even though the Labour government extended state subsidies in the mid 1970s, the ITBs relied on industrial profit; funding dried up in periods of recession, leaving industry short of recruits in subsequent periods of expansion. Finally, and most importantly, the system did not allow any overview of training as a whole; there were few or no mechanisms for co-operative training across different sectors and, by the early 1970s, there was an evident need to plan training according to longer-term requirements than the ITBs were capable of attaining.

In 1973, the Conservative administration developed a more positive national manpower policy. Thus was the Manpower Services Commission (MSC) born: the sole agency in British history whose original brief was to promote manpower planning in all sectors of employment. It was to revamp government placement agencies and training schemes, promote redeployment from declining to expanding sectors of the economy, foster recruitment of school leavers into areas where their services would be most needed and generally eliminate the high-tech skill shortages that continued to dog Britain's economic performance. Technological change and economic progress were moving faster than ever before, the public was informed. Training and retraining in the course of a working life were essential if labour market deficiencies were not to handicap growth. In its early years, the MSC promised a complete revolution in policy. The old employment exchanges were renamed Job Centres, were shorn of their old duty of benefit administration and given attractive new premises in high streets and shopping centres. By 1977, government placements had risen by 30 per cent. State grants were made available for courses and programmes run in universities, polytechnics and colleges to help cut skill shortages in key areas. What was so novel about the new policy in general and the Training Opportunities Programme (TOPs) in particular was that it did not aim simply at the unemployed, but sought to tackle the whole problem of labour market restructuring in order to anticipate future demand.

This did not last. What appeared initially to be a revolution in the making was subsequently readapted to cope with the rising tide of unemployment. This chapter will not document the fate of all the individual MSC schemes, a veritable alphabet soup of initials, which were set up in these years. MSC policy switched, away from strategies to cope with labour market problems in general, towards temporary solutions for the unemployment crisis in particular. The notion of government playing a major part in retraining and redeployment went by the board as state agencies reverted to their traditional, residual role. TOPs was scrapped; the Job Centres, like the employment exchanges before them, lost their influence on placement and reverted to being a source of low-grade, poorly paid jobs that employers otherwise found difficult to fill. By the late 1970s, unemployed school leavers were the chief client group of the MSC and the Youth Opportunities Programme (renamed the Youth Training Scheme in 1982 and extended from one year to two) dominated the agency's activities. In addition, the Labour government had introduced a variety of special employment programmes that offered employers state subsidies to stave off redundancies (by short-time working), gave local authorities funds for temporary employment schemes and boosted recruitment in areas of acute depression. Such measures saved around 130,000 jobs by 1978 at an initial cost to the Treasury of £1 billion (Bowen 1991). In the event, all these jobs – and more – were wiped out by the recession that hit the country in 1980–81.

While the cost of such measures was partly offset by savings in social security and sustained tax revenues, they were vulnerable to the criticisms listed in the previous section. There were constant worries about substitution effects; were subsidized workers effectively replacing unsubsidized workers? MSC schemes encouraged the substitution of labour for capital and did not promote the macroeconomic adjustment of the economy by raising productivity. Their effects on jobs were essentially temporary; targeted at disadvantaged groups (school leavers and the long-term unemployed), they did not affect the existing competition for jobs and hence – while not stimulating wage inflation – they did not help contain rising wages. To the incoming Conservative government in 1979, the activities of the MSC were an expensive waste of public time and resources. Special employment programmes were scrapped. Throughout the 1980s, manpower policies were dedicated to the programme for school leavers and schemes for the young (meaning under 25) long-term unemployed: the object being to raise competition for work and to cut wages. According to Conservative doctrine, this was the only way to extend the number of jobs on offer. However, the only reason for retaining the MSC was political: the government had to be seen to be doing something about – if not for – the unemployed.

By 1988, recovery appeared to be under way and the numbers of jobless began to fall. The Thatcher Government seized this opportunity to reduce its commitment to manpower training: which, ideologically, the Conservatives had long believed to be the responsibility of industrial employers and not of the state. The MSC was abolished and its functions reabsorbed into the Department of Employment. Responsibilities for training promotion, together with state subsidies to cover existing commitments to school leavers and the long-term unemployed, were passed to new Training and Enterprise Councils (TECs). Run by local businessmen on a local basis, with the training itself commercially provided, the TECs represented the privatization of training. No sooner had the transfer been completed than the government revealed its true motive by cutting state subsidies to the TECs, angering those businessmen who had been persuaded to run them. In spite of rising unemployment in the 1990–92 period, these cuts were never restored. TECs currently have few resources, little co-operation in local business communities, few qualified instructors and no means of monitoring the quality of training they offer. Moreover, places for all unemployed school leavers, as promised when school leavers' benefit rights were removed in 1987, are no longer available, leaving the 16–18 year old unemployed reliant on their families or, in cases when the family cannot or will not take on this responsibility, wandering on the streets of major cities, begging for their livelihood.

In policy terms, we have come full circle. Training and manpower questions are once again the provenance of the private employer. While government in the 1990s continues to make the same noises as governments in the 1950s about the need for employers to train, nothing is done to rectify the appalling record of private employers in the technical training field. We might question whether the government programmes have ever tackled the main issue. Public trainees have been hairdresser's assistants, typists and keyboard operators, garage forecourt attendants if they were lucky: check-out personnel, shelf stockers and floor sweepers if they were not. Skill shortages existed (and exist) for financial specialists, computer programmers, electronics engineers, not for semi-skilled, service sector personnel, of which there has long been a glut on the market. Scarcely any wonder then that the much discussed "qualifications" that state trainees were to receive on completion of their courses have had but marginal impact on the subsequent employment of their recipients. For a long time now, the primary purpose of these schemes has been to increase competition for work at lower rates of pay, replacing one job applicant with another, while, further up the scale, the absence of skilled personnel in key technologies continues to damage industrial investment and growth.

Conclusions: back to the future

Over the last half-century, the labour market has changed enormously. The spread of more informal modes of employment has been ascribed by many analysts to the advent of a post-industrial, "post-Fordist" age. Nowadays, goods and services are supplied by small, "flexible" and independent units, not by large conglomerates. These new firms need labour willing to work as and when required; they do not – and cannot – sustain permanent jobs. To view new modes of employment as simply the product of economic restructuring is, however, both partial and ahistorical. This explanation does not recognize the irregularity of employment in pre-war Britain: nor the results of the post-war Labour government's policies to promote full employment, job security and regular earnings. The reversal of this policy in the 1980s, the contraction in state-sponsored jobs and the government's encouragement of part-time work, has allowed old diversities in employment practices to reappear. Today, however, the characteristics of these diversities are not the same as in pre-war days, the gender and the location of "irregular" employees now being very different.

At the same time, cultural values stressing the centrality of work to personal identity and citizenship rights have strengthened since the war. In the 1970s, equal access to jobs was a major goal for both feminists and racial minority groups; political pressures to secure this end culminated in legislation to guarantee equal job opportunities for all. The growing influence of the women's rights movement has partly coincided with the labour market restructuring noted above. The spread of part-time work has allowed many married women, unable to take on full-time work, access to the job market. Government policy, social expectation and falling earnings, all have helped to drive increasing numbers to search for waged work. The number of households with two wage-earners has risen dramatically in recent years. How far the spread of female employment can be seen as the consequence of their rising social consciousness, and how far as the result of new opportunities and falling household earnings, is a matter for conjecture. Yet, at the same time, the overall demand for labour has begun to falter and the state has been increasingly less willing or able to stimulate economic expansion or create jobs.

Certainly it appears that state action has become much more circumscribed in this area in recent years. To understand why this is so, we have to look at the changing world economy: an aspect of the employment problem only touched on in this chapter. Keynesian economics encouraged state regulation not only in the domestic sphere, but in international trade and finance. Hence the Bretton Woods agreement in 1946 underwrote a long-term commitment to the promotion of trade and the provision of international financial liquidity. In this, the American role, as guardian of the free world against the Communist threat, was central. It was American finance that reconstructed post-war Europe and American policy that fostered the creation of a free trading area within Europe (the forerunner of the European Union). In the 1950s, in all developed countries, employment opportunities were increasing and growth was sustained. It was only in the early 1970s, thanks to multiple causes (the Vietnam war and the damage sustained by the US dollar, the formation of the OPEC cartel and so on), that international financial and commercial stability became less secure. The floating of national currencies in the 1970s, coupled with the impact of computer technologies on world financial markets, has allowed an unprecedented growth in financial speculation, which undermines the ability of individual governments to control their own economies. Financial speculation now influences national resources more than any trade deficit; governments have learned that any action liable to upset the money markets (meaning any departure from strict financial probity) affects investment, savings and general financial stability. Unilateral reflation is no longer a viable policy option. Hence neither Labour nor Conservative parties offer policies promising a return to full employment, nor even any appreciable extension in state welfare. The policies of the mid 1940s present something of a contrast to those pursued since the 1980s. Whereas the former aimed to shape the international economy in accordance with broader social and political objectives, the latter accepted international economic forces as given and aimed to create a labour market that conformed to them.

Thanks to the dominant influence played by the financial and insurance sector in the British economy, the effects of all this have been very strong in this country. Hence, although most of Europe is currently plagued by unemployment, the incidence and persistence of the problem in Britain has been peculiarly marked. The reasons for the dominance of our financial sector are rooted in the role of sterling as an international trading currency, a legacy of Britain's imperial past. The sensitivity of the City of London – and the Treasury – to any government policy liable to damage "confidence in sterling" has placed considerable constraints on all areas of domestic policy. In particular, post-war efforts to generate growth through expensive programmes – of job creation, of long-term training, of extensive state investment – have not been well received. In this, Britain is unique; in no other European country have the interests of financial trading been given such high priority. The problems this has produced for British industry in general and British exporters in particular can be witnessed in the statements issued by the CBI whenever the government raised interest rates to protect the currency during the 1980s. Since the war, every downward movement of the pound on the international exchanges has been viewed politically as a national disaster, instead of an opportunity for restructuring an economy that is sorely in need of substantial new investment. The very election of every post-war Labour government has tended to stimulate unrest in the City, thanks to their association with expansionist policies. Whether it is possible to continue to support a major trading currency on the back of a deteriorating economy is a political question that needs to be faced if Britain's economy – and British workers – want a return to state-sponsored expansion to secure full employment.

Suggested reading

The transformation of the government's role in employment policy in the post-war years is traced in Tomlinson (1987). Hawkins (1987) explores the recent rise in unemployment, its causes and possible cures, a perspective also covered by Dawson (1993). Although basically a study of the Engineering Industry Training Board, Senker (1992) provides a useful overview of training policy in post-war Britain. Showler (1976), thanks to its date of publication, establishes the rationale underpinning the creation of the MSC and Lee (1990) contains some useful essays evaluating the impact of MSC programmes on that agency's main client group.

CHAPTER 4
Spending more to achieve less? Social security since 1945

Alan Deacon

Any discussion of social security policy must begin with a striking paradox. Spending on social security has risen enormously in the post-war period, and it now represents nearly one third of all government expenditure. To meet this cost every working person effectively paid, on average, £13 every working day in 1993 (Lilley 1993). And yet the problem of poverty has not been solved. On the contrary, the numbers of poor people have risen sharply in recent years. The measurement of poverty is both technical and contro versial, but whatever definition is adopted the pattern remains one of wide spread and increasing poverty (Hills 1993). Why has this happened? Why has poverty increased despite such a high level of spending, and despite the creation of a government bureaucracy that employs over 70,000 civil serv ants and is responsible for more than a billion separate transactions every year? (Ditch 1993).

Explaining the paradox

Broadly speaking, the current literature offers six different answers to these questions.

The first answer is that the growth of poverty is due to a lack of political will on the part of successive governments. The problem is not the structure of the benefit system, but the reluctance of politicians to raise enough money through taxation to enable them to pay benefits at an adequate level. Those who argue this would also point to the importance of three other factors; the increase in the proportion of the population that is over pension age, the growth in the number of one parent families and – especially – the rise in long-term unemployment. The higher expenditure on social security, they claim, simply represents the costs of demographic change and of the failure of economic policies. As we shall see, these writers do not deny the need to adapt the benefit system to changing social and economic conditions, but they may conveniently be termed the "New Beveridge" group. It is a perspective that is represented by the publications of the Child Poverty Action Group (CPAG) and by recent books by Alcock (1993) and Donnison (1991).

The second answer is that the problem lies primarily in the structure of the social security system itself. Many benefits are paid universally, irrespective of the resources of those who receive them. This means that pensions are paid to people who also have generous occupational pensions, child benefits to households with high incomes and so on. It is argued that this is wasteful, and that poverty could be alleviated without extra spending if the benefits were directed to those who need them and withdrawn from those who don't. Those who advocate this approach are called here the "targeters", and they are represented by Dilnot et al. (1984).

The third answer is that of what are termed here the "marketeers". They argue that the problem stems not from the structure of the social security system but from its very existence. State provision is inherently paternalistic and inefficient. It would be much better to restrict the role of government to that of guaranteeing a basic minimum income, and to allow individuals to take out their own insurance against sickness, old age or unemployment. Everyone would be a consumer of a service from a private company rather than a claimant upon the state, and the discipline of the market place would ensure they enjoyed choice and value for money. This is advocated by Harris and Seldon (1979), and in Chapter 10 of this book.

The fourth answer is that of the "dependency theorists". They argue that far from relieving some forms of poverty, benefits may actually make the problem worse. This is because the benefits system generates "perverse incentives" that lead people to behave in ways that are attractive in the short term but lead ultimately to greater poverty. The two examples that are cited most often are the increase in long-term unemployment and the growth in the numbers of single mothers. The availability of benefits, it is claimed, reduces the pressure upon the unemployed to accept whatever jobs are on offer, while the position of especially the young lone parent is less onerous than it was in earlier years – and may be more attractive than working. The end result is the creation of a "dependency culture" and of an underclass trapped into a life of dependency upon benefits (Green 1992).

A fifth answer is that social security policies have failed to eliminate poverty because they have been gender blind. The scheme of national insurance introduced after the Second World War, for example, was designed on the assumption that women would give up paid work on marriage, and this was to have far-reaching implications. Moreover, the way in which poverty itself was viewed and measured assumed that income was shared equitably *within* households, and thus failed to recognize the concentration of poverty upon women. This "feminist" perspective has also challenged the notion of dependency put forward by the "dependency theorists", pointing out that they regard reliance upon a man as normal but reliance upon the state as a problem. The "feminist" perspective is represented by Williams (1989) and by the contributors to Glendinning and Millar (1992). The former has also written of the need to develop an anti-racist critique of welfare, and there is a growing recognition of the extent to which black ethnic minorities are particularly vulnerable to poverty and are disadvantaged by the regulations governing entitlement to some benefits (Morris et al. 1993).

The sixth and final answer to our question is that poverty is simply inherent in capitalist societies, which are characterized by the concentration of wealth and economic power in relatively few hands and the dependence of the mass of the population upon wage labour. This, of course, is the answer of "Marxist" writers such as Novak (1988). Under capitalism, they argue, social security serves the needs of the labour market, and the relief of poverty is less important than the maintenance of work incentives and of labour discipline. This is also emphasized by "post-structuralist" writers such as Squires (1990) who draw upon the theories of Michel Foucault to analyze what they see as the "essentially disciplinary" role of social security.

The above categories are not, of course, exclusive or clear cut. The "New Beveridge" writers, for example, would claim to have incorporated much of the "feminist" critique. Nor do the categories correspond in any simple way to political parties. It will be seen, for example, that Thatcherism drew upon the ideas of "targeters", "marketeers" and "dependency theorists". In some cases, however, the contrasts are sharp and illuminating. Whereas the increase in one parent families is seen by the "New Beveridge" group as an additional burden upon the social security system, it is viewed by the "dependency theorists" as a product of that system.

The central point, however, is that debates about social security are ultimately debates about values. The objective of the "New Beveridge" group is to reduce social inequalities and to restore a sense of community and mutual care in society, and they believe that this will be fostered by benefits that are paid for and received by everyone. For the "marketeers" and "dependency theorists", on the other hand, the goal is to reinforce personal freedom and responsibility. This, they believe, is undermined by state benefits that are paid indiscriminately and thus too readily protect individuals from the consequences of their own decisions and behaviour. This is why arguments about the definition of poverty are so central to the policy debate. "What commentators mean by poverty depends to some extent on what they intend, or expect, to do about it" (Alcock 1993), and it will be seen that the policies advocated by "targeters", "marketeers", or "New Beveridge" writers rest on different assumptions about the nature of the problem they are addressing.

The importance of values also means that the debate is often a highly polarized one. Social security has long been a subject on which one either hunts with the hounds or runs with the hare, and arguments tend to be exchanged from fairly fixed positions. In view of this the reader should be clear about the position from which the present chapter is being written. The author belongs to the "New Beveridge" camp (Deacon & Bradshaw 1986), although he has recently argued that those within this tradition should be more willing to debate the influence of benefits upon the labour market (Deacon 1993).

It is from this perspective, then, that the remainder of the chapter provides an inevitably brief review of the policies that have been adopted in the post-war period and of the values and assumptions that have underpinned them.

Beveridge and his world

Social security changes gradually. New developments usually take the form of amendments to existing provisions. It is for this reason that even the briefest summary of post-war policies must start with the Beveridge Report of 1942 (Cmd 6404). Very little of Beveridge's plan has remained unscathed, but it is essential to understand the nature of that plan – and the flaws within it – in order to make sense of what has happened since.

The centrepiece of Beveridge's proposals was the extension of national insurance (NI) to almost everyone in work. All would pay contributions, and all would be eligible for benefits that would cover them against loss of earnings due to sickness, old age, unemployment or any other anticipated contingency "from the cradle to the grave". Contributions would be flat rate: they would not vary with earnings. Benefits would also be flat rate, but they would be sufficient for subsistence: they would be enough to live on. More over, everyone who was receiving benefit would have established a right to that benefit through the payment of contributions, and so the amount they received would not depend upon their other resources or those of their families. It was this that made Beveridge's report so popular. He seemed to have devised a practicable way of banishing both the fear of poverty and the spectre of the means test (Deacon & Bradshaw 1983, Lowe 1993).

The euphoria that greeted the Beveridge Report also owed much to the climate of opinion created by the Second World War. This was a time when the public seemed eager for social reform, and most of Beveridge's recommendations were speedily implemented by the wartime coalition and subsequent Labour governments. There are, however, two very important points that should be made here.

The first is that Beveridge had a very clear view of what was and what was not the responsibility of governments. His scheme was designed to eliminate want, and Beveridge believed that this could be achieved by redistributing income over an individual's lifetime; people paid contributions when they could work and received benefits when they could not. Of course the government and employers also paid contributions, but Beveridge did not seek to redistribute income from the better off to the poor any more than was necessary to ensure a minimum income for all. In politics Beveridge was an old-style liberal not a socialist. This was also why he proposed flat rate contributions and benefits. People who could afford to pay more should be encouraged to make further provision for themselves, but he believed that this should be done through private insurance and that it would be "an unnecessary interference with individual responsibility" if the government were to compel them to do so. Moreover, Beveridge was anxious that his scheme should not stifle incentives to work and save. He tried to ensure that even the lowest paid workers were better off than they would be on benefit, and for this reason urged that all those in work should receive a weekly family allowance to help meet the costs of their children. Similarly, he recognized that there would have to be a non-contributory, means tested scheme to provide for those who did not qualify for insurance benefits. He expected that relatively few people would have to claim such assistance, but was emphatic that assistance be made less attractive than insurance in order to safeguard the contributory principle.

The second point relates to the assumptions Beveridge made about the nature of post-war society. The NI scheme would only work if unemployment remained low. The Minister for National Insurance, James Griffiths, admitted candidly that the "disaster" of mass unemployment would "break" the new scheme. "If we were – God forbid that we should – to allow ourselves to drift back to the mass unemployment of the inter-war years, this scheme would be sunk – indeed the whole nation would be sunk" (Hansard 1946).

Beveridge, then, assumed that the great majority of people of working age would be in regular, full-time employment, and that even the lowest paid would earn enough to enable them to pay the contributions that were necessary to fund subsistence benefits. Equally crucial were Beveridge's expectations regarding the structure of the family. He took it for granted that the end of the war would see a return to pre-war trends and conditions. Divorce would be rare, few babies would be born outside marriage, and, crucially, women would give up paid employment after they were married. The NI scheme assumed that married women would not be contributors in their own right and would be eligible for benefits only as a dependant of their husbands. Beveridge's vision of a family in which the wife remained at home to serve the needs of her husband and children has made him "the arch-villain in much feminist writing" (Williams 1989). It also meant that the insurance scheme was ill suited to a world in which a majority of mothers with dependent children were in full-time or part-time work, in which one marriage in three was expected to end in divorce or separation, and in which nearly one fifth of all families with children were headed by a lone parent.

The result has been the growth of so-called "new poverty"; that of those who have been unable to establish an entitlement to contributory benefits. Prominent amongst these are lone parents, young people, and people with disabilities (for whom Beveridge made no specific provision). All are wholly dependent upon means tested assistance (unless, of course, they have an alternative source of income such as that of a cohabiting partner or maintenance payments). This group also includes the long-term unemployed because although Beveridge proposed that unemployment benefit be paid indefinitely it has always been subject to a time limit and following the budget of November 1993 it ceases after 6 months. Anyone out of work for longer than this – or experiencing recurrent spells of unemployment – is similarly forced to rely on assistance.

In addition very large numbers of people have come to receive assistance as a supplement to insurance benefits. Despite Beveridge's recommendations, contributory benefits were not fixed at levels that were sufficient for subsistence when the insurance scheme was introduced in 1946. The detailed story is an extremely complicated one, but the most important point is that the success of the wartime assistance scheme persuaded the Labour government that it would not be a serious problem if at least some claimants were to receive a means tested supplement to their benefits (Deacon 1982). The overall effect of the post-war legislation, then, was that assistance benefits were paid at a higher rate than the corresponding insurance benefits in the majority of cases. This meant that those receiving insurance benefits would need to apply for additional assistance, unless they had other resources. As the numbers particularly of pensioners rose in the 1950s and 1960s, so more and more people became eligible for such "top-up" payments.

The combined effect of all this was that means tested assistance came to play a much greater role within the social security system than Beveridge had ever envisaged. These trends were all the more significant because of the change that had taken place in the way in which assistance was perceived. In the late 1940s assistance benefits were seen by politicians and academics as something that lifted people out of poverty. In the words of one junior minis ter, the assistance scale provided "an appreciable margin over bare subsistence" (Hansard 1948). National assistance (NA), then, was something that solved the problem. Subsequently, however, it came to be seen as part of the problem rather than part of the solution. This turnabout was due in part to the discovery that not everyone who was eligible for NA benefits was willing to claim them. It was also due, however, to changing perceptions of the standard of living provided by assistance. Increasingly those who were receiving assistance benefits were believed to be actually living in poverty rather than having been rescued from it.

This shift in attitudes towards assistance was just one consequence of a broader change in prevailing ideas about poverty that was to transform the debate about social security policy. The nature and impact of that change is discussed in the next section.

The "rediscovery" of poverty

We have seen that there were some differences between the social security scheme proposed in the Beveridge Report and that introduced by the post-war Labour government. These differences, however, did not reflect any disagreement about the objective of the scheme. For both Beveridge and the Labour ministers social security was to eliminate "want", and was to do so by providing benefits that were at least adequate for subsistence. But what was subsistence? For an answer to this question Beveridge turned primarily to the work of Seebohm Rowntree. In essence Rowntree defined poverty as an income that was insufficient to maintain bodily health and to sustain a minimum level of social participation. He arrived at his "poverty line" by calculating what different types of household would need to spend on food, clothing and rent. This is the absolute definition of poverty, so called because it appears to be based upon an objective assessment of physical needs.

In fact Rowntree's approach was considerably more sophisticated than this, and his budget included an amount for items such as tea that had no nutritional value but that were "conventionally necessary" (Veit-Wilson 1986). The important point here, however, is that this absolute approach was almost universally accepted in the 1940s and early 1950s, and the available evidence seemed to show that the new benefits had all but abolished poverty. In 1951, for example, Rowntree claimed that the proportion of the population in poverty had fallen from 17.7 per cent in 1936 to 1.66 per cent in 1950 (Rowntree & Lavers 1951).

Rowntree's findings reinforced the combination of pride and complacency that was to characterize public attitudes towards the welfare state in the 1950s. As early as 1952, however, a few isolated critics had begun to question Rowntree's approach. Peter Townsend, for example, pointed out that once Rowntree had included some items as conventionally necessary, it was difficult to decide where to draw the line (Townsend 1952). In subsequent years Townsend went on to develop the argument that what constituted poverty was always relative to the standards of living experienced in the wider society. People were in poverty, he claimed, when they lacked the "resources to obtain the types of diet, participate in the activities, and have the living conditions and amenities" that were customary in the societies to which they belonged (Townsend 1979).

It is important to recognize, however, that the wider acceptance of such "relative" definitions of poverty was a slow and uneven process, and that the debate continues today. A crucial question is how relative poverty is to be measured. In 1965 Abel-Smith and Townsend published *The poor and the poorest*. In this they used the level of National Assistance benefits as the basis for calculating the poverty line, and claimed that far from falling the proportion of the population in poverty had increased from 8 per cent to 14 per cent between 1954 and 1960 (Abel-Smith & Townsend 1965). Even more striking was their finding that the largest group in poverty were not the elderly but the so-called "working poor": people who were in full-time employment but whose take-home income was not enough to keep the household out of poverty. On Abel-Smith and Townsend's definition there were more than two million children living in poverty in 1960.

More than any other single event the publication of *The poor and the poorest* marked the rediscovery of poverty, and it had an enormous impact upon the debate as to the nature and extent of poverty. The details of that debate are beyond the scope of this chapter, but there are three points that should be made at this stage.

The first point is that *The poor and the poorest* provided an extremely crude measure of the extent of poverty. In particular their use of benefit rates as the basis of the poverty line was widely criticized as illogical. (Strictly speaking it meant that a government that made benefits more generous in order to improve the circumstances of claimants would find that it had raised the poverty line and thereby increased the numbers who were defined as being in poverty). To avoid such anomalies subsequent studies have used a range of measures. These include the development of behavioural or lifestyle indicators to assess the proportion of the population that is excluded from customary activities, and the formulation of standard budgets as a way of calculating the level of income that different households need in order to participate fully in the wider society. A full account of these and other measures is given by Alcock (1993).

The second point is that the redefinition and subsequent rediscovery of poverty was part of a sustained attempt by a group of academics led by Richard Titmuss to demolish what they saw as the dangerous myth that Britain had become a more equal society. They "set out to challenge the comfortable assumptions of the day. Their research was explicitly political: they were setting out to reshape [the] policy makers' interpretation of their environment" (Banting 1979). For Titmuss and his colleagues the solution was to adopt a more redistributive strategy; in effect they had a "New Beveridge" agenda. Others, however, interpreted their data quite differently. The "targeters" and the "marketeers" had kept their heads down immediately after the war because public opinion seemed to be so firmly in support of universal benefits. Now, however, it had been shown that the Beveridge system had failed. Surely, they could argue, the answer was not to devote more resources to it but to replace it with something that would work better (Deacon & Bradshaw 1983).

The third point to emphasize, then, is the way in which the "rediscovery" of poverty precipitated a far-reaching debate about the purpose and scope of social security. If the Beveridge scheme could work at all, it would only be for as long as poverty was understood in minimalist, absolute terms. Once the objective was raised to the alleviation or even prevention of relative poverty, then a new strategy would be required. This was the starting point of the "universality versus selectivity" debate that dominated the policy agenda – and student textbooks – of the 1960s and 1970s.

Policy developments: 1946 to 1979

Benefits for children

One of the most striking features of this period was the decline in the value of the support provided to families with children by the tax and social security systems. There were originally two sources of such support. First, parents of dependent children were allowed to receive some of their earnings free of tax in recognition of their extra responsibilities. Secondly, a weekly family allowance was paid in respect of second and subsequent children. Neither family allowances nor tax allowances, however, were increased in line with the rise in earnings and prices. In 1946, for example, the total child support for a family with three children was equivalent to 27 per cent of average male manual earnings. Thirty years later the proportion was only 11 per cent, although it did recover slightly to 13 per cent in the early 1980s (Deacon & Bradshaw 1986). It is not easy to explain why family support was allowed to decline so sharply. Undoubtedly, however, it owed much to the fact that both Labour and Conservative Chancellors of the Exchequer found it easier to increase tax revenues by failing to raise allowances than by the more open method of increasing the actual rates of tax. (Nor would it have escaped their notice that less than one third of voters have dependent children.)

Whatever the reasons for the decline in child support, its effect was to lower the living standards of families relative to those of single people and childless couples at every income level. The impact was greatest, however, upon those on the lowest incomes, and it created the "working poverty" highlighted in *The poor and the poorest*. One response to the problems of the working poor would have been to raise wages. Even the most enthusiastic advocate of a statutory minimum wage, however, did not suggest that it would be possible to increase even the lowest wage to a level at which even the largest family would be free from poverty. The policy debate, then, focused upon two issues; to what extent should wages be supplemented to take account of family responsibilities? and what form should that supplementation take?

In the broadest terms there were two possible approaches to the problem of family poverty. The first was to increase family allowances. This was the option favoured by the group that had rediscovered poverty and it would be at the centre of any "New Beveridge" strategy. The advantages of higher family allowances were obvious. As a universal benefit, they contributed to the costs of children in all families and raised no problems of low take-up or of disincentive effects (see below). The drawback, of course, was that they were extremely expensive. One way of offsetting the costs of an increase in family allowances was to make a corresponding reduction in tax allowances (which would take more from the better off who paid tax at a higher rate). This was the basis of the so-called "clawback" scheme of 1968. Clawback, however, served to highlight the contentious issue of to whom the benefit should be paid. Family allowances were paid at the Post Office to the caring parent, usually the mother. This had the advantage of giving some independent income to a mother who was not in paid work, but it meant that in the majority of households a switch from tax allowances to family allowances would take money from the man's pay packet in order to pay it to the mother at the Post Office. It was this issue that dominated the replacement of family allowances by child benefits in 1976. Unlike family allowances, child benefits were not taxed, but their introduction was financed by the withdrawal of all tax allowances for children. At the last minute the Labour cabinet feared that the impact upon the take-home pay of many male trade unionists would jeopardize their co-operation with the government's policy of pay restraint, and the new scheme was eventually introduced in stages (Macarthy 1986).

The alternative approach was to restrict the additional child support to those on low wages. One proposal that was much discussed in the 1960s was that of a negative income tax. The idea here was to use the machinery that already existed for the assessment and collection of tax to also calculate entitlement to negative tax that would be paid as a supplement to low wages. This was much favoured by the "marketeers" who saw it as a means of redistributing sufficient income to the low paid to enable them to participate in private markets for pensions and health care. To date, however, it has proved impossible to devise a workable scheme, although the idea still has its supporters (Hill 1990).

In practice the means tested alternative to family allowances was the family income supplement (FIS). This was introduced as a temporary measure in 1971 but remained until it was replaced by family credit in 1988. FIS was a relatively small scheme. It was originally claimed by only 70,000 households and that figure had only risen to just over 200,000 by the mid 1980s (at which time child benefit was being paid to nearly 7 million parents with over 12 million children). Nonetheless, it attracted a great deal of attention because it illustrated very clearly the advantages and disadvantages of means tested benefits.

The attraction of FIS to policy-makers was that it was an inexpensive way of targeting help upon a small number of very low earners. Moreover, it was

81

particularly effective in helping lone parents in work because the amounts paid were the same for one parent as for two. There were, however, two major disadvantages. The first was that only around half of those eligible for FIS actually claimed it. Such low take up is common in means tested benefits. As Joan Brown has noted, means testing "may be wholly successful in withdrawing benefits from those above the means test line [but] it has never succeeded in delivering them to all those who are eligible" (Brown 1984). There are many reasons why people do not take up benefits. They may not be aware of their eligibility, they may perceive the claiming process as stressful and potentially humiliating, and they may expect their own circumstances to improve in the near future (Craig 1991). Whatever its cause, the fact of non-take up is a major constraint upon the further expansion of means testing. There is also some evidence that the take-up of benefits in the black communities is lower than amongst the white population, despite the higher incidence of poverty amongst the former (Cook & Watt 1992, Marsh & Mackay 1993).

The second disadvantage of FIS also applies to all means tested benefits. This is the disincentive effect, or "poverty trap". FIS made up half the difference between the claimant's gross wage and a specified prescribed amount. This meant, of course, that were someone receiving FIS to secure an increase in wages, then half of that increase would be offset by a reduction in FIS. Moreover, that person may also pay additional tax or insurance contributions and lose other means tested benefits. The net effect could be to leave the FIS recipient worse off after the pay rise. In practice the impact upon individuals may be less dramatic than this because their entitlement to benefit would not be reassessed immediately but after a period of up to 12 months, by which time the scale rates may also have gone up.

Nonetheless, this does not alter the fact that the combined effect of taxation and the withdrawal of means tested benefits is to all but equalize the net income of people earning very different gross wages. It has recently been calculated, for example, that a couple with two children and living in rented housing could double their gross income from £100 to £200 a week and yet find it made very little difference to the money in their pockets (Hills 1993). This situation would provoke an outrage if it applied further up the income scale.

Returning to family support, the dilemma that confronted the incoming Thatcher Government in 1979 was that it recoiled from the cost of increasing support for all children, but knew that were it to means test child benefits, then many poor families would either not get the money they needed or would face marginal tax rates that the government would never consider imposing upon high earners.

Pensions

In contrast, the key issues in pensions policy appeared to have been resolved by the late 1970s. The dominant influence upon policy-makers was the steady increase in the proportion of the population that was over pension age. This was – and remains – crucial because national insurance was never funded on a strict actuarial basis. The contributions paid by individuals established an entitlement to future benefits but they were not invested in order to generate the income needed to pay those benefits. Instead the costs of the pensions and other benefits paid out in any one year was met out of the contributions paid in during that year, the so-called "pay as you go" system. With such a system a rise in the ratio of pensioners to contributors would increase the burden upon contributors even if the rates of pension stayed the same.

Faced with just such a prospect in the 1950s, the Conservative government abandoned Beveridge's flat rate principle and introduced a graduated pension scheme. Contributors were now to pay an additional earnings related contribution in return for which they would receive an enhanced pension on retirement. The extra income from contributions meant that the scheme was excellent for the Exchequer, but it was a disaster for the contributors because when they came to draw their pensions they found that they had been rendered all but worthless by the rise in prices in the intervening years. The lesson of the graduated pension scheme, then, was that if pensions were to be earnings related, they had also to be protected from inflation.

Two further earnings related schemes were developed by Labour and Conservative governments in the following years. The details were too complicated to outline here but the differences between the two schemes reflected the conflicting priorities of the "New Beveridge" approach and that of the "targeters" and "marketeers". Labour's "National Superannuation" plan of 1969 emphasized state provision, and incorporated a redistributive formula that gave a disproportionately higher pension to lower paid workers. The state also guaranteed to inflation-proof pension entitlements by revaluing them in line with the level of earnings at the time of retirement. In contrast, the Conservative scheme of 1973 was designed to encourage the growth of occupational pensions and would have provided those who were not in occupational schemes with a relatively low pension through a residual State Reserve Scheme.

There was, however, one further aspect of the Conservative proposals that was implemented and that was to prove enormously important in later years. Under the scheme a basic state pension would still be paid at a flat rate, augmented in most cases by occupational benefits. This flat rate pension, however, would now be paid for by wholly earnings related contributions. The effect was to transform national insurance contributions (NICs) into a tax. It was a tax, however, without the complex reliefs that operated within income tax. Moreover, NICs were only earnings related up to one and a half times national average earnings, after which point the amount of NIC remained the same however high the earnings. This introduced a massive distortion into the tax system because it meant that the combined rate of tax and NICs paid by an individual actually dropped once his or her earnings reached this level. (From April 1994 this occurred at £430 a week.)

A third scheme finally made it to the statute book in 1975, the State Earnings Related Pension Scheme (SERPS). This was a Labour measure but at the time it received all-party support. It was something of a compromise because it incorporated a redistributive element, most notably in favour of women with interrupted work records, but it also included a generous provision whereby those in occupational schemes could partially opt out of NICs. The compromise, however, rested on somewhat shaky foundations. The scheme worked on a Pay As You Go basis and in effect SERPS promised generous pensions in future on the assumption that future contributors would be willing to pay higher NICs than current contributors (who would, of course, be the ones to enjoy the higher pensions in the future). This rested in turn on some optimistic assumptions regarding future unemployment and earnings growth. These chickens were to come home to roost in the 1980s.

Social assistance

It was noted earlier that means tested social assistance played a much greater role in the social security system than Beveridge had envisaged. A central theme of post-war policy has been the attempts of successive governments to adapt assistance to this enlarged role. The paradox is that the numbers dependent upon assistance rose at the same time as the weaknesses of the scheme were becoming increasingly apparent.

Evidence emerged in the 1960s that many old people were failing to claim national assistance (NA), as it was then called, and it was believed that it was due to the stigma attached to the benefit and to the intrusive manner in which it was administered. An Act in 1966 introduced the new name of Supplementary Benefits (SB) along with a greater emphasis upon the claimant's right to benefit if the income conditions were met. Even so SB was still sharply distinguished from national insurance by the amount of discretion retained by local officers, and particularly by their power to award additional weekly payments or lump sum grants to meet extra needs. The number of such payments grew rapidly during the 1970s and they became the chief focus of the fierce controversy that came to surround SB. On the one hand the emerging welfare rights movement was pressing for a reduction in discre tion and the payment of benefits as of right. On the other hand, the rising numbers of single parents and unemployed on SB fuelled popular fears of scrounging and calls for a more rigorous scrutiny of claims. The scheme seemed to many commentators to be close to breakdown and it was reformed again in 1980. The Act of 1980 changed the legal basis of the scheme. The unpublished rules that had guided officers in the exercise of their discretionary powers were now to be published as regulations that had the force of law. This was supposed to simplify the system and to give claimants a clear idea of what they were entitled to. At the same time the government expected that it would reverse the growth in additional payments by reducing the scope for welfare rights activists and other groups to pressurize local offices into making discretionary additions (Walker 1983).

The 1980 Act was a total failure. A genuine simplification of the system would have been expensive. It would have required a sufficient increase in the basic scale rates to permit the withdrawal of some discretionary additions without penalizing those currently receiving them. The new Conservative government, however, was adamant that there should be no additional expenditure; and so, hopelessly complex internal guidelines were published as hopelessly complex regulations. Moreover, the number of additional payments soon started to rise again as "claimants and their advisors learnt how to extract help from the system by using the structure of rules clarifying entitlement" (Hill 1990). The incoming Thatcher Government had inherited the broad principles of the 1980 Act from its Labour predecessor, but these were clearly issues to which it would return.

Benefits for people with disabilities

The social security benefits introduced in the 1940s included no specific provisions for people with disabilities or for the people who cared for them. Those unable to work, and hence to pay contributions, would have to depend upon NA. So too would those whose opportunities to work were restricted by their caring responsibilities. The overwhelming majority of the latter were women.

People with disabilities did receive discretionary additions to their NA benefits, but no other attempt was made to meet the extra costs arising from disability until the 1970s. The benefits then introduced included a mobility allowance (MA) for those unable or virtually unable to walk, and an attendance allowance (AA) for those who needed intensive care by day or night, or both. Invalidity Benefit was also introduced for those unable to work for more than six months, although this was effectively an extension to NI sickness benefit and consequently was of help only to those who had been able to work in the past. A Non-Contributory Invalidity Pension (NCIP) was also introduced, but this was paid at a very low rate. NCIP was also a striking example of the gender discrimination within social security at this time as it was only paid to a married woman who could demonstrate that she was unable to perform household duties. Similarly the Invalid Care Allowance (ICA) that was paid to people of working age who were caring for someone in receipt of MA or AA was withheld from married or cohabiting women until 1986. Indeed, there remains a general problem for carers that their entitlement to such benefits depends not upon their own status and circumstances but upon those of the person they are caring for.

Social security and housing costs

Benefits to meet housing costs have become an increasingly important part of the social security system (Hill 1990). There are two aspects to this issue. The first is the growth of rent and rate rebate schemes. In the immediate post-war period housing subsidies were directed towards local authority houses rather than the people who lived in them. The subsidy reduced the rent, but the rent for each property was fixed and did not vary with the circumstances of the tenant. After the mid 1950s, however, policy changed to one of allowing rent levels to rise and using the subsidies to provide rebates for poorer tenants. This process was boosted greatly by an Act of 1972 that required local authorities to increase rents and introduced a national system of rebates. The rationale was that of the "targeters": it was a waste of money to reduce the rent of every tenant; it was much more efficient to focus help on those who needed it. Nonetheless it is very important to emphasize that such rebates were seen as being primarily instruments of housing policy, rather than as income maintenance benefits. They were a means of widening access to housing, not of income redistribution. The White Paper that preceded the 1972 Act made clear that the rebates would not be restricted to those on the poverty line but would be available "to tenants with incomes above this level, if the rent of their home would otherwise impose an unfair burden on the family budget". (Another objective was to encourage owner occupation and readers in the mid 1990s might be surprised to learn that home ownership "satisfies a deep and natural desire [and gives] the greatest security against loss of home and price changes" [Cmnd 4728]).

The subsequent Labour government retained the rebate scheme despite the contribution it made to the growth of the poverty trap, and despite the increasingly serious overlap between it and the SB scheme. Those on SB, of course, had their rents met in full in the great majority of cases. There were, then, two systems of housing support; one for SB claimants and one for those in work or claiming NI benefits. There was no consistency between them. The rebate scheme provided help to households on incomes some way above SB levels, but was less generous than SB to working households on incomes comparable to the SB scale. Those responsible for the administration of SB were pressing for a unified scheme that would eliminate these anomalies and also remove housing costs from calculations of entitlement to SB. The Department of the Environment, however, was opposed. It recognized that a combined scheme would be either very expensive or very unpopular. It expected that the latter would be the case and that it would get the blame. This was to prove a prophetic assessment.

Thatcherism and social security

Many books have been written on the subject of Thatcherism. Most agree that the social and economic policies adopted after 1979 marked a radical departure from those pursued in earlier years. In general, the distinctiveness of Thatcherism as an ideology is believed to stem from its fusion of two strands of political thought. The first was conservative populism that emphasizes national identity and law and order, and the second was liberal political

87

economy that emphasizes individualism and the technical and moral superiority of markets over state provision. Hitherto these had been associated with different groups within the Conservative party but Thatcherism brought them together in the concept of the "free economy and the strong state" (Gamble 1983).

In the specific case of social security, the Thatcherite approach is seen as having been underpinned by four central ideas or themes. These themes reflect the influence upon the Thatcher Governments of the "targeters", the "marketeers" and the "dependency theorists".

The first theme was that it is the duty of government to encourage the creation of wealth, but that it should not concern itself with the distribution of that wealth. It should provide a minimum income for all, but no more. The second theme was that the government should not try to maintain a particular level of employment in the economy. Jobs occurred when labour markets worked properly, and labour markets worked properly when people were prepared to accept the work that was available. Government could facilitate the operation of the market by curbing the monopoly power of trade unions, by establishing training schemes that equipped the unemployed with the skills and attitudes required by employers, and by fostering a climate in which effort and enterprise were rewarded. What it could not do was to create jobs by spending money. That only led to inflation. The third theme was the need to restrict the scale and cost of government activity. Many tasks would be carried out more efficiently in the private sector, while lower spending would permit lower taxation and thereby safeguard incentives to work and save. The fourth theme became more pronounced after Mrs Thatcher's third election victory in 1987. This was the belief that the benefits system was beginning to foster the culture of dependency that "new right" critics had identified in the United States, and the consequent emphasis in government rhetoric upon the obligations as well as the rights of claimants (Deacon 1991).

The policy objectives that flowed from these ideas were clear; a reduction in the value of benefits for the unemployed and stricter controls on their administration, an expansion of means testing, a greater role for occupational and private provision and the simplification of the benefits system to facilitate its administration by fewer civil servants. If the objectives were clear, however, their attainment would not be straightforward. For a start, some were incompatible. Means tests, for example, were complex and required more staff, not less, while some of the tax reliefs and other financial incentives that were introduced to encourage people to switch to private sector provision were to prove very expensive. Moreover, some elements of the Conservatives' programme were to encounter opposition from unexpected quarters. Small businesses, for example, were to resent being required to administer sickness benefits, and Conservative women's groups were to see reductions in the level of family support as a threat to their identity as the "party of the family". The rigorous implementation of Thatcherism would not be easy.

Early measures

One of the first steps taken by the new government was to end the link between the level of NI pension and the growth in earnings. Henceforth pensions would be increased in line with the rise in prices. Earnings have since increased much faster than prices, and so the change in policy has meant that the standard of living of those dependent upon NI pensions has fallen further and further below that of those in work. By 1992 the pension was a lower proportion of average disposable income than it had been in 1948. Some indication of the significance of uprating policy is given by the fact that if the pension for a single person had been linked to prices since 1948, it would have been worth £23 in 1992 rather than the actual rate of £56.10 (Hills 1993). Other early measures included the transfer to employers of the responsibility for paying sickness benefit (they were reimbursed through rebates on their NI contributions) and the introduction of housing benefit. The latter was a classic "botched" affair. Rather than incur the cost of merging the two systems of housing support discussed in the previous section, the government effectively operated the two means tests side by side within a single scheme administered by the local authorities. The result was the emergence of further anomalies and administrative chaos in some areas (Hill 1990). The government quickly announced that it intended to conduct a further review of housing benefit, and in due course it launched further reviews of child support, pensions and social assistance.

The Social Security Act 1986

The reviews were completed in 1985 and their findings formed the basis of the Social Security Act of 1986. The Act can be understood in two ways. It sought to achieve the distinctive objectives of Thatcherism, but it also represented a further attempt to resolve particular issues and problems that had confronted earlier governments. This was especially true in the case of social assistance.

It was seen earlier that the 1980 Act had totally failed to curb the award of discretionary payments. The government's response was to remove the scope for additional payments altogether. Renamed Income Support (IS), the scheme would effectively consist of two basic scale rates, one for those aged under 25 and one for those over 25. These would be augmented by weekly premiums for specific groups such as families, the elderly or the disabled. Such a radically simplified scheme would be able to handle a larger number of claimants without the strains and staffing problems that had bedevilled SB, and would make it possible to control costs much more tightly. The problem for the government, however, was that the discretionary payments were there for a reason. There were a host of needs that claimants could not be expected to meet out of their weekly benefits and for which they would have to receive some form of lump sum payment. Moreover, the wide variations between local offices in the number of awards they made indicated that discretionary payments also served as a safety valve in some areas, and that their sudden removal would provoke an angry response (Walker & Lawton 1988). It was these considerations that led to the introduction of the Social Fund.

The Social Fund was to be quite separate from the main scheme. Social Fund officers were to have the power to make additional payments to meet exceptional needs. Those payments, however, would normally take the form of loans rather than grants. Furthermore they would be entirely at the discretion of the officer, there would be no entitlement to a payment and no right of appeal against a refusal of an award. Finally, the Social Fund was cash-limited; once the budget was exhausted for the month that would be that.

The operation of the Social Fund has aroused great controversy. From the government's perspective it has succeeded in limiting the number of additional payments and in thwarting the activities of welfare rights groups. At the same time, the replacement of grants by loans and the loss of appeal rights has undoubtedly exacerbated the hardship experienced by many claimants (Huby & Dix 1992).

In the case of child support, the issue was whether or not the government would introduce a means test for child benefit. To do so would save large sums of money and would mark a major advance for the "targeters". It would also make the poverty trap much worse, and almost certainly mean that many poor families would not receive money that the government itself said they needed. Means testing child benefit would also mean that it no longer contributed to the costs of children in all families and no longer provided an independent income to all mothers. In the event, the government backed off from means testing child benefit. Instead, the value of child benefit would be frozen and the emphasis was to be upon a new means tested benefit for working families – Family Credit (FC). In 1991, however, this policy was itself suddenly reversed; Child Benefit was uprated and a commitment given to safeguard its value in real terms. FC, however, remains an important benefit. It provides more help to more families than did FIS, and its introduction was part of a wider attempt to restructure means tested benefits.

Housing Benefit (HB) was cut back sharply by the Act, and is in effect now paid to those close to the IS level. In the terms used earlier it is now purely an anti-poverty measure rather than an instrument of housing policy. The changes to HB were significant in two respects. First, the withdrawal of HB from those on higher incomes was the largest single source of savings within the reform package. Second, the Act established a more rational relationship between eligibility for IS, HB and FC, and this has lessened some of the excesses of the poverty trap (Hill 1990). The changes, however, did little to improve take-up. In 1989, take-up of FC was just under 60 per cent and take-up of both IS and HB was around 75 per cent (DSS 1993).

The 1986 Act also made important changes to SERPS, although the details are too complex to outline here. The problem for the government was that not only were the projected costs of SERPS alarming, but the relative attraction of the state scheme was impeding the development of occupational pensions. The government's initial proposal was to abolish SERPS. This, however, aroused tremendous opposition, not least from the pensions industry, which recognized that the terms proposed by the government would not enable it to provide low paid workers with adequate pensions. The package that eventually emerged was to trim back the more expensive elements of SERPS, to encourage the growth of private pensions by giving rebates of NI contributions to those who took them out, and to lessen the financial risks to employers of starting occupational schemes. Overall, the effect was to shift significantly the balance between private and public provision. Indeed, pensions afford a striking example of the importance of non-state provision and of the cost of the tax reliefs given to it. By the end of the 1980s, the cost of the tax reliefs to private pensions was nearly one third of the direct cost of providing NI pensions (Parry 1991). There are now many pensioners whose standard of living depends as much if not more upon the performance of the financial markets as upon decisions in Whitehall.

Thatcherism: the outcome

Thatcherism brought a new agenda to social security, but commentators differ over the extent to which the Thatcher Governments were able to achieve their objectives. In some respects the policy changes were less dramatic than may have been anticipated from the rhetoric. The broad structure of NI benefits remained, child benefits were still paid to all families, and the social security budget kept on growing. At the end of 1993, a fourth Conservative government was still desperately seeking ways of cutting the cost of social security in order to reduce a public sector deficit then running at over £50 billion per year.

At the same time it is possible to identify areas in which a Thatcherite strategy was pursued with some success. There was a significant shift from public to private and occupational provision in pensions, benefit rights were withdrawn from those under 18 as part of an attempt to forestall the growth of a culture of dependency amongst young people, and unemployed people were subject to much greater pressures to seek work and to accept whatever jobs were on offer. This last objective was achieved by reducing the value of unemployment benefits and by strengthening the conditions that claimants had to satisfy in order to receive those benefits. Indeed, an authoritative study of social security since 1974 concluded that the most radical policy change in this period was the deliberate worsening of the position of the unemployed relative to earners that occurred in the 1980s (Barr & Coulter 1990).

It was noted earlier that the relative position of pensioners has also declined following the change in uprating policy in 1980. Indeed, it is important to emphasize that the increase in the overall cost of social security was due less to a rise in the level of benefits than to an increase in the number of people claiming them. This increase was itself the result of the growth in unemployment, and, to a lesser extent, the rise in the numbers of lone parents, pensioners, and people with disabilities. It has been estimated, for example, that if the provisions and uprating policies in 1989 had been the same as they were in 1979, then the total benefits budget would have been more than ten per cent higher (Millar 1991).

The changes to benefits were accompanied by substantial reductions in direct taxation that overwhelmingly favoured the better off. Figures given in the House of Commons in June 1992, for example, indicated that the richest 10 per cent of taxpayers received over half of the total given in tax cuts between 1978/9 and 1991/2, while the bottom 50 per cent – a far larger number of people – shared 15 per cent of the total. In terms of individuals, someone earning around one and a half times the national average received ten times as large a tax cut as the lowest paid, and for the highest earning group (over £50,000 p.a. in 1992/3) the tax cuts were worth 140 times as much each as for the lowest paid (CPAG 1993). The effect of all this was to throw into sharp reverse the post-war trend towards greater equality in incomes and wealth.

This, of course, is exactly what the Thatcher Governments had told the electorate they would do. They rejected the pursuit of equality as an aim of policy, and sought to create a tax and benefit system in which effort and enterprise would be recognized and rewarded. It was always expected that this would lead to a widening of the differentials between the incomes of the most successful and those of the rest of the workforce, and no apology would be made for that. This was not the whole story, however, because it was also expected that a more dynamic and productive economy would thereby be created, and that the fruits of this would eventually "trickle down" to the poorest. The poor, then, would also become better off, albeit at a slower rate than the rest of society.

This "trickle down" effect has simply not happened. The government's own data show that between 1979 and 1991 the poorest tenth of the population experienced a fall of 14 per cent in their real incomes after housing costs, compared with a rise of 36 per cent for the population as a whole and increase of 62 per cent for the richest ten per cent (Hills 1993). The figures on poverty are even more striking, whatever definition is adopted. One measure is the number of people living on an income that is less than half the national average (standardized for household size). On this basis the total in poverty has risen from 5 million in 1979 to 13.5 million in 1990/1. Moreover, there were 5.8 million people who were living in 1990/1 on incomes that would have been less half the average income in 1979. This, of course, is an increase on the 5 million who were living below that level in 1979. "Even from an 'absolute' viewpoint using a fixed measuring rod relative to 1979 incomes, the numbers affected increased despite a 36 per cent increase in overall incomes" (Hills 1993). Nearly two thirds of those living on incomes that were less than half the national average in 1990/1 were families with children. There were 4 million children in poor households in 1990/1 compared to 1.4 million in 1979 (Millar 1993).

This upsurge in poverty was the result of a combination of fundamental changes in the labour market and of the policies pursued by the Thatcher Governments. The most important of the former were the rise in long-term unemployment and the growth of low-paid and insecure employment. These made it impossible for more and more people to meet their needs through employment, but this in itself would not necessarily have led to more poverty. The needs generated by the lack of employment opportunities could have been met through the benefits system. It was the fact that these changes occurred at a time when the government was seeking to redefine and diminish the role of state provision that produced the increase in poverty. It is this that provides the context for the current debate regarding the scope and purpose of social security in the future.

What next?

By the end of 1993 there was scarcely a single aspect of the social security system that was not being subjected to a fundamental reappraisal or review. For many commentators this process was necessitated by the urgent need to reduce the level of government borrowing, which they believed had risen sharply in the early 1990s because of an unforeseen and unsustainable increase in welfare spending. For its part the government has pointed again and again to the underlying growth in the cost of social security and to the implications for future spending of the continuing increase in the number of old people (DSS 1993). Others, however, have argued that talk of a "demographic time bomb" is exaggerated, and that the recent increase in expenditure is primarily due to the recession. Hills, for example, has claimed the likely increase in welfare spending over the next *fifty* years due to the ageing population is less than that caused by the recession in the *three* years to 1992 (Hills 1993). Even amongst those who are most sanguine about future costs, however, there is a growing belief that it is necessary to radically reform the system in order to adapt it to current social and economic conditions. Indeed, such is the eagerness of think tanks, pressure groups, politicians and academics to think the "unthinkable" that it sometimes seems that the only policy option not on the agenda is the retention of the status quo.

The nature of the debate is such that it has led to some blurring of the distinctions between the different perspectives outlined in the introduction to this chapter. Nonetheless it is still possible to identify the policy options that flow from these positions. The centrepiece of a "New Beveridge" strategy remains a substantial increase in both child benefits and NI benefits. More generous NI benefits, paid for longer periods, would reduce the role of means tested income support but would also be very expensive. To meet the cost the advocates of a "New Beveridge" approach would remove the ceiling on NI contributions, introduce a more progressive structure of tax rates, and further reduce the tax reliefs on occupational welfare and mortgage interest (Sinfield 1993). The greatest obstacle to the implementation of such a strategy is, of course, the well-recognized reluctance of the British electorate to pay more in taxes, especially when the proceeds can so readily be presented as being spent on people who do not really need help. Moreover, advocates of a "New Beveridge" face something of a dilemma regarding the contributory basis of the NI scheme. On the one hand the contributory conditions have served to exclude important groups from benefit. On the other hand, it is the fact that NI benefits are paid in return for contributions – that claimants have established a right to them – which provides the firmest argument against means testing. They are forced, therefore, into a position of arguing that the payment of some contributions should establish a general right to benefit, but that the link between individuals' precise entitlement and their detailed record of payment should be broken or at least be made looser (Alcock 1992). Some "New Beveridge" writers have also begun to question the value of simply paying benefit to unemployed people and to consider a closer linkage between eligibility for benefit and the individual's willingness to participate in active labour market measures such as work or training programmes. This would introduce an element of conditionality into the benefits system that has hitherto been associated with "dependency theorists" and regarded with great suspicion in the "New Beveridge" camp (Piachaud 1993, Deacon 1993).

The policy priorities of the "targeters" are clear and unambiguous. The introduction of a means test for child benefits and for NI benefits, particularly pensions, would save large sums of money, some of which could be redirected to those most in need. There are, however, three obvious difficulties with this scenario. The first two are the well-established problems of low take-up and of the poverty trap. (The latter would be made far worse if child benefits was also withdrawn as an individual's income rose.) The third problem is that to means test pensions would be widely seen as a betrayal of people who had paid NI contributions all their lives in the expectation that they would receive a pension in return. In strict logic, of course, NI contributions are a form of direct taxation and individuals' past contributions do not in any way cover the cost of their current pension. Nonetheless, the popular belief that people have paid for their NI benefits and should in some way be better off than those who have not contributed is a major obstacle to the large scale means testing of NI benefits (Hill 1990). As the former Secretary of State for Social Services, Norman Fowler, told the Society of Conservative Lawyers in

October 1990, "What worries me about so many of the targetting proposals is that you end up penalising middle England and middle income families" (Fowler 1990).

The "marketeers" face similar obstacles. It was noted earlier that the precondition of a major shift towards private provision is a redistribution of income on a scale sufficient to allow the poor to purchase that provision. To date no workable scheme has emerged, and the response of the financial services industry to the proposal to abolish SERPS does not suggest that it perceives a ready market for private insurance against unemployment and sickness.

In contrast, the policy prescriptions of the "dependency theorists" could be introduced incrementally. Indeed, some already have. They advocate the withdrawal of one parent benefit that is currently paid in addition to child benefit, and would restrict the access of lone mothers to public housing (Green 1992). More generally, they would introduce much more stringent conditions governing entitlement to benefits. The purpose of provision would not simply be to relieve need, but to change the attitudes and behaviour of claimants in order to prevent the need arising again. They believe that it is essential to enhance the financial and social status of those who are or who become self-reliant and, if necessary, would impose sanctions upon those who continue to behave irresponsibly. In part the justification for such measures is a utilitarian one: they may operate harshly in some cases but those affected must suffer for the good of the majority. Even so, such an approach only makes sense in so far as poverty is caused by individual failing. If it is not, then the policy simply penalizes people for circumstances beyond their control. Indeed, this is inevitable in the case of measures to reduce the living standards of existing lone parents and their children, and the widespread reluctance to do this is the major obstacle that the "dependency theorists" have to overcome. As Joan Brown has put it, "I have never seen the social morality of storming the barricades over the bodies of living children. The reform of our society ought not to require the sacrifice of the 1.6 million children currently in one parent families" (Brown 1990).

The impact of the "feminist" literature on social security has stemmed primarily from the way in which it has documented the higher incidence of poverty amongst women (particularly amongst the elderly) and the assumptions about gender roles that underpin provision for carers. The most important single policy change that follows from a "feminist" analysis would be to base entitlement to means tested benefits upon the circumstances of the individual and ignore those of a partner. This would bring the benefit system into line with the tax system and would remove assumptions about income sharing within households. It would be very expensive, however, because it would mean that someone without an income of their own would be eligible for benefits such as income support even although they were living with someone in work. One estimate is that it would cost the equivalent of seven pence in the pound on income tax (Hills 1993). Any such change, of course, would do nothing to improve the circumstances of women who did not live with partners.

The implementation of any of these strategies, then, would encounter formidable obstacles; financial, administrative, technical and political. This indicates that the changes to the structure and finance of the benefits system that are likely to emerge from the current round of reviews may be less dramatic – less "unthinkable" – than might be suggested by some of the contributions to the debate. In any case the most important issue remains the adequacy of the benefits. No matter how streamlined the structure, how computerized the assessment, how customer-friendly the administration, if the amounts paid are not sufficient to enable those who receive them to participate fully in the society in which they live, then millions will remain in poverty.

Suggested reading

Hill (1990) is the best introduction to the major issues in social security between 1945 and the late 1980s, and pays particular attention to the implementation of policy. Alcock (1993) provides a comprehensive account of all aspects of poverty, and Hills (1993) is a clear and up-to-date discussion of the options for future policy. Lowe (1993) is an excellent history of the "classic welfare state" from Beveridge to the mid 1970s, and Barr & Coulter (1990) discuss the impact of policy between 1979 and 1990. The best introduction to the issues of Thatcherism and social security is Becker (1991).

CHAPTER 5
Health: from seamless service to patchwork quilt

Judith Allsop

Introduction

The National Health Service (NHS) provides a comprehensive service to the whole population at a relatively low cost. It is mainly financed from taxation and is substantially free at the point of delivery. Compared with many health systems, access to services is more socially equitable. The NHS has had popular support and, in the 1940s, was seen as a central plank of the collectivist welfare state. In 1944, Henry Willink, the Conservative Minister of Health, described the health proposals as representing the: "very root of national vigour and national enterprise . . . the biggest single advance ever made in this country in the sphere of public health" (Webster 1988). In the 1992 election campaign, all the major political parties claimed to be guardians of the principles of the NHS.

Yet despite its achievements and its popularity, since the 1980s the service has come under increasing strain. Conservative governments have seen the NHS as a burden on the economy. It was widely criticized for being professionally dominated, unresponsive to consumers and internally inefficient and ineffective in the use of resources. In 1990, against a background of fierce opposition, the NHS and Community Care Act introduced changes that have been seen as the most radical since the 1946 Act that created the service. The NHS remains tax funded and substantially free at the point of delivery but the central command and control model has been replaced by the introduction of a quasi- or internal market. At the local district level there is now a division between agencies that purchase services for their populations through annually negotiated service contracts from a variety of providers. One consequence has been a proliferation of agencies and a move from a planned NHS which aimed to provide a seamless service to "a patch-work quilt" (Webster 1991). Day & Klein (1991) have remarked: "In the context of the NHS culture, this move from the implicit to the explicit, from trust to contract, is truly revolutionary".

This chapter has two aims. The first is to describe the major policy shifts over the period against the background of changes in the population and the burden of disease. Following the themes, examples are given of how this relates to women's health and that of ethnic minorities. The second aim is to show that particular issues have been more or less dominant on the policy agenda of governments. Policies to deal with inequalities in health status have rarely surfaced, while issues of funding, value for money and organization have dominated. Some policies such as meeting the needs of vulnerable groups have been difficult to implement, while others such as policies for prevention and primary care were slow to develop.

The chapter is organized as follows: the first section focuses on the population structure and the burden of illness especially as it affects particular groups. In the second section, the dilemmas of providing health care are outlined. Demand for health care has increased and cost containment has been an overriding concern of governments. In the third section, policies for the organization and management of the NHS are examined. Especially recently, these have been driven largely by a search for efficiency. By the mid 1980s, the Thatcher Governments began seriously to address health service reform. The fourth section examines these reforms. The next looks at policies for primary care, prevention and consumer empowerment, while the final section draws out the main determinants of policy change.

Patterns and trends in the health of the population

Patterns of ill health and population structure

Over the period from the late 1940s to the 1990s, the health status of the UK population has improved for every age group. This means that more people in every age group are surviving (Social Trends 1993). For example, mortality rates in the first year of life (the perinatal mortality rate) are now very small for all groups. Dramatic improvements occurred in the first half of the century and more slowly since 1950. Life expectation at birth for men in 1950 was 67 and for women 71. By 1990, this was 73 for men and 78 for women. Improvements in mortality rates have been attributed to improved nutrition, housing and other environmental factors rather than expanding health care (McKeown 1976).

In terms of the incidence of various diseases, there has been a decline in infectious diseases but a relative increase in diseases of the heart and circulatory system, the cancers and accidents as the leading causes of mortality and morbidity. Susceptibility to disease in individuals is a complex mix of genetic, behavioural and environmental factors. In recent years, the study of biogenetics has developed so that it is possible to identify the presence of specific genes for an increasing number of diseases. However, social scientists concentrate on particular behaviours such as smoking and alcohol abuse and on environmental factors such as the work that people do, and the material conditions in which they live. These have been shown to have a major effect on health status, although there is considerable controversy about the relationship between these factors as well as about the appropriate ways to intervene to improve health (Lambert & McPherson 1993).

Increased life expectancy has led to changes in the age structure of the UK population that grew steadily from 1951 to 1971, from 50 million to 55 million. Thereafter, the growth was slower and in 1991 the population was 57.5 million. The proportion of children under the age of 16 has declined, while those in the pensionable age groups have increased. The number of those over 80 years old was three times greater in 1991 than 1951, 2.2 per cent of the population compared to 0.7 (Social Trends 1991). The "burden" of an ageing population has created continuing pressure on health care spending. Robinson & Judge (1987) estimated that each person over the age of 65 cost the NHS nine times more than the average.

Diversity of health status within the population

The overall improvements in health status disguise differences between the experiences of particular groups within the population. Variations between those living in different regions and in different material conditions have been most fully documented while those between men and women and various ethnic groups have received less attention. Through the activity of researchers and pressure groups, policy makers have been confronted with issues of inequities in resource distribution and inequalities in health status. However, governments have either found the issues intractable or they have not considered them a policy priority. Measuring health inequalities presents problems; attributing cause even more. Therefore, the most appropriate interventions to improve health are uncertain as well as contested.

Difficulties of measurement:
some key findings and policy problems

The main measure of health status is by mortality rates. Since 1839, the Registrar General has kept statistics on death, the causes of death and decennial studies of deaths by occupation. These can be linked with census data by enumeration district to calculate standardized mortality ratios (SMRs) for purposes of comparison. Data on sickness comes mainly from the *General Household Survey* that is carried out annually and covers a sample of about 10,000 households. It includes questions about short-term acute illness and longer term chronic sickness, and whether the GP has been consulted in the previous two weeks, among others.

Both these sources of data have limitations, but the main trends in relation to regional and socio-economic groupings are clear. Studies from the 1960s onwards have indicated that the health status, measured by SMRs, of those living in the more northern regions and in the unskilled and manual socio-economic groups, is worse than for those living in the more southern regions and from the managerial and professional groups. The 1980 Black Report on health inequalities (Townsend & Davidson 1982) and its sequel, *The health divide* (Whitehead 1988) demonstrated most fully the major differences. Using 1971 figures, the Black Report showed that health status followed a class gradient with men in social class V between 15 and 64 having a standardized mortality rate 1.8 times greater than men in social class I.

In reviewing changes ten years later, Davey Smith et al. (1990) concluded that differentials on a number of mortality measures, such as death rates at different ages and life expectancy, have tended to increase. The same trend is indicated in sickness rates. For example, the *General Household Survey* data show double the rates of long-standing sickness among unskilled manual working men than professional men. This may reflect perceptions of illness and a willingness to report as well as need. Overall, there is strong evidence of an association between poverty and ill health but also of health status improving along with income and relative affluence (Quick & Wilkinson 1991, Wilkinson 1992). However, data on utilization suggest that lower income groups make greater use of health services (Hills 1993). But what is not known is whether this is relative to need.

Data are less readily available to examine the effect of other social divisions such as gender and ethnic group. In relation to women, a major problem arises in the recording of women's occupations.[1] In comparison to men, women have a greater life expectancy but, largely due to women's role in reproduction, women consult health practitioners more. Pregnancy and childbirth tend to be treated as illnesses. Women also consult for contraception, abortion, fertility treatment and problems associated with the menopause. McFarlane (1990), in a detailed analysis of women's health, argues that once the consultations for pregnancy and childbirth and diseases of the male/female genito-urinary systems were excluded, the differences between male and female consultation rates virtually disappeared. Mortality from these events is now very small. However, there are differences between women's and men's death and morbidity rates for particular diseases depending on age.

In relation to inequalities between women in different socio-economic groups, it is apparent that women's health status too is affected by material circumstances. For example, a study by Moser et al. (1988) showed that high mortality among women was associated with working in a manual occupation, living in a rented house and having no access to a car. Where these indicators were combined, the authors found that mortality rates were two or three times higher than for women with none of these disadvantages. Arber (1990), in a secondary analysis of recent *General Household Survey* data, found that women in the professional classes have less long-term sickness than other groups but the clear class gradient for other groups is less marked. This may reflect the fact that women's health is subject to more complex influences than that of men.[2]

The health divide concludes: " research is only just beginning to unravel the complexities of inequality in health in women" (Whitehead 1988). Examples are studies of the higher incidence of mental illness in women (Brown & Harris 1978) and the relationship between smoking and ill health (Graham 1990). Graham argues that health behaviour, and most importantly smoking behaviour, varies with social position. She states that "the risk factors associated with heart disease and cancer tend to be more common among those living in working class households in the north of England. Three times as many women in unskilled manual households smoke cigarettes as those in households classified as professional". She also suggests that those in higher income brackets eat a healthier diet than households on low incomes.

Data about the health of ethnic minorities, and especially by gender and class within this category, are scarce. Routine statistics do not record ethnicity. Until 1991, for example, the Census only asked questions about the country of birth. Recording membership of an ethnic group is more useful as it reflects cultural history and ways of life. Balarajan & Raleigh (1993) provide a summary of current data on ethnicity and health. The 1991 census showed that 94 per cent of the population was white and the largest ethnic minority was Indian at 1.7 per cent. Other Asian groups were 1.6, Black Caribbean 1.0. However, in Brent, the local authority in Britain with the highest ethnic minority population, 45 per cent of the population were from minority groups.

Balarajan & Raleigh also show, using routine population registration data based on country of birth, that men born in the Indian sub-continent tend to have higher death rates from heart disease than the white population. Both Asian and Afro-Caribbean men are at greater risk of stroke and, for Asians, this is particularly marked in the younger age groups. Also, babies of ethnic minority mothers are twice as likely to die in the first year of life than the average. Conversely, the death rates from heart disease and cancer are lower than the average for women in ethnic minority groups. In relation to mental illness, small scale studies have suggested that Afro-Caribbean males have higher admission rates to hospital and are much more likely to be diagnosed as having a serious mental illness than the population as a whole. The causes of these differences can currently only be speculated upon. For example, it has been suggested that the lower deaths rates of women in the ethnic minority groups may be due to low smoking rates. Higher levels of mental illness in certain groups have been attributed to a range of factors such as the stress of migration, the effect of cultural and social mores on behaviour, the response of service gatekeepers to particular groups, racism and poor material conditions.

While in the 1970s governments began to address problems of inequities of resources distribution through equalizing regional funding allocation according to weighted populations, there have been few direct attempts to tackle inequalities. As suggested earlier, this is partly due to the complexity of the issues and partly to uncertainty about where to intervene. However, the individualist values of the "New Right" also played a part. In 1979, the incoming Conservative government ignored the Black Report. Subsequently, Ministers tended to blame individuals for their ill health. However, recently, there are examples of greater responsiveness to pressures from minority groups. For example, as a consequence of their inquiry into maternity services, the Expert Group on maternity services recommended that women giving birth should be offered greater choice (Expert Maternity Group 1993). Health authorities have also been encouraged to respond to the needs of ethnic minorities.

Dilemmas in health care

Increasing demand

The changing pattern of disease and the socio-demographic structure of the population has led to rising costs due to the larger numbers in the older age groups. In addition, expectations of what constitutes good care have risen and innovations in biomedical science have been applied to clinical practice. Most notable of these have been the development of immunization and vaccination; techniques that allow earlier and more accurate diagnosis; the introduction of antibiotics, drugs to treat heart disease and digestive disorders, and advances in surgery which permit not only organ transplants but also less invasive procedures that reduce post-operative recovery time and therefore length of stay in hospital.

Once available, the existence of a national service has created pressures for a diffusion of new treatments. From the perspective of governments, the problems of containing costs and how to make choices between different areas of health care is a major problem. In the 1980s, these problems became intense as Conservative governments gave a priority to cutting public expenditure.

Containing health care costs

One way of meeting demand is to increase the amount of resource available; another is to use what is available more efficiently and effectively; yet another, to ration health care by devices such as increasing waiting times, developing eligibility criteria or simply not providing a service. Since the 1950s all three strategies have been used by governments.

From its inception, the NHS faced financial problems. The Conservative party, then in opposition, claimed that the country could not afford the NHS and must introduce charges. In 1953, the Guillebaud Committee was set up to investigate. It concluded that "Any charge that there is widespread extravagance in the National Health Service, whether in respect of the spending of money or the use of manpower, is not borne out by our evidence" (Cmd 9663). On the basis of this, the Committee rejected the introduction of further charges. The decision was crucial in legitimating a tax based service.

It was not until the economic crises of the mid 1970s that NHS funding again became a serious problem. Until then, there was steady incremental growth to cover increasing demand, meet inflation and allow modest new development. This led to gradual service improvement. However, funding mechanisms based on historic costs and NHS internal politics perpetuated inequalities in resource distribution between regions. Hospital care grew at the expense of primary care and, within hospitals, the stronger specialisms such as surgery and general medicine were favoured compared to geriatrics, mental illness and mental handicap. Inequalities were increased by the additional capital investment in the 1960s hospital building programme. Many of the large new hospitals were built in London in relatively close proximity to each other, creating a problem which, in 1994, still awaits a resolution.

Anyone discussing NHS costs faces a paradox. Funding has risen, yet there are claims of resource starvation. There has been a constant search for efficiency, yet the NHS has low costs compared to other systems. The background to the debate is now considered.

The proportion of GDP spent on health and the size of the NHS workforce have both grown, although not always steadily. In 1950, NHS expenditure in the UK took 4 per cent of GDP. This had risen to 4.7 per cent in 1970 and in 1990 to 5.2 per cent. This can be expressed differently in terms of spending on each person in the population. In 1980, per capita health spending was £162 per head. By 1990, it was £425, a 78 per cent increase in real terms (Office of Health Economics [OHE] 1992).

The number of staff employed has also grown. In 1951, the NHS employed 407,000 in the UK; In 1970, 699,000 and by 1990 over one million (OHE 1992). A slightly rising proportion of staff have been in the medical, dental or nursing category. However, the numbers of administrative and management staff increased following the health care reforms by a reported 30,000 (Timmins 1993). For example, the amount spent on "managers'" salaries increased tenfold between 1987 and 1991: from £25.7 million to £251.5 million (Department of Health [DoH] 1992a).

Compared to other health systems, the UK spends less of its GDP on health care than all but one other OECD country – Greece. The UK's total health care spending remains one quarter below the EC average (OHE 1992). Since the mid 1970s, to keep expenditure within limits, governments have introduced a variety of measures to achieve the three Es: economy, efficiency and effectiveness. In the 1970s, the service was cash limited, although this brought conflicts with groups of NHS staff who withdrew labour in pursuit of higher wages. In the 1980s, there were a variety of efficiency-saving exercises. Many districts were forced to reduce activity to keep within allocated funding (Allsop 1989).

Considerable achievements were made in improving efficiency in the hospital service. More patients were treated using fewer hospitals and less beds. Since the 1940s, the number of hospitals has fallen steadily and so have the numbers of beds available. On the eve of the NHS, there were 544,000 beds in Britain. By 1971, in the UK, there were 526,000. By 1989, this had fallen again to 373,000. Despite the decline in the number of beds, the numbers of inpatients and outpatients treated has risen steadily. This is due to the substantial reductions in the average length of stay and, in recent years, the increase in outpatient and day patient activity. Between 1981 and 1991, the number of inpatient cases increased by 17 per cent. The average number of staffed beds available fell by almost 25 per cent, yet the number of patients treated per available bed per year increased by more than two thirds (Social Trends 1993).

The above discussion suggests that the NHS has achieved greater efficiency. More have been treated for less and administrative costs are low. But demand has tended to outstrip supply. The needs to be met by the service are not finite. The means for assessing interventions have been and remain, inadequate. The main engine that governments have used to achieve savings has been through the management of the service and to this we now turn.

Managing the service:
the years of consolidation and growth 1948–74

A major aim in establishing the NHS was to improve and modernize the "patchwork quilt" of services that had grown in an unplanned way over the previous hundred years.[3] All health services were brought under a central ministry; the hospital service was nationalized; the family practitioners, including GPs, were under contract to local bodies, the Executive Councils; while the local authorities ran public health, community and certain social services under a medical officer of health. The structure, as Figure 5.1 shows, was tripartite.

Each section of the service had a different line of accountability and source of funding. Individuals had access to the service free at the point of service, bringing new freedom from the anxiety of sickness. Before the war only limited sections of the population, mainly working men, were covered by the national insurance scheme. The costs of illness fell heavily on all but the very rich. The uneven distribution of services added to the costs of obtaining treatment.

Figure 5.1 Organization of the National Health Service (NHS) in England and Wales 1948-74.

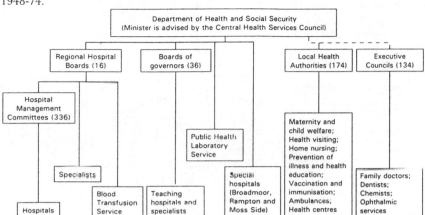

——————— Direct responsibility

- - - - General supervisory powers

Note: The Ministry of Health became the Department of Health and Social Security in 1968. *Source:* J. Allsop, *Health policy and the NHS* (London: Longman 1984).

By the early 1970s, concerns had surfaced not only about the costs of health care but also about the discontinuities in both service planning and patient care created by the tripartite structure. There was also a growing concern about the care of patients in long-stay institutions, following mishaps that led to a series of public inquiries. The solution to these problems was seen to lie in service reorganization, centralized planning and priority setting.

Reorganization and centralized planning 1974–82

In 1974 the NHS was restructured to bring the community health and hospital services under district management. Districts were then grouped under Area Health Authorities whose main function was to plan service delivery for particular groups and services. An elaborate planning system was established to plan services for groups such as elderly, physically and mentally disabled people. Community Health Councils (CHCs) were set up to represent the consumer and act as a watchdog over local services. At the centre, policies were developed to achieve a more equitable distribution of resources

107

Figure 5.2 Organization of the NHS 1974–82.

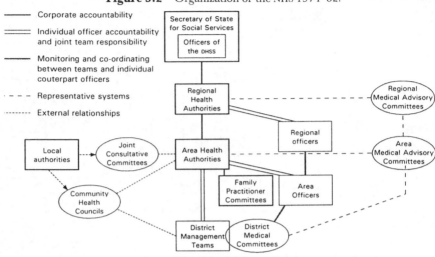

Source: Kings Fund Library Service.

according to weighted populations and priority was given to developing services for care in the community. Figure 5.2 shows the NHS structure in 1974.

By the mid 1970s it was acknowledged that the reorganization had failed to achieve its objectives in a number of respects. It proved difficult to change the flow of resources from hospital services to community care, as key spending decisions were made by powerful clinicians in the hospital sector. The planning mechanisms were time consuming and unwieldy. CHCs tended to resist any service change or rationalization. In addition, price inflation in the latter part of the 1970s was rapid.

The search for effective management

In 1982, a new management structure was introduced following the White Paper *Patients first*. The structure was simplified through the abolition of the area tier. The districts became responsible for both planning and operational matters. They were managed by a group representing different interests including administration, nursing, medicine and finance, who were required to agree local policy collectively. However, the Conservative government was now looking to private sector business for ideas about how to run public services and, in 1983, the management of the service was to change again.

In 1983, the Management Inquiry chaired by Roy Griffiths (now Sir Roy) reported. Griffiths was appointed for his success in private sector management as a director of Sainsbury's. It was still believed that the gap between supply and demand for health care could be narrowed by better management. His recommendations, in the short and succinct report, aimed to achieve a change in the ethos and culture of NHS managers. Consensus management was abandoned. Instead, a single general manager was to be appointed at each level in the NHS to take clear responsibility for leading the organization. At the centre, a Management Executive (NHSME) was made responsible for the day-to-day running of the service. Ministers were to determine general strategy through a Policy Board and were thus distanced themselves from decisions. To reinforce the point, the NHSME was set up in Leeds while the Department of Health remained in London.

Griffiths aimed to make the NHS more businesslike, and general managers were to focus on improving the quality of care for patients. He placed an emphasis on obtaining better information on which to base decisions and recommended cost-centred budgeting to involve clinicians in management. Incentives for managers were increased through the introduction of personnel practices such as individual performance review and performance related pay.

Although the Griffiths proposals were implemented quickly, the government's overriding priority was not service quality but reductions in expenditure. On the basis of their research in 1987–8, Harrison et al. (1988) found that while managers were remarkably successful in containing the conflicts, few were positively leading their organizations in the manner envisaged by Griffiths.

Towards the 1990 reforms

The crisis in health care funding

In the 1980s Conservative governments held expenditure back tightly. In the eyes of the "New Right", the main enemies to economic growth were inflation and a bureaucratic and insatiable public sector. Welfare was seen as a "burden". Because NHS funding is determined by Treasury allocations, governments can, and did, control the share of public expenditure going to the NHS. Growth was at a lower rate than the previous decade. In 1986, the Social Service Select Committee drew attention to the relative shortfall thus:

Taking into account efficiency savings, on the most favourable interpretation of the Government's own data for the last five years, the
Government has done no more than half what, by its own admission, should have been done: resources for the hospital and community service ought to have grown by two per cent in volume terms,
but they have actually grown by only one per cent since 1980–81.
The most telling way of representing the shortfall is to say that
between 1980–81 and 1985–86 the cumulative total under-funding
on the Hospital and Community Health Services current account
was £1325 billion at 1985–86 prices, after taking full account of the
cash-releasing cost improvements. (HC Social Services Committee
1986)

The consequence of underfunding was a sense of crisis. Beds were closed,
waiting lists grew and public dissatisfaction increased (Bosanquet 1988).
Despite government efforts, by the end of the 1980s there were almost a million people waiting for treatment, mainly for elective surgery.

The growth of private health care can be taken as a symptom of dissatisfaction with NHS services. The number of people covered by private insurance,
after remaining relatively static, rose rapidly during the 1980s. In 1955, 1.1
per cent of the population were covered. By 1970, this had risen to 3.6 per
cent. By 1990 it had almost trebled to 11.6 per cent (OHE 1992). Although the
numbers of individual subscribers increased slightly, most of the growth came
from employer-led schemes encouraged by tax concessions. A recent study
by Calnan et al. (1993) showed that the people surveyed had a mixture of
motives for subscribing to private insurance. Concern about loss of time and
dissatisfaction with NHS care were important demand-side motives but many
joined because it was a business "perk". They remained committed to a tax
based NHS. In Britain private insurance tends to be used for short-term
episodes rather than life threatening and chronic long-term care. As these
are more expensive, the NHS indirectly keeps private insurance costs low.

Ideas that influenced the 1990 health care reforms

By the mid 1980s, a number of barriers to efficiency were identified by those
advising government. Enthoven, a visiting US economist, suggested that the
NHS was in a state of gridlock (Enthoven 1985). He proposed that large
health authorities should hold budgets to buy services from health care

providers. His view of the NHS was echoed by Nigel Lawson, the then Chancellor of the Exchequer, who wrote in his memoirs that he found the NHS "highly inefficient and fundamentally flawed" (Lawson 1992). The criticisms of the NHS made at the time can be summed up as follows:

First, those providing health care at the interface with the patient, the GPs, hospital consultants and nurses, made the spending decisions and their knowledge and expertise was a jealously guarded aspect of professional judgement. However, as a consequence, the final cost of treating any particular patient was unpredictable.

Second, ministers of health and managers within the service had their freedom of manoeuvre curtailed by powerful interest groups, represented by professional associations and unions. Pay, conditions of service and issues of service delivery had to be negotiated centrally.

Third, the NHS lacked good information. Except in the case of pay beds, it did not have to identify the costs of treatment in order to bill patients. For example, although there were data on the number of people entering and leaving the hospital there was little information on how patients were treated, what the treatment cost and how effective it was.

Fourth, little attention was paid to the outcomes of health care interventions. The efficacy of many health care interventions was untested. Treatments were often determined by custom and fashion rather than scientifically validated knowledge.

Fifth, despite this uncertainty, and not surprisingly given the burdens that illness brings, people's enthusiasm for medical care was high. In a centralized UK, health ministers were held accountable in the media and in parliament for deficiencies.

Sixth, central resourcing reduced the incentive to be efficient as those who treated more patients were not rewarded. Indeed, the reverse could occur. A unit that carried out more cataract operations might simply attract more patients for which it did not receive additional funding.

Seventh, the NHS had been starved of capital. Much hospital stock was old and major equipment outmoded as technologies continued to advance.

By the mid 1980s, a sense of crisis had developed. Health care professionals were vocal in their criticism and there was public dissatisfaction, particularly over waiting lists. The media highlighted the shortcomings. It was in this atmosphere that alternative means of funding the NHS through insurance were investigated; but, significantly, these were rejected.

In 1988, the Prime Minister set up a review team to propose changes for the NHS and in the same year her Efficiency Unit (1988) published a report,

The next steps, which provided a critical review of the civil service. The recommendations provided a synopsis of government thinking. The aim was to reduce the size and scope of government by contracting-out services. The report recommended the setting up of quasi-autonomous self-regulating agencies responsible for fulfilling contracts and meeting performance targets set by ministers. These views echoed the writings of management theorists who argued that a distinction should be made between the core functions of an organization and those which could be hived off to the periphery. Drucker (1989), a US management theorist, summed up contemporary thinking when he argued that large organizations needed to "unbundle" to survive into the 1990s. Organizations, he suggested, should have fewer layers, be knowledge based, smaller and leaner.

The immediate political context provides some clue to the timing of the reforms. One week after the review White Paper, *Working for patients* (Cm 555), the Conservatives, embarking on their third term of office, decided to gamble. *The Independent* newspaper recorded that David Willetts, who worked for a Conservative party policy think tank, asked a senior civil servant what he would do about the NHS. He received the reply: "I'd either leave it entirely alone, because it is too politically dangerous, or, I'd destabilise it and see what happened" (Timmins 1989).

Working for patients and the 1990 NHS and Community Care Act

In the event, *Working for patients* recommended the introduction of an internal or quasi-market and, most crucially, the introduction of a split between those with budgets who purchased services for their populations and those who provided them. A costed contract at district level replaced a relationship that had previously operated on custom and trust. The command and control model of the large, centralized NHS with top–down directives was replaced by a system where local purchasers negotiated contracts with providers. Considerable emphasis was placed on the introduction of clinical audit and better monitoring of performance, although the arrangements operated within the framework of a tax-funded NHS.

Where *Working for patients* was radical was in the change in incentives and relationships implicit in contracting. Purchasers (the districts) would have to determine what services they wanted and from whom they should be bought. This meant trading cost against quality and deciding on priorities.

Providers (of hospital and community services) had to calculate costs including capital costs and so, in effect, competed with each other and the private sector. After the first year of operation, providers who did not receive sufficient contracts to sustain their activity would have to scale down or even close. As a consequence all those employed in a provider unit would have an interest in its survival, whether manager or clinician. Doctors would no longer be able to distance themselves from management, indeed the aim was to draw them in so they could not ignore the financial consequences of their decisions. Market theory indicated that costs would thus be driven down as providers had an incentive to seek innovative rather than habitual ways of doing things. The "hidden hand" of the market would operate.

The key recommendations of *Working for patients* were introduced in the 1990 Act. Districts as purchasers now receive a budget based on a weighted capitation. They draw up contracts annually for services to meet the needs for health care of their population. Those agencies offering services, the provider units, tender for services on the basis of a block, cost and volume contract or a cost per case contract. Where patients require urgent treatment outside the contract, this is funded by the purchaser as an extra contractual referral. Money, therefore, follows the patient. The greater the activity of the hospital, the more revenue is earned.

The 1990 Act introduced a further element into purchasing: GP fundholding. GP practices above a certain size, initially 11,000 patients although this was later reduced, may hold funds to purchase a limited range of services directly from the hospital or community unit. Research suggests that a range of entrepreneurial activity has ensued (Glennerster et al. 1992). By April 1994, about a third of all patients will be in practices covered by GP fundholders (DoH 1993). Figure 5.3 shows the structure.

Since the Act, greater independence has been offered to provider units who can opt to become trusts, rather than units directly managed by the District. By 1994, more than 90 per cent of NHS services of all hospital and community units had become self-governing through 440 Trusts (DoH 1993). Trusts may cover hospital or community services or both. They are financially responsible for their own affairs and must survive by winning contracts of service from purchasers. They may hire and fire staff and set their own salary structures. Competition from trusts for key specialists may drive up pay which is low by international standards. In 1993 further changes in NHS structure were announced which removed the regional tier. Figure 5.4 shows the new NHS structure from 1993.

Figure 5.3 Structure of the NHS 1993.

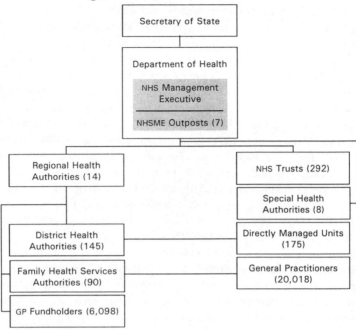

Source: Department of Health, *Managing the new NHS (*London: HMSO 1993).

Figure 5.4 New structure of the NHS 1993 to date.

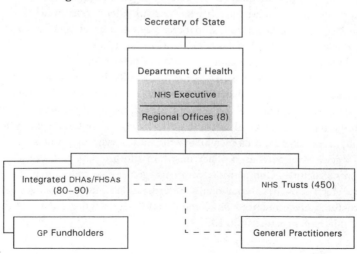

Source: Department of Health, *Managing the new NHS (*London: HMSO 1993).

Criticisms of the 1990 Act

There was fierce opposition to the 1990 reforms from professional groups through lobbying and media campaigns (Butler 1992). While overt opposition has subsided, critical comment continues. This relates to the effect of a market approach on health care; the lack of evaluation; issues of accountability; the difficulties with implementation; funding issues; and issues of equity.

It has been argued that competition is not appropriate to health care. The introduction of markets has created instability and uncertainty and the lack of planning will undermine the commitment to a comprehensive service. Good health care depends on continuity of staff and, in the case of hospitals, on the quality of capital stock and equipment. The requirement to contract annually creates uncertainty. Furthermore, purchasers may chase cheap rather than good quality care. GP fundholding, which was introduced almost as an afterthought, makes planning by purchasers impossible as they cannot predict what fundholders will do. Fundholding introduces inequities as these practices can buy priority for their patients irrespective of the severity of their condition.

On the other hand, Le Grand & Bartlett (1993) argue that NHS changes have *not* created competition and major problems arise in introducing a market. In some geographical areas, either providers or purchasers may be in a position of monopoly. In the first case, a Trust may put up wage costs or decide to provide community services that would put a weaker community unit out of business. Equally, a purchaser, in the context of a large number of providers, may push down prices to the point where the unit becomes unviable and has to close. Such shifts could have dire effects on local services that patients are unable to influence.

Sabin (1992), a visiting US academic, comments both on the uncertainty and lack of accountability in the new arrangements. In drawing up contracts Districts are expected to consult with their local populations. This may be with pressure groups, voluntary agencies, GPs and the Community Health Council. However, there is no mechanism through which purchasers are held accountable to local populations for their decisions. They are only accountable to their Board which consists of managers and a small number of non-executive members appointed by the Secretary of State. Furthermore, despite the rhetoric of patient choice, individuals have little control over where they go and how they are treated. Choices are still made by GPs or consultants on their behalf.

In the first year of implementation, agencies were asked to keep to a steady state; that is, to enter into contracts that reflected past practice. "Freer trading" began in 1993–4. In some areas, for example London, where the high costs have brought a shortfall of contracts for the present levels of activity, this poses immediate financial problems and a threat to the survival of hospitals with additional teaching and research roles. Short-term gains or survival in a market situation may take precedence over planning for the longer term.

Another criticism has been the way in which the 1990 Act has been implemented – about the speed with which the reforms were introduced. The timescale and preparation were minimal for such a major change. Rules have been developed as problems occurred but there has been little time to evaluate and learn from mistakes (Allsop & May 1993). Sir Roy Griffiths in his 1991 Audit Commission lecture also made clear that he would have preferred different implementation priorities. Major policy issues were left uncovered. " There was no attempt to establish objectives at the centre and no concentration on outcomes" (Griffiths 1992).

In some areas, such as assessing population needs and drawing up specifications and contracts, there has been a lack of expertise to carry out what in any case is a difficult task. Osborne & Gaebler (1992), whose text on entrepreneurial public sector management, *Reinventing government*, is acknowledged as a major influence on UK government, spell out the pitfalls. While contracting is a common method of injecting competition into public services, on the basis of US experience they suggest that it is one of the most difficult methods an organization can choose. Writing and monitoring contracts requires a great deal of skill.

Another more fundamental criticism of the NHS reforms is that they do not address the issue of funding. Webster (1988), the official historian of the NHS, argues that successive governments have pinned down health expenditure to unrealistically low levels. The reforms themselves have brought additional costs. Salary costs have risen and there has been heavy investment in data collection and in utilization and associated human capital as a result of costing and pricing.

A final area of criticism is the lack of a central commitment to plan priorities and ensure equity in distribution and access to services. This has become even more vital as authorities fragment into a variety of separate trusts and purchasing authorities. There are issues of equity in access to services, in their distribution and service standards. Questions arise as to whether the decisions of a variety of purchasing authorities will result in an appropriate range of general and specialist services that reflects also the needs of teaching and research. Currently, it is the job of regions to fulfil this role. In October 1993, it was announced that the number of regions would be reduced from 14 to eight and in two years they would be abolished altogether (DoH 1993). It remains to be seen whether the NHSME will be able to steer local level agencies without detracting from the gains that may accrue from their greater autonomy to manage.

In relation to the criticisms of the "old" NHS that were outlined in the third section, it should be noted that changes in the dominance of structured interests have been achieved by the internal market with great rapidity. What is not known is whether the disadvantages and their overall effect on patient care will outweigh the advantages of greater management control.

Policies for primary care, the prevention of ill health and the empowering of the consumer

Running in parallel with the health care reforms there have been major policy initiatives focusing on areas hitherto neglected in UK health policy: primary care, preventive health care and giving a voice to the consumer. From the 1940s until the 1980s, despite the rhetoric, the emphasis in UK health policy was on the growing and most expensive sector of care, the acute hospital services which accounts for about 70 per cent of NHS expenditure. Critics said that the NHS was concerned with illness, not health, and by the late 1970s, it had become apparent that Britain had a poor record in dealing with the major causes of deaths before their time (National Audit Office 1989). Conservative governments in the 1980s had a two pronged strategy. They aimed to improve general practice, which was seen as a key sector in illness prevention, and in 1990 a general strategy for health began to develop.

Policies for primary care

GPs and their staff provide first line care in a variety of ways from small singlehanded practices to large health centres. They do so under contract to Family Health Service Authorities.[4] A recent Audit Commission report (1993) showed that 90 per cent of illness episodes are treated wholly in general practice and the fact that GPs act as gatekeepers to the hospital is one of the reasons why British health care costs remain relatively low. About 30 per cent of NHS spending is on primary care (that is community health and family practitioner services). Of this, about 30 per cent goes to GPs and their staff while 46 per cent is attributed to the prescriptions written by GPs for medicines. Although cheap, at about £100 per head of the population in 1992, spending on general practice was not cash limited until the late 1980s. Furthermore, remarkably little was known about GP activity. The studies that had been done showed considerable variation in aspects of practice, such as referrals for hernias or hysterectomies, which could not be readily explained (Coulter et al. 1990). The quality of GP practice was also known to vary considerably. Many deprived areas had a high proportion of poor quality practices (Bosanquet & Leese 1989).

Primary care became the focus of attention for three reasons. First, it was believed that strengthening this sector would be cost effective. The drift to the hospital could be halted and more services could be provided by the GP at a lower cost. Secondly, there had been long-standing problems in co-ordinating the community health services and general practice. This could be approached by encouraging GPs to employ more staff. Thirdly, preventing the onset of serious illness had become an important issue. As, on average, people consult their GP four times a year, and 98 per cent of the population have an NHS GP, intervention at primary care level was thought to be the most effective way of screening for risk factors and providing health education.

In 1987 the White Paper, *Promoting better health* (Cm 249) placed GPs firmly at the centre of primary care. In 1990 a new contract for GPs was introduced (DoH 1989). This brought a form of performance related pay to promote what the government defined as good medical practice. Targets were set for vaccination, immunization and screening, and those who met the targets received bonus payments. Patients over 70 and new patients were offered health checks and GPs received 70 per cent of the costs of employing practice nurses. They were also given incentives to hold specialist clinics and carry out minor surgery on their premises. A recent report from the Audit Commission (1993) indicates that additional resources have been devoted to medical services. Although there is still a long way to go before all practices are well managed, the numbers of staff employed and practice activity has increased dramatically since the mid 1980s.

Policies for prevention

Also separately from the reforms, the government has developed a health strategy for the separate countries within the UK. Published in 1992, *The health of the nation* (Cm 1986) reviews the health status of the population in England and sets targets for reducing the incidence of risky behaviour. The health authorities at various levels are responsible for working together with other organizations to promote a healthy public policy. The part of the UK that has developed its strategy furthest is Wales which began the Welsh heart programme, Heartbeat Wales, in the mid 1980s. The programme involved the establishment of a variety of healthy alliances across the public and private sectors, while the level of public knowledge was raised through mass media campaigns. *The health of the nation* is an important landmark in focusing on health and the target-setting approach adopted is a useful way of focusing activity and assessing progress. However, in policy terms, the focus on individual behaviour accords with the "New Right" view that while governments should inform people of the risks, the responsibility for healthy living then lies with them. This avoids the issue of the effect of material conditions on behaviour and health status.

Policies to empower the consumer

In the UK, the theme of empowering the service user has gathered strength since the 1970s. The Citizen's Charter Unit initiative, launched by John Major in 1991, is a ten year programme designed to enable consumers to play their part in making the internal market work. By 1993, 33 charters had been published. The Patient's Charter (DoH 1992 [b]) outlined patient's rights and standards to be met by the NHS. The latter were quite specific and, for example, outlined target waiting times for getting an ambulance and waiting for an operation. Great stress was placed on giving users greater opportunities to voice their desires, opinions and grievances.

The Citizen's Charter First Report (Cm 2101) claims:

> The principles of the Citizen's Charter, simple but tough, are increasingly accepted. They give the citizen published standards and results; choice and competition as a spur to improvement; responsiveness; and value for money to get the best possible service within the resources the nation can afford. They give more power to the citizen and more freedom to choose.

The passage illustrates the change of rhetoric but also the user's place as an aid to managers in running "their organizations in a way that best meets their customer's priorities" (William Waldegrave in Tritter 1994).

Politically, the Charter initiative provides some counterweight to criticisms that the NHS, in common with other public sector services, has become increasingly undemocratic. Citizens now have less representation on Trust and health authority boards. Regulation by central agencies controlled by ministers has been used as a way of overseeing the much larger number of peripheral agencies. While contracting and fundholding has the potential for consumer involvement, past experience suggests that matters of finance tend to dominate decision-making.

There is a tension between the "New Right" focus on the consumer and participative and pressure group activity. Like policies for preventive care, the focus is on the individual. However, the individual is unlikely to affect policy unless activity is harnessed through a group which can apply pressure. While British society has grown increasingly diverse, minority groups have been effective in areas of policy such as maternity care, disability and the care of those who are HIV positive.

Factors that have influenced UK health policy

In this final section, I will focus on the major factors that have influenced UK health care policies. In the introduction to this chapter, I suggested that governments have been the major driving force in setting the policy agenda. Their agenda has been dominated by concerns about funding health care which, in turn, has been driven by the state of the economy and an ageing population. This is inevitable in a centralized service where 80 per cent of health funding comes from taxation. Health, therefore, has to compete with other areas of public expenditure. However, governments have had to contend with the internal politics of the NHS in implementing their policy agenda and that agenda itself has changed in emphasis with succeeding administrations.

Taking the long view over the decades from the 1940s to the 1990s, the period can be divided into two. Until the 1980s, there was consensus about a command and control model of the NHS and incremental change. The Thatcher Governments brought a radical shift. What changed was government's attitude towards policy priorities and towards interest groups in health care. Day & Klein (1991) suggest that the centralized NHS was based on an implicit "concordat" between governments and the professional interests. Incremental growth of the acute hospital sector was in the interests of the professions who in turn exercised an informal rationing system to contain spending within allocated funding. There was a general ethos of commitment to the NHS and the state was accepted as the monopoly employer. In return, governments did not encroach on issues of concern to the professions such as control over the supply of medical manpower, the appointment of medical staff, the exercise of clinical judgement or issues of self-regulation. Changes that affected pay and conditions were discussed prior to policy announcements.

However, an indirect consequence of this arrangement was that certain policies were not implemented. For example, in the mid 1970s, the attempt to divert resources to services for mentally ill, handicapped and elderly people was largely ineffective. Sometimes concerns for minority groups rose up the agenda through a well publicized scandal, a significant piece of research or the activities of a pressure group, but actual resource reallocations were small. Nevertheless, over time, services slowly developed in the community.

A radical policy shift occurred in the 1980s, as a consequence of the policies and priorities of the "New Right". There was a determination to reduce public spending, achieve greater value for money in health care and distance the government from NHS management. Like the restructuring of any business, this led to opposition from the workforce and, in the NHS, breaking the gridlock of professional dominance. In the run-up to the NHS reforms, the usual channels of consultation were bypassed and, for a time, changes were resisted fiercely by the health professions. There are interesting parallels between 1946 and 1990. On both occasions, radical changes were resisted by professional groups but implemented through the political process, reflecting current political values. In 1946, the movement was towards a comprehensive centrally controlled service, in 1990 away from this towards devolution and local diversity.

The period of consensus politics, as well as slowing down policy implementation in areas that were not the concern of dominant interests, kept other issues off the agenda altogether. The UK has been slow to develop a strategy for primary and preventive care in spite of their importance in relation to the changing burden of disease. However, by the mid 1980s broad support had developed for these sectors, in part perhaps because they accorded with the individualistic ideas of the "New Right".

This account of UK health policy has implicitly taken an explanatory approach that views social policy as a product of a structured pluralism in which governments are the strongest force. An alternative explanation for recent health policy developments is possible. It could be argued that the breakup of the NHS, through privatizing support services and then opening up Trusts to competition from the private sector, is designed to increase the opportunities for the private sector. An underfunded NHS will not only provide opportunities for profit but will also boost contributions to private insurance and direct payments for health care. Curtailing public expenditure provides a stimulus to private investment and therefore suits the interests of capital.

Conclusion

Whatever the motives, recent government policy with its concern for economy, its espousal of a business approach to welfare and the value of market forces in increasing choice and driving down costs, has hastened the deconstruction of the seamless web of the NHS. There is now considerable organizational diversity with a patchwork quilt of agencies. Purchasers combine over different geographical areas, Trusts cover a variety of services, there is a major split between health and social care.

Pausing to consider the question, a patient or family member may well wonder who is responsible for what and find accountability difficult to pinpoint. Under the "old" NHS there was a general commitment to meet all presented health care needs, albeit that in practice rationing was paternalistic and covert. In the "new" NHS, responsibility is devolved. What is provided may vary with priorities of purchasers, whether or not a patient's GP is a fundholder, and if a fundholder, how well those funds are managed.

There is nothing in the health reforms that will dampen demand for health care. The critical awareness of consumers has been growing; information, knowledge and the ability to manipulate health care systems is unequally distributed between people and this may affect their access to, and use of, health services. Furthermore, although the reforms maintained a tax based system, they did not tackle the problems of under funding. The last Thatcher Government rejected alternative forms of funding but the issue may well return to haunt future governments.

Notes

1. A women's occupation can be recorded as her own at death or that of her husband as head of the household. If she is not married and has been economically inactive, no classification will be given at all.

2. For example, once set by qualifications and occupation, men's social status and career pathway may vary less than that of women.
3. See Webster, C. (ed.) *Aneurin Bevan on the National Health Service* (Wellcome Unit for the History of Medicine: University of Oxford).
4. These were called Family Practitioner Committees until 1990.

Suggested reading

Ham (1992) provides a comprehensive review of British health policy since 1948 and how it has been made. Klein (1989) examines the politics of interest groups in health care. Ahmad (1993) has a series of chapters on the health of ethnic minority groups and provides up-to-date statistics. Davey & Popay (1993) discusses competing objectives in contemporary health care issues. OECD (1992) provides a review of the strengths and weaknesses of European health care systems. Beck et al. (1992) provide a critical analysis of 1980s health policies in key areas. Roberts (1990) contains a series of chapters analyzing available data on aspects of women's health.

CHAPTER 6
Housing: on the edge of the welfare state

Alan Murie

Accounts of the nature and development of housing policy in Britain refer to nineteenth-century measures to deal with the problems of the health of towns and a succession of measures to replace slums, improve dilapidated dwellings and build model houses and model estates (see, for example, Merrett 1979, Malpass & Murie 1994). Policies relate to the supply, standards and condition of housing; to rents and housing costs; and to ownership and control. During the present century there has been a transformation of housing provision, and the contemporary description of the condition of the dwelling stock and of levels of overcrowding and sharing reflects a dramatic change in living conditions within the life experience of households. The restructuring of housing tenure has also been dramatic with the near monopoly position of private renting being replaced by a dual tenure system in which home ownership was the senior partner and council housing the junior.

These dramatic changes in the housing system and the housing situation have been the product of incremental changes rather than comprehensive reorganization or nationalization. The impact of war on housing was profound and involved a dramatic scaling down of new production and the introduction of rent controls as well as severe damage to the housing stock through aerial bombardment. However, wartime measures did not include the nationalization of ownership and the post-war policy framework was not dramatically different from the pre-war period. There was no reorganization of policy and provision comparable with that in education, health or social services, and housing remained on the edge of the welfare state. By the 1970s the mixed economy of housing policy included a considerable public sector presence. Some one in three dwellings were owned by the state. But the state did not seek to guarantee citizens' rights in housing. The philosophy of the Ministry of Housing in the early 1960s was *laissez-faire*. It left local housing authorities to decide what their local need was and how far, if at all, they would meet it (Griffith 1966). Legislation did not place a statutory duty on housing ministers to ensure that the community was better housed and did not require the same degree of scrutiny or control as in school building or even road building (Griffith 1966). This *laissez-faire* approach operated against a background in which local housing conditions and housing markets varied markedly. Housing provision related directly to a physical dwelling stock that remains in use for a long period of time. The legacy of past building as well as the scale of new building and replacement determine what housing stock exists. The stock changes slowly and incrementally and in response to speculative and private sector investment as well as state provision and regulation. The language of universality of provision, unification of administration and uniformity of benefit rates and conditions has not been apparent at this edge of the welfare state. The state has been inextricably bound up in a system that delivered unequal benefits and rewards with periodic innovation through projects and initiatives substituting for major reorganization and universalist programmes. This environment was one in which political disagreements have remained. While there was a post-war consensus around reconstruction and the need for a major housebuilding programme, there was considerable room for disagreements at both national and local level. Consequently, the consensus at the edge of the welfare state began to break up earlier than was apparent in other services. Disagreements over the respective roles of public and private sectors were apparent from the outset, became more profound and spilled over into strategies for demunicipalization and privatization. Fiscal and other measures designed to encourage home ownership began to dominate housing policy. With post-war housing shortages largely removed, equity and redistribution became less apparent in policy aims and housing policy was increasingly linked to individual choice, reward, accumulation and enterprise.

An overview of change

At the outbreak of war in 1939 Britain's housing situation reflected considerable advances related to public policy and economic development. Housebuilding between the wars had not eliminated severe problems of house condition, overcrowding and sharing but there was a rough balance between the number of households and the number of dwelling units and steps had begun to be taken in relation to slum clearance and improvement.

The impact of war set this situation back dramatically. An accumulating housing shortage built up, complicated by bomb damage, evacuation and homelessness and the redeployment of labour and materials away from housebuilding and repair. A total of some 3,745,000 houses in the United Kingdom were either damaged or destroyed. In certain cities, Plymouth, Hull, Coventry and London, for example, the proportion was higher than average. At the extreme, in London, only about one house in ten escaped some kind of damage and in Bermondsey only four houses in every hundred were undamaged. Titmuss (1950) states "the vast majority of the millions of people who continued to live in these 3,500,000 or so damaged houses emerged at the end of the war with a lower standard of accommodation and poorer equipment".

Repairs on these dwellings were generally carried out in two or three stages and were often temporary patching. In addition, "undamaged" dwellings, including those previously scheduled for slum clearance, had by 1945 gone for six years with only limited maintenance. Some 50,000 dwellings had been requisitioned and converted for non-residential use. In the same period, some 155,000 new houses had been completed. A population increase of a little over a million was competing for a smaller housing stock (some 700,000 fewer than in 1939) in poorer physical condition.

In spite of the deterioration in the housing situation, there was no major enquiry into housing. There was no equivalent of the Beveridge Report for housing. Beveridge, in his foreword to *The rehousing of Britain* by John Madge (1945), stated

> The provision of good housing for all the people of Britain is the most urgent and the most important of all our domestic problems . . . It is the most important problem for three distinct reasons. First, variations in housing standards represent the greatest inequalities between different sections of the community and afford, therefore, the greatest scope for raising the standard of living. Second, expenditure of our energies and our money on getting good housing is the most practical immediate contribution that we can make towards winning full employment, by the radical route of social demand. There is no question that for years to come we can use all the man-power that can be spared from other essential tasks in bringing about the revolutionary progress that is needed in the housing of the

people. Third, good housing – far better housing than we have at present – is the indispensable foundation for health, efficiency and education. It is a waste of money to build hospitals to cure disease if families are forced to live in houses that breed disease. It is a waste of money to build schools for children who must return every night to squalid, crowded, unhealthy homes.

Beveridge went on to state that good housing meant a house in the right surroundings, fully equipped to save labour and promote health, and proclaimed that the time had come for a revolution in housing standards:

> We now have new materials and new methods of construction, new ideas on planning towns and preserving country, new means of transport, new understanding of all that the State can do to place good homes within the reach of all by lowering the rate of interest and so lowering rents, by bulk buying of material and equipment, by substituting a vast orderly programme of expansion for the destructive meaningless fluctuation of building in the past. We need only the will to use our new powers as means to serve our common accepted purposes. Squalor in Britain, no less than Want, is a needless scandal. (Madge 1945)

The Beveridge report itself identified squalor as one of the five giants on the road to reconstruction but was not delegated to propose how to attack it. The report grappled with the problem of rent but withdrew somewhat the worse for wear. The wide variation in rents threatened the adequacy of recommendations about uniform levels of benefit. Such uniform benefits would not be adequate to meet average rent levels in London, or some one in three rents in England and Wales, in 1938. As the Beveridge report stated,

> These practical conclusions are suggested to make the best of a difficult situation . . . The extreme variation of rents, between regions and in the same region, for similar accommodation is evidence of failure to distribute industry and population and of failure to provide housing according to needs. No scale of social insurance benefits free from objection can be framed while the failure continues. In this, as in other respects, the framing of a completely satisfactory plan of social security depends on a solution of other social problems. (Cmd 6404)

While it would be wrong to imply that there were no innovations and initiatives in policy there was no comprehensive reassessment of housing policy sufficient to meet this agenda. After the end of the war there was no nationalization of defined sectors of the housing stock, and any municipalization proceeded on the basis operating in the past. There was no nationalization of land or of the building industry. The nationalization of development rights (under the Town and Country Planning Act 1947) was designed to remove problems of speculation and profiteering, but was a substantial retreat from Labour's earlier commitment (Merrett 1982). This initiative in planning policy and the start of apprenticeship and adult training schemes are the nearest thing to a new framework for policy that emerged under Labour between 1945 and 1951. As Headey (1978) states, Labour "bungled its chance to control the supply of land". He also says

> A great opportunity was missed to impose governmental social priorities in the housing field. The public had grown accustomed to planning in wartime, and probably would have accepted after the war far greater control over the housing sector than was actually exercised . . . attempts made to regulate the supply of the factors of production required for housing – capital, land, labour – were inadequate . . .

In an environment of reconstruction and radical reorganization, in housing Labour chose to work with existing structures. Bevan, as Minister of Health, stated "if we are to plan we have to plan with plannable instruments, and the speculative builder, by his very nature is not a plannable instrument . . . we rest the full weight of the housing programme upon the local authorities, because their programmes can be planned" (cited Donnison 1967). But there was no reorganization of the building industry to make it a plannable instrument.

To augment traditional building, prefabricated dwellings had been started in 1944. By the end of 1948, 124,455 "prefabs" had been completed. These, the repair programmes for war-damaged dwellings, continued requisition of property (up to 1948), and the provision of some 20,000 temporary huts, represented only emergency action. A series of enactments established the main directions of post-war policy, particularly in relation to subsidies, and the use of local authorities to spearhead the housing programme before the general election of 1945.

The crucial decisions taken by the Labour government in 1945 were to maintain controls over private building and to rely on local authorities to carry out the government building programme. The government maintained the subsidy system that had developed between the wars. Legislation in 1946 raised the flat rate of exchequer subsidy paid annually (for 60 years) for each council dwelling. A rate contribution was also required and low interest rate loans were available to local authorities from the Public Works Loans Board. Other measures, and particularly planning legislation, speeded up land acquisition, clarified compensation terms in the event of compulsory purchase and set such compensation at existing use value rather than market value, thus taking a potential cost off the Housing Revenue Account. These measures sparked off an unprecedented rate of building of high quality council housing for the working class.

The New Towns Act 1946 provided for the setting up of development corporations to found and run new towns. This was a break with the policy of local authority responsibility that operated elsewhere. The new-town development corporations went on to build over a quarter of a million houses for "overspill" population from urban areas, and to play a role in regional policies.

The priority for houses to rent involved a different role for local authorities than existed before 1939. Aneurin Bevan explained:

> Before the war the housing problems of the middle-classes were, roughly, solved. The higher income groups had their houses – the lower income groups had not. Speculative builders, supported enthusiastically, and even voraciously, by money-lending organizations, solved the problem of the higher income groups in the matter of housing. We propose to start at the other end. We propose to start to solve, first, the housing difficulties of the lower income groups. In other words, we propose to lay the main emphasis of our programme upon building houses to let. That means that we shall ask Local Authorities to be the main instruments for the housing programme. (Hansard 1946)

Bevan also commented on the disadvantages of allowing local authorities to build houses for only the lower income groups, and private speculators to build houses for the higher income groups. In 1949, a new Housing Act introduced grants for improvement or conversion of dwellings in the public and private sector. In these ways, the early post-war measures established a wider role for local authorities and government in housing. Policy was concerned not just with the poor or the working class and not just with new building, or even renting.

The post-war priority given to high quality council building was steadily eroded after 1950. In 1951 the Labour government reduced "circulation space" and subsequently the Conservative government reduced living space and equipment in order to achieve more units of output. However, this was accompanied by higher subsidies and the higher building targets set and achieved still related to good quality housing. The relaxation of controls on private building was more important in shifting the balance, and after 1954 the restricting of local authority building to slum clearance replacement, and the relaxation of rent controls represented a marked shift from the post-war pattern. Private renting, now reviving, also justified changing arrangements for local authority borrowing and rising rents.

In 1954 Harold Macmillan said, "Local authorities and local authorities alone can clear and rehouse the slums, while the general housing need can be met, as it was to a great extent before the war, by private enterprise" (cited Samuel 1962). This return to the pre-war role of local authorities formed part of a more general "market" philosophy in housing. The temporary and extraordinary shortages occasioned by war were now thought to be remedied. Problems were thought to arise because of misallocation of resources rather than absolute shortage. The market was seen as the best mechanism to reallocate: local authority action was needed to meet the peculiar circumstances of slum clearance. The view that "a national sufficiency of housing existed and a return to economic rents would allow housing policy to be directed at real problems instead of a larger and artificial and spurious shortage occasioned by rent restrictions" (Howe & Jones 1956), was indicative of Conservative views.

Both Labour and Conservative governments continued to support major public sector housing programmes until the 1980s. The framework of central policy determined the focus of these programmes (general needs, slum clearance, improvement), types of development (high rise and systems building or traditional), and rent levels. However, the volume of building was sufficient to maintain a steady growth in the public sector stock even after 1954. At this stage the expansion of council housing was not incompatible with other policy priorities relating to the private sector. The policies of the 1950s designed to revive private renting met with mixed success. While many landlords preferred to sell, others exploited loopholes in the law and the powerlessness of their tenants. In spite of relaxation of rent controls (and because of it) the private rented sector continued to decline. Sales to sitting tenants as

130

well as open market sales added to slum clearance related losses. New measures to regulate private renting were introduced in 1965 to respond to problems of "Rachmanism" and to the Milner Holland Report (Cmnd 2605) without recourse to general municipalization.

While strategies for reviving private renting proved flawed, home ownership emerged as the preferred housing option and Labour and Conservative governments competed to be its main proponents. The most notable development was the increased importance of tax relief subsidy to owner occupiers. As owner occupation has expanded and has embraced a greater proportion of the population, and as rising incomes brought more people within the tax net and so eligible for tax reliefs, so the impact of measures introduced a long time before has become more marked. The maintenance of a policy that was so crucial in the financial advantages offered to home ownership was accompanied by other mechanisms to increase the attractions of home ownership. These included improvement and repair grants, capital gains tax relief, the abolition of Schedule A tax in 1963 (on the imputed rent income of an owner occupied dwelling), leasehold reform and option mortgages. Systems of fiscal welfare and direct public provision have operated alongside each other to represent the organization of two welfare states in housing. As the welfare state developed after the 1950s, it was fiscal welfare that grew most strikingly.

By the late 1960s a new pattern of household behaviour was emerging in response to this development. This involved increasing social differentiation between and within tenures. Households with lower incomes, out of employment and less able to obtain mortgages, were increasingly funnelling towards council housing as the private renting alternative declined. As the financial advantages associated with home ownership increased, so those who could afford to buy did so. The social profile of tenures changed and the social mix that had marked council housing declined (Murie 1983). Council housing, which had ended the 1940s as the most modern and best equipped and was therefore attractive to affluent households, ended the 1970s with an image tarnished by an ageing stock and problems of design, maintenance, repair and management. And within the council stock there were real issues of segregation relating to race and other aspects of bargaining power (Malpass & Murie 1994). To the extent that the worst housing and the worst estates were increasingly the only choice for those with least bargaining power, council housing was failing in the terms set by Bevan. Its capacity to contribute to the redistribution of life chances was flawed by this and by the wider context of a housing finance system that was regressive in impact.

As state support shifted from council housing and the working class and towards home ownership and the cohort of affluent younger households, other policy developments had a major impact. Powers to introduce rent rebate schemes had been introduced in the 1930s and their steady growth in use was consolidated in 1972 with the introduction of a mandatory system. As rents rose and the social profile of tenants changed, so the experience of council housing changed towards one of means tested assistance with housing costs. The need for assistance with rents, identified as a problem by Beveridge and obscured by general exchequer subsidies for much of the postwar period, became increasingly apparent in council housing. As housing benefits succeeded rent rebates, and as exchequer subsidies were reduced and rents increased in the 1980s, so issues of dependency on means tested benefits and the poverty trap were increasingly associated with council housing (Hills 1993).

Alongside this development, and consistent with the dual tenure system emerging, an increasing proportion of new council tenants were those with limited resources. The decline of private renting meant that those unable to buy sought to rent from the local authority. Increasing homelessness in the 1970s aroused public concern and contributed to new legislation. However, the increasing proportion of households subsequently entering council housing homeless was less the result of this legislation than of underlying trends in access to housing, social, economic and demographic change and a changing housing market. The creation of new housing associations and the development of policies to enable public subsidy of an alternative to local authority landlords can also be seen in this context.

Thus far the story of housing policy is one of low level concerns and *laissez-faire* attitudes in central government. Local housing markets developed very differently, reflecting local political and economic factors as well as the legacy of the past. The sharp break with this situation came in the legislation of 1980. Government from the mid 1950s has pursued an increasingly residual policy towards council housing. As the Labour government of 1965 stated:

Once the country has overcome its huge social problem of slumdom and obsolescence, and met the need of the great cities for more houses let at moderate rents, the programme of subsidized council housing should decrease. The expansion of the public programme now proposed is to meet exceptional needs; it is born partly of a short term necessity, partly of the conditions inherent in modern urban life. The expansion of building for owner occupation on the other hand is normal; it reflects a long term social advance that should gradually pervade every region. (Cmnd 2838)

The ambitious aims of the 1940s had given way to a more restricted vision for council housing. But it remained a positive vision in housing old and disabled persons and those unable to buy. By the mid 1970s government regarded the problem of housing shortage as solved. However, the 1970s saw major disagreements over the way forward. The Conservatives' Housing Finance Act of 1972 aroused considerable opposition and was replaced by Labour in 1975. The Community Land Act of 1975 marked a new attempt to manage the land market and government embarked on a Housing Finance review and new proposals for subsidies. In 1980 a new Subsidy Scheme similar to one proposed by Labour was introduced. But at the same time the Conservative government embarked upon major cuts in public expenditure and on a privatization programme. These steps represented a significant break with the past. They were implemented by a newly interventionist and centralizing government with increasing power and control and what has been referred to as a nationalization of policy. Council housing began to decline in size and became the government's largest single programme of asset sales. Cuts in expenditure had been made consistently since 1975 but the changes from 1980 onwards were much more dramatic. In the climate of the period after 1979 public expenditure decisions on housing were based on "what the country could afford" rather than on calculations of what was needed. Need itself was regarded as a moving target and the aims of policy were concerned with the promotion of market processes, incentives, choices, self-help and the redistribution of wealth through council house sales. Rather than being based on a redistributive welfare state approach, with priority given to homelessness or housing stress, and subsidy directed to those in greatest need, housing policy was intended to promote a property-owning democracy giving "freedom and mobility and that prospect of handing something on to their children and grandchildren".

The final phase of policy emerged in 1987 and legislation of 1988 and 1989. It related to further dismantling of the council sector through tenants choice measures, voluntary transfers of stock on the initiative of councils and a Rent to Mortgage Scheme designed to add to the sale of council houses. The operation of the Right to Buy would continue to lead to sales of council properties as rents rose and mortgages proved an attractive alternative. Alongside the tenant's charter, a new emphasis on individual rights, the encouragement of tenant's management, the favouring of housing associations, the emphasis on an enabling role, requirements for compulsory competitive tendering for housing management and an impending reorganization of local government, the presentation of public policy involved little to encourage local authorities to make the positive contributions of the past. While continuing to promote the merits of home ownership, government began to erode the fiscal advantages associated with Mortgage Interest Tax Relief. MITR has a long history and drew in increasing numbers of owners as the tenure expanded and as tax thresholds rose to embrace more people (Forrest et al. 1990). In 1974 a ceiling of £25,000 was placed on the size of mortgage that could attract tax relief. This ceiling was raised to £30,000 in 1983 but not raised subsequently. Although the Conservative Party Manifesto in 1992 referred to maintaining MITR there was a steady erosion of the picture. The 1988 budget had removed home improvements funded by mortgages from eligibility for tax relief and eliminated the opportunity for joint purchasers to obtain double tax relief by attaching the limit on MITR to the dwelling rather than the purchaser. With assistance through income support rising from £71 million in 1980/81 (Supplementary Benefit) to £353 million in 1989/90 and £1,143 million in 1992/3, and in an environment of fiscal crisis and mortgage costs significantly reduced by falling interest rates, successive Chancellors of the Exchequer announced reductions in MITR. In 1991, MITR was pegged to the standard rate of tax and the announcement of a reduction to a 20 per cent tax band from 1994/95 (March 1993 budget) was followed by an announcement of a 15 per cent band from 1995/6 and reductions by 5 per cent in each of the next three years to phase out MITR in 1998/9. This shift in assistance with housing costs involves a significant and rapid change to a system widely attacked as inefficient and inequitable. Arguably, however, its greatest impact will be on lower income tax payers rather than the high income groups that had been the main recipients in earlier years. For some, however, policy had come full circle with the dramatic growth of homelessness and the emergence of visible homelessness and sleeping rough as an indication of problems of housing shortage. Initiatives in relation to homelessness, mortgage rescue schemes and management initiatives on council estates were evidence of the failure to consolidate the achievements of the early post-war years.

Ringing the changes

Accounts of policy changes in housing identify a range of key actors. In the early period following the war, national politicians and parliamentary legislation dominate with Bevan and then Macmillan as key figures. The aftermath of war, of shortages and bomb damage dominated the language and imagery of policy and created a core identity that was more powerful than differences over how best to achieve results. The subsequent period was one more marked by fragmentation. The record building rates of the late 1960s are associated with Crossman but the influential figures include those associated with scandals (Rachman) and the chairs of committees set up to investigate major problems (Milner Holland, Francis). Municipal leaders who pioneered city centre redevelopment or other policies such as council house sales also figure more strongly.

However, most accounts of the changing policy environment for housing would emphasize other elements. There has been a consistent ideological disagreement centring on the role of private renting. The Conservatives in opposition and latterly in government have revived the conviction that if the market was freed of regulation private landlords would provide. In more recent years the association between council housing and high rise and other failed housing solutions has contributed to an anti-municipal stance and a view that council housing was part of the problem rather than the solution. Finally, there has been a steady assertion of the intrinsic merits of home ownership and its role in maintaining the family and community. These tenure issues have sometimes been presented in terms of financial necessities or prudent housekeeping but the changes in housing finance do not stand up to scrutiny in terms of reducing expenditure. Rather, what has emerged is a shift in subsidy to fiscal measures aimed at home ownership. In this context it also appears that building societies and other private sector interest groups have become more powerful and effective influences on policy. With the disenchantment with local government, their influence and that of trades unions and other traditional bodies has diminished, and been replaced by financial and private sector influences and a new generation of "quangos" including the Housing Corporation and its equivalents, Scottish Homes and Housing in Wales.

The final element in explanations of change in housing is one that relates to electoral politics. Housing had a major importance in the election campaigns of the post-war years and there were votes to be lost by deviating from the reconstruction programme. By the 1980s housing had very limited electoral importance and few votes were at risk. In the general election of 1979 the Conservative party regarded pledges relating to the sale of council houses as important in electoral success. This and the maintenance of mortgage tax relief remained important electorally. The electoral calculations had changed. With the elimination of major problems of shortage and slum housing the agenda shifted to one about rents and tenure. With the increasing dominance of home ownership even rents carried little electoral weight. A nation of home owners was not, apparently, to be stirred by problems of the minority in poor housing conditions, homeless, or faced by rent increases or a poverty trap.

Residual problems

The housing problem in the post-war period and the major measures designed to address that problem were couched in terms of the population structure as it was then. The emphasis in housing policy has continuously been on families with children and on local housing needs. In the post-war environment of full employment, households who did not have priority for housing were usually able to find accommodation in the relatively open access private rented sector. However, increasing problems were apparent as the private rented sector declined and as both employment and households changed. Private landlords had always discriminated on various grounds and examples of the exclusion of Irish or Polish tenants were common.

The first waves of immigration from the new Commonwealth and Pakistan were economic migrants who were forced to settle in cheaper inner city areas of renting. The refusal of some landlords to house black persons and the lack of access to other tenures left these immigrants exposed to exploitation with high rents for poor quality housing. Problems of discrimination and access existed in all tenures. While legislation had an impact on direct discrimination, indirect discrimination in housing remained. It was particularly apparent in the way that residential qualifications and minimum registration periods restricted effective access to council housing. While these practices were changed, the way that allocation policies were organized meant that black households disproportionately found housing in less popular estates (Henderson & Karn 1987).

Council housing allocation policies tended to discriminate against lone parents as well as minority ethnic groups. However, minority ethnic groups, lone parents and female headed households were increasingly evident in the council sector in the 1980s. As more council house allocations have gone to the homeless, to lone parents and to those from minority ethnic groups so the investment in new building of council housing has declined and the best of the council stock has been sold off. The context in terms of properties, neighbourhoods, rents and benefit has changed. The experience of the current generation of new council tenants (with their very different social and ethnic profile) is less favourable than that of the 1940s and 1950s generation in most respects. Homeless households do not have to wait interminably on waiting lists (although they may have done so prior to becoming homeless). However, they are likely to experience unsatisfactory temporary housing before being provided with permanent but often less popular housing.

Council housing that had started as highly desirable housing attractive to the affluent working class had become a second best housing sector from which tenants were encouraged to exit through various routes: the Right to Buy, Rents to Mortgages, and choosing a new landlord. The residual stock of dwellings was ageing, and, as the properties were sold, increasingly consisted of flats and non traditional dwellings. The sector still predominantly represented good housing with high standards of maintenance and management. Nevertheless, it was increasingly a sector for the elderly, the unemployed, female headed households and those with no choice, and stock characteristics were changing.

Conclusions

In the last 50 years public policy in relation to housing has moved through various phases. Following the emergency wartime situation, post-war reconstruction placed council housing and local government at the centre of an attack on squalor. In the subsequent phases government developed a more complex approach using a wider range of organizations and mechanisms to contribute to meeting housing need and improving housing conditions. Improvement grants and encouragement of housing associations, private landlords and home ownership formed part of an increasingly comprehensive approach. By the mid 1970s, however, success in solving the most visible housing problems coincided with a consensus about the superiority of home ownership, the delegitimation of council housing and a new fiscal and ideological orthodoxy. While the approach to housing remained complex, council housing and local government ceased to have a central role in providing housing.

Housing associations that came to be preferred to local authorities were incorporated into the private sector with a financial regime more exposed to risk and private funding. The private sector and the private housing industry dominated provision mainly through home ownership.

In the 1990s this market dominated system operates in an environment of wider social inequality. The end of full employment and the erosion of benefit rates has contributed to changing demographic trends and created a wider gap in incomes (DSS 1992). In this situation council housing has increasingly become a welfare sector for low income and benefit dependent households. The partitioning of the housing market has been accompanied by a partitioning of subsidy, with more funds channelled to better-off home owners than to tenants in general. At the same time the inability of lower income households to meet housing costs has resulted in increased social security provision directly related to housing. The inadequacy of other benefit rates meant that tenants were increasingly dependent on housing benefit. Housing policy decisions were inextricably bound up with social security matters from the outset and in the 1990s the problems for low income tenants and the poverty trap became fundamental to the experience of council and housing association housing in particular. The failure to resolve these problems of the link between housing and social security, the damaging dominance of issues of housing tenure in the debate on housing in recent years and the inequities associated with it should not, however, detract from the advances made in housing. Because of its long life the legacy of past decisions about building have a continuing impact. The improvement in housing conditions are direct evidence of the general success of policy and the satisfaction with the bulk of housing built by councils (whether the 2 million dwellings sold by local authorities and new towns or the 4½ million still in the stock) are direct evidence of the quality of council housing.

Between 1938 and 1981 local authorities and new towns in England and Wales built some 4.4 million dwellings. In the years 1914–38 they had built 1.1 million. On a pro-rata basis the post-1938 achievements were much higher. In the period 1939–60, 2.3 million dwellings were built; and in 1960–75, 1.6 million. It is in the period since 1975 that the contribution has been most limited. There can be no doubt that the public sector made a major impact on housing supply. Private sector speculative house building was held back by licensing between 1945 and 1951 but in the whole period 1938–75 new building for owner occupation was 3.9 million dwellings: the same as by the public sector. In the 1980s, when council house building was severely restricted, the private sector failed to achieve building rates in excess of 150,000 dwellings a year. It has nowhere near regained its own highest levels of investment, let alone those of the public sector; and in the 1990s problems in the home ownership market led to a fall in private sector completions. The construction industry has indeed been highly dependent on the activities of local authorities in housing investment.

Changes in family size as well as housing investment have contributed to a marked reduction in overcrowding (from 664,000 households in 1951 to 15,000 in 1976). The total housing stock has increased more rapidly than the number of households and a crude deficit of 800,000 dwellings in 1951 turned into a crude surplus of 500,000 in 1976. The condition of dwellings in the stock has also improved with slum clearance, improvement and new building. In 1981 there were 18.1 million dwellings in England. Of these, 1.1 million were unfit (almost certainly on a more generous definition), 0.9 million lacked basic amenities, and 1 million required repairs costing more than £7,000. While problems of unfitness and lack of amenities had been enormously reduced, those of disrepair were growing (DoE 1982). Between 1951 and 1981 the percentage of households that did not have sole or shared use of a fixed bath fell from 37.6 per cent to 3 per cent and of a water closet from 7.7 per cent to 3 per cent. Although the minimum standards of new building have fluctuated they have consistently been an improvement on older stock.

These statistics of housing supply and condition are only one perspective on the impact of policy. Households' changing experience of housing, the role of council housing in providing access to modern well equipped housing and then to home ownership are also significant, as are the effects of legal and financial measures contributing to security of tenure in all parts of the market. The expansion of home ownership has involved a major growth in personal sector wealth and affected the profile of housing costs paid through the lifecycle.

The successes of housing policy in the period since 1940 have been considerable but reflect the lack of a consistent and sustained comprehensive approach. The preoccupation with privatization and demunicipalization has prevented the continuing benefits of council housing accruing to those in greatest need. The lack of a clear and consistent vision and switching political agendas form part of the explanation of failure to achieve more. Part of the explanation also lies in the shortcomings of central and local administration and management and the role and fallibility of technical and professional advice. But the remaining and increasing problems in housing bear strongest testimony to the impossibility of developing a housing sector insulated from problems of social inequality elsewhere in society. Inequalities in housing do not simply reflect other inequalities but interact with them. However, housing programmes cannot be expected to overcome inequalities generated through other social processes. Inequalities in income and employment have dominated housing and the limitations of social security benefits have had a continuing effect. In practice, inequalities in housing have added to the problems of households disadvantaged elsewhere.

Finally, it is important to reiterate that the development of state intervention in housing has been consolidated in two welfare states: a system of direct public provision built on concepts of need but drifting from an ambitious universal role; and an increasingly important system of largely fiscal welfare that became an essential component in the operation of the principal sector of state sponsored private provision. There was and is no consensus over the necessity to maintain both these forms of welfare. Commentators who argue that provision could be made wholly through the private market have rarely suggested that housing should cease to form part of the welfare state. They have tended to defend fiscal welfare provision although recent developments, including the reductions of fiscal support and increasing costs falling on housing benefit and income support (for mortgage interest payments), present the possibility of housing becoming simply an aspect of social security policy.

This development is of considerable importance. Housing policy has ceased to be mainly about supply and housebuilding and a residual social security policy would be consistent with a withdrawal from direct roles in housing provision. The prospect is of increasing inequality in housing and a range of problems in each tenure. The possibility of transferring ownership of remaining council housing to other landlords would alter labels but not alter the associations between housing and other inequalities. In this sense the successes of housing policy in breaking links between low income and poor housing are likely to be further eroded. The lessons of the post-war period are that a comprehensive housing policy with interventions in production, consumption and exchange and involving a wide range of public and private sector agencies is necessary but not sufficient. It is not sufficient because the absence of a framework of other policies, related to employment, training and education, incomes and poverty, limits what can be achieved.

Suggested reading

Holmans (1987), Malpass & Murie (1994) together with Malpass & Means (1993) offer an introduction to housing policy and its implementation. Housing finance is discussed in Hills (1991) and Wilcox (1993).

CHAPTER 7
Urban policy in post-war Britain

Paul Burton

Introduction

Sixty years ago, as Britain began to emerge from the Great Depression of 1929–32, the disparities in prosperity and prospects between the South and Midlands on the one hand and the North, Wales and Scotland on the other became impossible for government to ignore. They embarked on two courses of action which, over the years, have been seen many times both alone and in combination. First, they designated the depressed northern regions as "special areas" and appointed commissioners to stimulate the regional economies through public investment programmes. Secondly, they launched a study in the form of a Royal Commission to examine the *Geographical distribution of the industrial population*. The Barlow Commission examined the causes of regional disparities, considered the consequences of uneven development and made recommendations for improving the situation (Cmd 6153). The Commission reported in 1940 and, following the end of the Second World War, the government began to legislate on the basis of this and other reports on the patterns and processes of urban change in Britain. The legislation enacted in the immediate post-war years laid the foundations for a system of town planning that has survived remarkably intact to the present day.

However, other aspects of urban policy-making have changed dramatically over the last half century. The most significant has been the identification of an "inner city problem" and the focusing of urban policy on trying to deal with it. Alongside this has been a concerted attack in recent years on the very notion that planning, by governments local and central, can make a positive contribution to solving urban problems. In her foreword to the government's booklet on inner city policy, *Action for cities*, Margaret Thatcher talked of cities trying to adjust to change, "All too many have had their problems intensified by misguided post-war planning and development which had the best of intentions but the direst results for the people living there" (Cabinet Office 1988).

Since the 1980s a much greater role has been given to market mechanisms in attempting to revive the inner cities and greater responsibility has been given to private sector agencies and institutions in this process. At the same time there has been a revival, especially in government circles, of looking at the apparent deficiencies of certain groups of people and certain areas to explain the causes of problems. Most recently this has involved using the shorthand term "underclass" to signify a group of poor people who, through their dependency on welfare benefits, have allegedly disengaged from the values and behaviour of mainstream society and contributed to the persistence of "the inner city problem". The notion of underclass came to prominence in the USA where the process of blaming the victims has been most pronounced and particularly damaging to blacks and other minority ethnic groups. In Britain it has not been quite so vivid, although racism in particular has been a powerful driving force for urban policy since the 1960s, both in trying to deal with the problem of racism and in treating black people as part of the inner city problem.

The rest of this chapter consists of three main parts: the first describes the main changes that have taken place in the development of urban policy since the end of the 1940s; the second considers different views of what has driven urban policy-making, while the final section offers an overall judgement of the effectiveness of urban policy, speculates on where it seems to be going in the future and suggests where it might go instead.

Changing urban policy

Since the 1940s urban policy in Britain has been concerned with the consequences of uneven development, in other words with the problems caused by rapid economic growth in some areas and rapid decline in others. In the immediate post-war years and in the period up to the 1960s policy tended to be more concerned with the management of physical rather than social development at a national and regional rather than a local level. This is not to say that social problems were ignored or that local planning was not practised, but there was an underlying assumption that local social problems

143

could, to a very great extent, be alleviated by the national and regional management of economic and population growth.

Drawing on this assumption, the Labour government that took office after the Second World War embarked on a programme of building new and expanded towns around the major conurbations. Following the New Towns Act of 1946, some 14 new towns were designated in England and Wales, mostly around London, beyond the newly created "green belt" which was intended to control the suburban growth of the capital.

Political control of these new towns highlighted what has remained a critical element of urban policy development: the balance between local democracy and national interest. In recognition of what is now known as the "nimby" principle – I am in favour of this proposal in principle but I don't want it located in my back yard – development corporations were established to bring the new towns into being and to manage them until they had reached a point of maturity. As Hall put it, "In building the new towns, freedom for managerial enterprise and energy had to be given priority over the principle of democratic accountability" (Hall 1975).

In addition to the new towns programme, a variety of other measures were introduced after the war in an attempt to control urban change in Britain. Industrial Development Certificates were required by firms over a certain size when expanding existing premises or developing new ones and were used, not with any great success, to steer industrial activity away from London and the Midlands. Of much greater significance was the nationalization of development rights enshrined in the 1947 Town and Country Planning Act. This required all prospective developers, from domestic householders wishing to build an extension to their home to multinational property companies, to obtain planning permission from the local planning authority. Decisions were to be made in accordance with development plans drawn up by these planning authorities and endorsed by the government.

This new system of spatial and economic planning, operating at both central and local levels, assumed a relatively slow pace of change and a dominant role for public sector developers. In fact the pace of economic and social change after the war was much greater than anticipated and the significance of private sector developers much greater. Thus, by the early 1960s it had become apparent that the pattern of development across the country was not as it had been anticipated 20 years before; the need for national, regional and local planning was greater than ever but the limitations of the planning system were increasingly obvious. Not the least of these limitations was the lack of an effective regional tier of government or of planning.

It had long been recognized that effective urban planning had to be based on reasonably extensive city regions rather than on more tightly defined city boundaries. In the 1960s this became increasingly apparent as census data revealed a movement of population away from the old inner areas of cities towards their suburban fringes. Plans to accommodate and to manage this change needed to be able to embrace both core and suburban areas and this often proved difficult as local authorities of different political complexions struggled to co-operate in finding mutually beneficial solutions to rapid social and economic change in their areas.

An important element in these developments was the changing social composition of urban core areas, later to be known as the inner city. The spatial mobility seen in the continued growth of suburban populations was inextricably linked to social mobility in that it tended to be the younger, more affluent households that moved out of the old core areas to the suburbs, leaving behind those who were older, poorer and with fewer opportunities for improving their circumstances. Of course there were important variations to this simple process, not least in the decanting of poorer families to new towns and to suburban council estates and the retention of wealthy households in enclaves of urban affluence.

Of even greater significance in this process of social change in urban areas was the impact of the latest wave of immigration from the former colonies, in particular from the Indian subcontinent and the Caribbean. Previous waves of mass immigration to Britain, from Ireland and from central and eastern Europe, had highlighted ethnic differences but in this post-war period the skin colour of those arriving was often of greatest significance. In the late 1940s and early 1950s this migration was driven primarily by economic factors and usually involved men. Subsequent phases were prompted also by the desire to reunite families and by changes made to the nationality and immigration laws that often provoked concentrated bursts of migration to beat newly imposed deadlines. In short, different groups and countries of origin have been prominent in patterns of black immigration at different periods of time over the last four decades (Saggar 1992).

What these black and Asian migrants found however was not a country in which employment opportunities abounded and in which they were welcomed socially and culturally. Instead they found hostility and discrimination in most walks of life: job prospects were limited beyond a very narrow range of relatively unpopular and poorly paid sectors; decent housing was difficult to afford and social housing denied because of residency requirements; social facilities were often unwelcoming, even to the point of specifically excluding black or Asian people. These forms of discrimination and hostility contributed to a degree of spatial concentration among black populations that in turn fuelled anxieties among the more vulnerable sections of the white population. While violence towards black people was commonplace (and always had been), more systematic political opposition developed in the 1960s (Fryer 1984 & 1988). "Race riots" in Nottingham and Notting Hill in 1958 had brought racial violence to national prominence and, in parts of London and the Midlands in particular, local politics became racialized as the mere presence of black people became a rallying point for right wing politicians. Indeed, on the national stage intense debate took place about the need for more stringent controls on black immigration and the supposed problems associated with black settlement (Solomos 1989).

It is significant that this political debate ranged from the highly racialized notions of what constituted the "British character" and whether it could accommodate the introduction of other cultures to the impact of black migrants on housing conditions, the welfare state, crime and other social problems (Solomos 1989, Gilroy 1987). In short, the discussion of social problems with an urban dimension began to take on a highly racialized character, a phenomenon that has not diminished to this day. Indeed, the association between black settlement and urban problems illustrates the historic tendency to conceive of urban, and later inner city problems, in a spatially bounded or contained way (Smith 1989).

Following the relatively prosperous post-war economic boom and the planning problems of containing and channelling growth, the 1960s saw a "rediscovery" of poverty or, perhaps more accurately, a growing acknowledgement that there were distinct pockets of deprivation among a generally more prosperous population (Edwards & Batley 1978). Alongside racialized and indeed racist explanations of these pockets of deprivation were notions of groups of people unable to cope with change or unable to take up the opportunities of growth. These explanations are often termed "pathological" in that they concentrate on the inadequacies of the groups or areas in question, individualizing and internalizing the causes of problems rather than looking for explanations in external or structural factors. MacGregor (1990) has summed up this view in saying, " inner cities are perceived as 'deviant' communities, areas that need to be turned around and brought back into the mainstream, a mainstream that requires little or no restructuring or reform".

This captures the way in which the definition of the problem contains within it a particular view of how it ought to be tackled, in this case by focusing policy measures on "turning areas around" and reintegrating them with the mainstream of society. The measures developed in practice involved the targeting of resources to these pockets of deprivation or areas of special need revealed by statistical indicators. Housing Action Areas, General Improvement Areas, Educational Priority Areas, Community Development Projects and the Urban Programme were all introduced as compensatory mechanisms designed to give the residents of targeted areas opportunities equal to those enjoyed by the mainstream majority of society.

One of these initiatives, the Community Development Projects (CDPs) established around the country by the Home Office as part of the Urban Programme, contained a specific element of research into the causes of deprivation in each of the chosen localities and an assumption that the findings of this research would feed into local policy-making (Edwards & Batley 1978). Twenty-five years after they were introduced, the CDPs are now remembered as the most prominent critics of small area compensatory programmes and as among the most fervent advocates of a more economic analysis of the causes of urban deprivation. They are also remembered for the tensions and hostility generated between the local teams and the sponsoring department, the Home Office. It was not to be the last time that relations between centre and locality were strained in the development and implementation of urban policy.

At the same time as the CDP experiment was drawing to a close, urban policy development had become much more clearly the responsibility of the relatively new Department of the Environment. Having commissioned major studies of the inner areas of Lambeth, Liverpool and Birmingham a new orthodoxy began to emerge and found expression in the 1977 White Paper, *Policy for the inner cities* (Cmnd 6845). Deakin & Edwards (1993) have summarized this orthodoxy

> . . . whatever the manifestation of deprivation, such as concentrations of the poor, deprived and dependent, the reason for these concentrations was socially selective population loss from the inner cities, leaving high proportions of the dependent . . . and the decline (and sometimes collapse) of the economic infrastructure of the areas.

Again, the definition of the problem suggested an approach to tackling it. The local economies of inner city areas had to be strengthened by preserving existing jobs, supporting indigenous growth and encouraging inward investment. On the back of these measures selective outmigration would, it was assumed, be halted and the living standards of those who remained

147

would rise. In addition to these economic measures, environmental improvement schemes would make the inner areas more attractive places in which to live and to invest, and social projects, not dissimilar to those developed under the CDP, would deal in a more selective or targeted way with the remaining social problems.

The White Paper and the subsequent Inner Urban Areas Act of 1978 saw a prominent role for local authorities in this new process of inner city regeneration, albeit in partnership with central government, with voluntary and community sector groups and with the private sector. The Act also saw a significant increase in the budget for inner city policy measures, from £29 million in 1977–8 to £165 million in 1979–80. The bulk of this spending occurred in newly created Partnerships and Programme Authorities. Seven Partnerships were established, covering the most deprived areas of the major conurbations, which drew together the district and county councils, central government departments and other relevant bodies including the health authority, police and organized voluntary sector. Each Partnership committee was chaired by a Minister and drew up an Inner Area Programme (IAP) that was to act as the strategic framework for tackling local deprivation on a three year rolling basis. Programme Authorities represented a second tier of the policy and initially covered 15 local authority areas with less extensive problems than the Partnerships.

The optimism associated with these new arrangements was soon tempered when a new Conservative government took office in 1979 and the Secretary of State for the Environment, Michael Heseltine, announced a review of urban policy. Four months later, however, he revealed his plans to retain the Partnership and Programme arrangements while simplifying some of the grant approval procedures. Overall spending on the programme was to be maintained at about the same level and there was to be a greater voice for private sector interests in developing local programmes. In retrospect we can see that the philosophy and the measures introduced in 1978 had been sufficiently geared to local economic development and the encouragement of enterprise to survive the arrival of what was shaping up to be a radical Conservative government. However, Heseltine's policy statement of September 1979 also heralded the establishment of new agencies to tackle the special problems of inner city regeneration in the docklands of London and Merseyside.

Urban Development Corporations (UDCs) were to be introduced in these two areas, modelled on the New Town Development Corporations with powers of planning, land assembly and disposal, development and infrastructure provision. The main reason given for the introduction of these new agencies, which would override the relevant powers of the existing local authorities, was the need for "a single minded determination not possible for the local authorities concerned with their much broader responsibilities" (DoE 1979).

Since then a total of twelve UDCs have been established in England and Wales, including a fourth generation UDC in Birmingham in the area known previously as Heartlands, while another one is currently planned for the former naval dockyards in Plymouth.

For over a decade UDCs represented the flagship of government urban policy. They enjoyed relatively high levels of financial and political support from central government often at the direct expense of other urban policy measures such as the Urban Programme (Imrie & Thomas 1993, CLES 1990). But the very level of resources required by each UDC has meant that they have been limited to a small number of areas. For the remaining parts of the country that have continued to demonstrate persistent physical, social and economic problems a series of other policy measures were developed.

The Urban Programme was maintained at a fairly stable level in cash terms throughout the 1980s and early 1990s and acted as the most extensive programme of supporting local action to create and retain jobs, improve the environment and housing conditions and support more general community development activities. Although its effectiveness has been criticized (Lawless 1988, Sills et al. 1988) the Urban Programme did act as a vehicle for supporting measures designed to meet the needs of black and other minority ethnic groups. A measure more focused on this group was introduced in 1986 with the announcement of a first round of eight Task Forces, doubled in the following year. Task Forces consisted of small teams of civil servants and secondees from business and the local authority, each with an annual budget of around £1 million and an anticipated life of around five years. They were charged with stimulating the local economies of the targeted areas and with ensuring that local residents were in a position to benefit from any improvement. Although the government was always circumspect in acknowledging any connection between urban civil disorder and the development of new policy measures and in giving much significance to "race" or ethnicity in the selection of Task Force areas, other commentators have made these connections. Deakin & Edwards (1993) suggest, " there can be no other adequate explanation for the creation of the Task Forces than the civil unrest that had preceded their announcement".

The need for greater local co-ordination had been acknowledged one year earlier when five City Action Teams (CATs) were set up in 1985. These represented another attempt at achieving more co-ordination and co-operation among the growing range of agencies with an interest and a responsibility for local regeneration activity. Although a critical report from the Audit Commission demonstrated, four years later, that there was still an element of complexity and idiosyncrasy in the relationship between local players (Audit Commission 1989), the CATs continued until the announcement of new integrated regional offices in late 1993.

In the face of sustained criticism from many quarters of its battery of urban policy measures, the Department of the Environment commissioned at the end of the 1980s a review of area based approaches to regeneration. Early in 1991 a new measure was announced that put local authorities back in the orchestrating role in developing local regeneration schemes. City Challenge introduced three new bywords – co-operation, concentration and competition – to go alongside the three Es of economy, efficiency and effectiveness that had characterized policy in the 1980s. Co-operation was intended to break down the barriers between the various institutions and programmes operating locally; concentration was to overcome the problem of resources being spread too thinly across the country; and competition was to be the mechanism by which the most imaginative local schemes were to be selected. It was a sign of the times that while the local authorities initially voiced their hostility to the principle of competition, the paucity of mainstream resources available led all invited authorities to submit bids.

City Challenge proposals were put together by partnerships of local statutory bodies, community groups and business interests for clearly defined localities. Unlike the traditional arrangement of selecting the most deprived neighbourhood, City Challenge was targeted on those areas that not only suffered deprivation but demonstrated some scope for improvement. The principle of public money levering in additional resources from the private sector continued with the initial public sector contribution in each area totalling £37.5 million over a five year period. Again, in line with what had become a trend in urban policy, these resources were not net additions but were drawn from existing programmes. It is still too early to judge whether City Challenge has succeeded in giving a boost to regeneration in the chosen areas, but it was extended to a further 20 areas in a second round of bidding in 1992.

Looking back over the post-war period we can see a high degree of superficial change in urban policy, but an underlying continuity. Policy is still based on the aim of both stimulating and channelling growth and trying to deal with the consequences of uneven development; special measures continue to be targeted on localities, although the number and the scale of these areas have changed over time. The balance between property-led approaches and those relying on more people-centred notions of community development continues to change and with it the level of resources devoted by government and the private sector. The next section looks more closely at some of the reasons for change.

Reasons for change in urban policy

So far we have made passing reference to factors that appear to be driving the development of particular urban policy measures. Can we identify any more enduring trends and patterns in these factors when looking at the whole of the post-war period? Three lines of argument stand out in accounts of change and development in this period: pragmatic, party political or ideological, and structural. They can be summarized as follows. Pragmatic arguments suggest that policy changes in the light of rigorous scrutiny of what works best and of changing circumstances. The party political line emphasizes the importance of maintaining party and ideological difference, while the structural argument builds on the notion of policy constantly struggling to deal with the consequences of uneven development.

Of course in practice it is likely that elements of all three lines will be interwoven in any plausible account of change. Moreover, there is a high degree of continuity in post-war urban policy, especially in the broad aims and underlying rationale if not in the institutional arrangements and funding regimes (Hogwood 1992). Nevertheless, we can see that elements of each line of argument do serve to illuminate different aspects of change over the period.

In so far as urban policy is associated with the planning profession, the principles of objective analysis, rigorous appraisal of options and constant monitoring and evaluation have always been important. The application of scientific method to the analysis of urban problems and the development of appropriate policy responses was a touchstone of the planning profession, at least until the 1970s. The major reports commissioned after the war that provided the basis for statutory town planning, the regional plans devised in the 1960s, and the inner area studies carried out in the 1970s all reflect a belief in objective analysis that is the hallmark of pragmatism.

In the last two decades the importance of monitoring and evaluation has been stressed in all new urban policy measures, which again suggests that

151

policy change is driven by the results of such work. Latterly, though, it has become hard to reconcile the development of some new measures with the results of policy evaluation, and the significance of ideology and party politics have become more prominent.

Before moving on to this second line of argument, it is worth considering one particular aspect of pragmatism in urban policy: the response to racism. As mentioned already, urban policy from the early 1960s has been connected, both positively and negatively, with racism. In positive terms, a number of urban policy regimes such as the Urban Programme and Task Forces have provided resources for local initiatives designed to counter racism and its effects. In negative terms, the presence of black people has been a *de facto* indicator of urban deprivation used in targeting policy measures. It can of course be argued that when policy resources are targeted in this way it is assumed that racism or racial inequalities are the focus. It would, however, be more plausible, and indeed more effective, if such considerations were made more explicit and were clearly part of a more concerted programme of tackling racism and institutionalized inequalities.

The ideological or party political line of argument can be seen to have influenced policy in two main spheres, in the debate between market-led and planned approaches to the management of urban change, and in the persistent tensions between central and local government. Any form of state intervention in the sphere of urban development has always attracted the ire of those committed to the free play of market forces. The nationalization of the right to develop land introduced in the Town and Country Planning Act 1947 had always presented difficulties to those Conservatives who believed in the virtues of untrammelled market forces. Since 1979 they have succeeded in limiting the scope for state intervention and increasing the influence of private sector interests. Thus, while maintaining some compensatory social elements, the main thrust of urban policy since 1979 has been to reduce the "burdens" on businesses in cities and to stimulate an enterprise culture.

The changing state of relations between central and local government has also been a persistent influence on urban policy development. The New Towns programme relied on autonomous development corporations to overcome alleged parochialism and act in the national interest, and the UDCs likewise were often introduced in the face of opposition by local authorities. Nevertheless, the tensions that have always existed between central and local government increased significantly after 1979 as they have taken on a more persistent party political dimension.

In the face of successive Conservative victories in general elections, the Labour and Liberal (Democrat) parties have succeeded in increasing their control of local authorities. During the 1980s this fuelled a bitter war between central and local government that continues, although with slightly less public prominence now (Stoker 1988). The impact of this on urban policy was profound as local authorities found themselves ousted from their position as the natural orchestrators of local regeneration and relabelled as one of the causes of inner city decline. Thus, many of the measures described in the previous section were put into effect by new institutions designed by central government to exist outside the traditional realm of local government. Not only were local authorities portrayed in a pragmatic manner as less effective than the new institutions of urban policy, they were also accused of clinging to a bankrupt ideological position that would do nothing to help the plight of their deprived citizens. Michael Heseltine articulated this view most clearly in a Commons debate on UDCs when he said, "It was not red tape and inaction, but pure, prejudiced socialism that was broken through by the London Docklands Development Corporation" (Hansard 1982).

The third line of argument represents the most theoretically developed view and derives from a more abstract notion of the role of state intervention in urban development (Dear & Scott 1981). Drawing on Marxist conceptions of the process of capital accumulation and its tendency towards crises, not least in the unevenness of development it stimulates, the state is seen to play a contradictory role of regulation and service provision. In the realm of urban policy it tries to regulate the externalities, such as congestion and pollution, created by private development while at the same time trying to stimulate and channel growth. As both the legitimacy and the effectiveness of its actions are challenged it resorts to an endless process of institutional tinkering in an attempt to preserve the impression that it is able to manage. While this line of argument has the merit of considering broader processes of urban change and state intervention, it is weakened by its tendency to degenerate into a rigidly deterministic view of the world in which there is no scope for local agency.

It is, however, possible to combine all three lines of argument in analyzing the development of urban policy over the years. Structural accounts provide an essential context and highlight the contradictory pressures faced by government in trying to manage urban change; in short, they demonstrate the need for constant change and development. Pragmatic lines of argument put the focus more clearly on the performance of particular policy measures and help to identify the impact they have in attempting to deal with urban problems. Party political or ideological analyses concentrate more on the specific factors leading to policy change and help us to understand why change happened when it did.

Effectiveness and future directions

In this final section we move on to consider three questions: how effective has been the plethora of urban policy measures developed over the post-war decades? where does urban policy seem to be going in the near future? and where might it go in the future if it were to be more effective in tackling the urban problems of Britain?

Has urban policy been effective?

It is commonplace to preface the answer to such a question by asking for clear definitions of the aims and objectives of policy, for it is only against these that questions of effectiveness can be answered. While this approach is clearly sensible in principle, in the case of urban policy evaluation it is somewhat difficult. This difficulty lies in the relationship between the activities carried out under the mantle of urban policy and other changes taking place in the urban environment. In other words it is always difficult to isolate the effects of urban policy measures and hence to judge whether they have contributed to wider patterns of change (National Audit Office 1993).

There are other factors to take into account when trying to evaluate the effectiveness of urban policy. Policy goals are not always specified to a level of detail that makes it easy or indeed possible to judge whether or not they have been reached. To take the case of UDCs, their overall aim is "to secure the physical, environmental, economic and social regeneration of their designated areas with the maximum amount of private investment" (Cm 2207), but the notion of regeneration is not defined in any further detail. To be sure, there is ample description of what will be done to secure it – reclaiming derelict land, servicing sites and selling them on to developers, improving social facilities and so on – but not of what regeneration actually means. It is sometimes suggested that regeneration is like an elephant, difficult to describe but obvious once you see one. This may be so but it does not make the task of policy evaluation any easier. It is also the case that while it is relatively easy to see the impact of physical measures, it is more difficult to know what to look for when trying to spot social regeneration. It is impossible in this chapter to present a detailed evaluation of the effectiveness of the full range of urban policy measures developed since the Second World War, but we can make more general observations on some of the successes and failures of the period.

The new towns clearly succeeded in relieving population pressure on the major conurbations and making a significant contribution to checking the pace and pattern of suburban growth. It is not so clear that they have succeeded in creating viable local communities in which the majority of their populations were happy to live, work and play, although the passage of time is making this more clear. Moreover, it is not clear now that the impact of selective outmigration to the new towns from the cities has been good for the cities, let alone for the new towns themselves.

The policies developed to channel business growth away from London, the South East and the West Midlands in favour of the depressed regions met with some success, but also with failure. Many firms took up the carrots offered by the development areas and depressed regions but the question remains as to whether they would have located in these areas anyway. In the growth areas, firms wishing to expand did not find the restrictions set by Office Development Permits and Industrial Development Certificates particularly difficult to avoid. Despite these difficulties, the endurance of regional development policies, now on a European scale, suggests a continuing belief in their efficacy among government bodies.

Turning to the compensatory programmes that constituted urban policy in the 1960s, we can again see a degree of resilience that is not entirely congruent with the evidence of their effectiveness. The problems described above of isolating the policy effect and knowing the precise aims of the programme again apply, but perhaps the most significant factor in the evaluation of compensatory programmes has been the extent to which they reach those in most need. While targeting has become a touchstone of welfare policy in this latest period of fiscal austerity, in the sphere of urban policy it has always been beset by the fact that greater numbers of the poor or deprived have always lived outside the areas targeted with special or compensatory programmes than within them. In some areas it was also the case that only a minority of residents of the defined area could be said to suffer deprivation of one sort or another. In these respects area based programmes have always been vulnerable to the criticism that they miss the majority of their target population and offer some benefits to those who do not in fact need them (Townsend 1976b).

But the most pertinent criticism of the compensatory programmes developed in the 1960s and continued in various forms to the present is that they are often time limited. This would not be a problem if the factors they are compensating for were also time limited, but they have tended to be rather more persistent. The more comprehensive area based programmes developed since the late 1970s represent an attempt to overcome this problem by aiming for self-sustaining regeneration whereby the need for compensatory measures would diminish over time. The key issue in evaluating these measures has now become the period over which it is reasonable to expect to see such changes. Clearly, government, whether central or local, needs to set time limits to the programmes it develops in order to review progress and to consider shifts in emphasis. Urban policy measures have often had relatively short lifespans, although the Urban Programme was launched in 1968 and is only now being wound up. In some cases projected lifespans have been exceeded while in others programmes have been cut short or subsumed into new measures. A continuing point of debate in urban policy has centred on the need to find new sources of support for schemes introduced and developed under particular grant regimes such as the Urban Programme. The assumption that successful local schemes or initiatives would be taken into the main spending programmes of local authorities once their period of support under the Urban Programme expired has proved difficult for authorities struggling to stay within central spending targets.

Some centrally supported measures have however benefited from a greater degree of flexibility in the time allotted to them to do their job. The first generation UDCs were given a decade in which to achieve their regeneration objectives, although they were not slow in flagging the need to adjust timescales in the light of changing market circumstances. The second and third generation UDCs were expected to be able to complete their task within five to seven years, but some have either scaled down their stated ambitions within this period or have obtained extensions to their lifespans. Nevertheless, the National Audit Office (a statutory body that scrutinizes the effectiveness and value for money of government policy measures) recently noted the likelihood of UDCs being unable to demonstrate their impact on the local area during their own lifetimes (National Audit Office 1993).

Finally, it must be recognized that central government has been somewhat hesitant in commissioning or carrying out research into the overall effectiveness or impact of many of its major urban policy measures. While there are significant methodological difficulties in dealing with vague objectives, distinguishing primary and secondary effects and relying on information supplied by others, it is noteworthy that the Department of the Environment did not begin to consider the ways in which UDCs might be systematically evaluated until 1993, twelve years after the first generation were established and rather too late to have any profound effect on their current direction.

Where is urban policy going at the moment?

Towards the end of 1993 the Secretary of State for the Environment, John Gummer, announced a series of measures directed at improving government services in the sphere of regeneration and economic development. Inner cities and even urban policy were not mentioned in the announcements, which were intended to bring "a new localism" to proceedings and "to shift power from Whitehall to local communities and make Government more responsive to local priorities" (DoE 1993).

On the surface, these measures heralded a major shift in the attitude of central government towards local regeneration and can be seen as a direct response to sustained criticism that power had been centralized over the previous decade while the number of local agencies had proliferated to an unhealthy level (Audit Commission 1989). A more careful reading of the proposals prompted a less sanguine view. Twenty spending programmes spanning five Departments will contribute to a single budget for regeneration that will be managed by newly integrated regional offices accountable to Parliament through a new Cabinet Committee chaired by the Lord Privy Seal.

"The new single budget would mean that priorities were set locally, in the light of local needs, and not in Whitehall and would give local people more influence over spending priorities." In practice it is anticipated that local partnerships, assembled and perhaps led by local authorities, would bid for resources "to improve education and training, to tackle crime, to meet ethnic minority needs and to improve run-down housing" (DoE 1993).

It is difficult to detect anything dramatically different in this list of measures, or in the notion of local partnerships bidding for resources from the centre. In fact, the proposals reflected a high degree of continuity with existing measures: there was to be no new money, local partnerships were to remain the main vehicle for the development of local strategies and untapped private sector money would be mobilized by relatively small amounts of public money. Even the new regional offices, integrating the staff of the Departments of Trade and Industry, Transport, Employment and the

Environment, had been prefigured by the CATs introduced in the mid 1980s to co-ordinate central government activity within the conurbations.

Since the financial and ideological commitment made to UDCs at the start of the 1980s, the pattern of urban policy development has been one of institutional turbulence against a background of public expenditure constraint. Partnership has remained an important principle, although the prominence given to different partners has changed over time. Private sector investment and enterprise spirit have been pursued relentlessly, although with varying degrees of success.

There are no signs that this pattern will change significantly in the remainder of the decade. Fiscal austerity will continue to give prominence to the role of private investment in partnership with public support, and institutional change will continue to give the appearance of activity and development. Nor are there any signs that enduring problems in the fields of housing, employment, education, crime or the environment will be solved to the extent that they no longer demand policy attention. Recent political debate, especially within the Conservative party, has focused again on the alleged inadequacies of particular groups and individuals in explaining social problems. The identification of single parent families and the lack of appropriate male role models as the cause of unacceptable pressure on welfare budgets and on social housing suggests a return to pathological conceptions of social malaise. If this continues, it is unlikely to provide the context for any radical change in the direction of future urban policy.

Where should urban policy be going in the future?

Most analyses of the development and impact of urban policy in recent decades reveal a remarkable consistency in the underlying principles, the institutional arrangements and the policy measures adopted. The principles involve the offer of compensatory measures or "carrots" alongside the application of occasional restrictions or "sticks", the notion of partnership or joint working and a belief in the value of spatial targeting. The institutional arrangements usually embody the partnership principle although special agencies are introduced periodically to boost progress, and the policy measures match a relatively unchanging set of activities. Local economic development is stimulated through direct grants and the provision of serviced premises; new housing is built or existing housing improved; new social facilities are provided and community development initiatives encouraged;

landscaping measures are taken to improve the physical environment.

There is nothing intrinsically wrong with any of these principles, arrangements or measures. To be sure they are sometimes applied crassly and with no apparent connection to local circumstances, and sometimes changed for reasons of political expediency rather than practical efficacy. The most significant criticism of them, and hence the basis for any future revisions to their application, is in the claims made for their impact and the expectations raised on the back of these claims. We now know, although we still find it difficult to acknowledge, that our capacity to intervene in processes of urban change is extremely limited. We also recognize that many of these processes have global dimensions that severely constrain the potential for effective local intervention. This is not to say that all local action is ineffective or that local government and other actors can have no impact on the prosperity or prospects of their areas: simply that many changes manifest at the local level are the product of global forces, although played out in conjunction with local circumstances (Judd & Parkinson 1990). Processes of economic restructuring represent perhaps the most obvious illustration of this: where, for example, the enterprises on which a locality depends for its jobs are subject to investment decisions by multi- or supranational owners. Local action can be taken in an attempt to influence those decisions, but it must be recognized that they are being taken elsewhere by people with different attachments and commitments to particular localities (Cooke 1986).

In addition to recognizing the limitations of local action and directing valuable resources to those areas where it can make a difference, there is a need for much more careful evaluation of what works locally and why. The notion of learning from mistakes as well as successes is not well established in public policy development generally, and urban policy is no exception. Of course there will always be political debate about the logic and the impact of particular courses of action and about the levels of resources needed and given. But urban policy measures benefit above all from stability and continuity and are least effective when faced with flux and uncertainty. Change based on careful analysis is more sensible than change for its own sake or change introduced merely to create the impression of action and commitment.

Finally, urban policy will have to become more modest in its ambitions and its claims if it is not to lead to widespread cynicism among those charged with putting it into effect and those for whom it is intended to bring benefits. There are sufficient examples from around the world of the awful consequences of breakdowns in confidence in local or national government for us to be extremely wary of allowing anything similar to develop in the inner cities, outer estates or other areas of deprivation in Britain. There has been a marked absence of serious political debate about the scope and the direction of urban policy in post-war Britain. Without such a debate it is likely that urban policy will continue to consist of a series of relatively disconnected measures, developed in response to local urban crises and ideological predilections, which serve only occasionally as effective sticking plasters on an ailing body politic.

Suggested reading

Lawless (1989) gives a thorough account of the development of inner cities policy from 1977 to 1988. For the periods before and after this, Edwards & Batley (1978) and Deakin & Edwards (1993) provide a combination of descriptive detail and analytical rigour. For a contrasting account of the development of urban problems and policy responses in the USA, Mike Davis (1990) provides a fascinating study of Los Angeles. Robson (1994) provides a major evaluation of urban policy over the last decade in research studies carried out for the Department of the Environment.

CHAPTER 8
Individual welfare: locating care in the mixed economy

Introducing the personal social services

David Gladstone

Services for individual welfare, known as the personal social services, have had a much lower profile in the welfare state than the National Health Service or the income maintenance services of Social Security. As a statutory sector of welfare, they have also had a shorter and more diverse history than the other services discussed in this book.

It was only in the mid 1960s that the term "personal social services" came into popular usage to describe a set of services which, from the 1940s, had been located in different departments of local authorities. The creation of unified Social Services Departments (SSDs) following the Seebohm Report (Cmnd 3703) in 1968, and the Local Authority Social Services Act 1970 represented a significant organizational change. This is usually represented as the replacement of smaller departments with specific responsibilities (e.g. for children) by larger generic or all purpose management units. In addition to administrative change, and, more recently, the increasing tendency towards diversity in the organization of SSDs, there have also been significant changes in policy since the early 1970s. Two recent Acts of Parliament significantly redefine the role of SSDs. They are the Children Act 1989 and the Community Care part of the NHS and Community Care Act of 1990 that came into effect in April 1993.

This section will review both the administrative and the policy changes in individual welfare. Its aim is to provide a context for the more detailed discussion of services for children, disabled and older people that occurs later in

161

the chapter. It begins by constructing a typology as an aid to understanding the diversity of the personal welfare sector.

Defining the individual welfare sector

The ingredients of a working definition have recently been suggested by Lawson (1993). But her formula underplays the diversity of the sector, especially in relation to suppliers, and is silent about the varying objectives of the personal social services.

> The personal social services are concerned with a range of services for children, for elderly people and for those with physical disabilities, mental health problems and learning difficulties. Local authority social services departments (SSDs) are the principal providers of these services, which include social work, domiciliary and day care and residential care . . .

The typology to be developed here both reinforces and goes beyond Lawson's definition. It consists of four dimensions, the first of which is suppliers. Of all the services of the welfare state, the personal social services best exemplifies what is called the mixed economy of welfare. By this is meant that a variety of suppliers may be involved in the process of individual welfare in addition to the local authority SSDs whose service provisions are designated by Act of Parliament. Studies of this sector of welfare have indicated the role of family, friends and neighbours or what can be termed "informal" networks of care, as well as the contribution made by voluntary organizations "outside the state", and the private market that has become increasingly important in areas such as the supply of residential care for older people.

Many statutory responsibilities for individual welfare have developed from earlier voluntary initiatives. Roy Parker's discussion of child care policy, later in this chapter, locates one influential strand in its development as the mixed motives and activities of the voluntary child welfare agencies of the nineteenth century. But it applies equally to services for disabled and older people. In relation to both these groups, voluntary organizations continue to offer a wide range of services and to represent the interests of their client groups. Increasingly, disability organizations have developed a positive anti-discrimination position. They are organizations *of* rather than *for* disabled people. But, in practice, the help given to disabled people living at home tends to be delivered "by a variety of professionals from a range of organizations . . . These include district health authorities, local authority social services departments and voluntary agencies, both national and local" (Barnes 1991).

The combination of statutory and voluntary services (and in many cases after 1948 much of the former's responsibility was devolved on to the latter) is complemented by two other suppliers. Care provided by members of the family of a dependent individual has crucially raised the issue of equal opportunities for women who are disproportionately the carers in a family setting. In the developing context of community care during the 1980s the double equation had much repetition: "community care = care by families = care by women" (Finch & Groves 1980). More recent studies have begun to address the situation of the male role in caring. But until very recently, men have been "the forgotten carers" (Arber & Gilbert 1989).

Care provided by the private market constitutes the fourth source of supply. The major part of care in this sector is that provided for older people in residential homes. In the mid 1970s local authorities still met demand for residential care principally from their own stock of residential accommodation. By 1990 the major provider of such care was the private sector. This change in the balance of supply over the previous 15 years is usually explained by reference to three factors. First, the increasing numbers of older people in the population. Secondly, the reduction in local authority spending on residential care that occurred from the mid 1970s. Thirdly, the changes in the social security system after 1980 that underpinned the private supply of residential care with public funding. Social security payments to homes in the private and voluntary sector that had totalled only £10m in 1979 had increased to £1000m ten years later (Glennerster 1992). An increase of this magnitude not only created problems for a government concerned to reduce the level of public expenditure: it also created a "perverse incentive" towards residential care at a time when much government rhetoric was directed to community care. Both these factors, and the continuing demographic issue of present and future numbers of old and very old people, begin to explain some of the changes introduced in April 1993. These will be discussed later in this section; but, in the context of the present discussion, one important change is the transfer to the SSDs of the Income Support element in residential care. Since most of that budget is already committed, however, its transfer cannot, of itself, give the SSDs the resources they need to create a more flexible service.

The individual welfare services not only come from a variety of suppliers, including the SSDs. They are aimed, secondly, at particular groups of clients or users. As subsequent sections of this chapter describe, the statutory social services are supplied especially to children, disabled and older people. In this respect, although the organizational structure may have changed, the modern SSDs are the inheritors of the Poor Law tradition.

By the 1834 Poor Law Amendment Act local Boards of Guardians were responsible for providing workhouse accommodation for the poor: "these included a growing number of elderly who had no independent means, children and the homeless" (Glennerster 1992). In the early part of the present century the categories of those being removed from the Poor Law meant increased local authority responsibilities. Thus, in 1913 local authorities were given the responsibility of making provision for ascertaining and providing institutional and community facilities for all mental defectives (people with learning difficulties) in their area. Legislation in 1920 required them to prepare registers of blind people and devise arrangements for their welfare, such as workshops and home visiting. In both these cases not only were categories of people being removed from the Poor Law, but local authorities were increasingly required to supplement the work of the already established voluntary organizations (Parker 1965).

Such origins in the Poor Law and in the work of voluntary organizations has, in the opinion of several writers, created a situation of "stigma by association" from which the modern SSDs have struggled in vain to free themselves. It is an image reinforced by a number of other factors. First, unlike the publicly provided health and education services that most of us will use, "the majority of us will not expect to use social services and probably will not do so". Secondly, those who use such services voluntarily "are likely to come to social services in times of distress", when vulnerable and experiencing threats to their wellbeing. Thirdly, there are also involuntary users for whom "social services is an unwelcome intervention in their life; they have constraints imposed upon them when, for example, their children are taken into care" (Clough 1990). This final point emphasizes the often uneasy combination of caring and controlling aspects of SSDs. This will be noted again in considering their objectives.

The services of the SSD can be provided in a number of different settings. This constitutes the third aspect of an evolving definition of their purpose and task.

Paradoxically, the largest part of the SSDs budget is still devoted to residential services despite the rhetoric and practice of community care. Residential care had its origins in the workhouse accommodation of the nineteenth-century "New Poor Law" and was reinforced especially in the residential provisions for older and homeless people in the 1948 National Assistance Act. Indeed, the contrast with the community care orientation of contemporaneous developments in children's services has been described as "striking". "Here residential provision was only provided as a last resort when boarding out was not possible" (Hall 1976). This, of course, raises the question of why at the time residential accommodation was regarded as an appropriate form of welfare for some such as older people, while children were, as far as possible, to be offered the alternative substitute of family life.

Services offered by the SSD outside residential care cover a wide range. These include the home care/home help service, meals on wheels, aids and adaptations designed to enable older or disabled people to live at home with as much independence as possible, as well as the specific counselling support, assessment and gatekeeping functions of social work professionals. In relation to children there is a considerable emphasis on preventative services. These include pre-school playgroups, day nurseries and the more recent trend towards family centres.

In a sense each of these services falls within the ambit of community care, broadly defined. But, as several writers have argued, especially in relation to disabled and older people, this term is itself ambiguous and often complicates rather than simplifies the analysis of social care settings. "The real distinction is actually between the institutions and home, and services are normally available either in the institution or *from* home (in the case of day care) or *at* home (in the case of domiciliary care)" (Higgins 1989).

The fourth and final element that needs to be considered is the objectives of the statutory services for individual welfare. In view of the diversity that has characterized the preceding discussion of providers, users and settings, "it is extremely difficult to identify one overarching goal that unifies the aims of the sector" (Evandrou et al. 1991). Evandrou et al. distinguish between social control (reminding us that "the whole debate about the creation of the personal social services began with concern about juvenile delinquency"), social protection (as, for example, in the case of child care) and social integration of those who would otherwise be marginalized in an unprotected competitive environment (such as people with disabilities and those who have never had the opportunity to earn resources for themselves). Social control is also one of the three basic functions that Webb & Wistow (1987) identify for the personal social services. The others are "the promotion of change in individuals, in social relationships and in the social environment" and what they term "social maintenance" which is essentially about offering or facilitating support to people in order to preserve "an individual's status quo or even the management of deterioration with dignity".

These discussions of objectives make clear that the intervention of the statutory personal social services is directed both at vulnerable individuals (a "care" function) and at protecting society from deviant, distressing and difficult situations (a "controlling" function). Professional social work staff, therefore, tread a difficult and delicate balance between these sectors of their work. It is perhaps not altogether surprising that they have been subject to vilification in the press in recent years both for what they have done and failed to do, especially in situations of child protection and child abuse. At the same time as social workers have been the subject of increased media attention, the departments in which they work have been the scene of much internal reorganization and a redefinition of their responsibilities. It is to these aspects that we now turn.

Administrative and organizational change

Over the past 50 years, the pattern of administrative change in the personal social services has been from fragmentation via generic all purpose SSDs to an emerging bifurcation consequent on more recent legislation relating to children and community care.

The period of administrative fragmentation in individual welfare occurred between 1948 and 1970. It was a consequence of three separate Acts of Parliament, passed during the 1940s, each containing an individual welfare component, and the different departments of local government to whom administrative responsibility was assigned.

> The Children Act 1948 provided for "a comprehensive service for the care of children who have not had the benefit of a normal home life". The National Health Service Act, that came into operation in 1948, placed certain powers and duties upon local health departments such as maternity and child welfare services, services for the mentally ill and subnormal, together with home nursing, health visiting and home helps. The National Assistance Act 1948 laid the foundations of the local authority welfare department's services by making the county and county borough councils responsible for providing accommodation and other services for the elderly, the physically handicapped and the homeless. (Hall 1976)

166

Hall (1976) and Cooper (1982) have explored in considerable detail the process by which this administrative fragmentation became part of an agenda for greater rationalization and change, especially during the 1960s. In that process the Seebohm Report on Local Authority and Allied Personal Social Services (Cmnd 3703) published in 1968 played a major part. But the Seebohm Committee was itself established as the result of changes and debates that were already in progress. These included the emergence in the early 1960s of an increasingly common identity among the previously disparate strands of the social work profession, as well as emergent debates surrounding the development of a family service not least in the context of juvenile crime. A Labour party study group on that subject, chaired by Lord Longford, reported in June 1964 only four months before the Labour party was returned to power at the General Election. Seven members of Longford's committee "took influential posts in the Labour administration and would ensure that the proposals were not forgotten" (Hall 1976).

The proposals may not have been forgotten but, although appointed in 1965, the Seebohm Committee did not report until 1968. When it did so one of its critics regretted that it had not made out "an unremitting and unambiguous case for a major new service to take its place alongside health, education and social security . . . Much of it gives the impression of recommending only a modest operation to tidy up anomalies and overlap without incurring greatly increased costs" (Townsend 1976).

The unification that the ensuing legislation of 1970 brought about in 1971 created new and larger SSDs in the major units of local government: the counties and the county boroughs that were themselves to be involved in a major reform of local government in April 1974. At the time of their creation there was "a mood of optimism, a feeling that great things were going to happen and that SSDs were going to transform the plight of the disadvantaged" (Challis 1990). The new, integrated departments represented not only a "single door" for users, but a higher profile service capable of bidding more effectively for financial resources against the well established major spending departments of local authorities.

Over the next 20 years Challis (1990) suggests the hopes that SSDs created turned "first to disenchantment and then to despair". It was also in this period that SSDs themselves attempted, by means of a series of internal restructurings, to resolve issues that had been created by the unified SSDs. In the process the organizational structure evolved into one of progressive diversity and in each case "the new tensions have piled on top of the old ones and the old ones have taken on new forms" (Challis 1990). Three major tensions can be identified.

The first is the place for specialist skills and workers in a generic department. The increasing emphasis on community care raised, secondly, the tension between field and residential care staff, the two principal sectors of operation in SSDs. In the early 1980s the SSDs "tried to neutralise the effects of becoming large bureaucratic organizations by 'going local' " (Challis 1990). Decentralized area or neighbourhood offices and the development of "patch" principles in social work practice are the responses that characterize this third tension.

More recently the 1989 Children Act, which extended local authorities' powers to help prevent family breakdown, and the quasi or internal market that has been introduced into community care contain considerable implications for the organization of SSDs. Increasingly, the pattern is one that clearly demarcates the management responsibilities relating to children from those tasks of assessment, contracting and regulation that the new community care legislation has imposed. These changes will be discussed in the next section.

Continuity and change in policies for individual welfare

Subsequent sections of this chapter will discuss in more detail policy changes relating to particular groups of users. This conclusion examines in more general terms the changing responsibilities of SSDs in the context of the 1989 Children Act and the community care changes introduced in April 1993. There are certain elements that these measures have in common. Both impose upon local authorities strategic responsibilities for identifying and estimating child care and community care needs. The common assumption is that "a rational planning approach is desirable; that the development of services will be needs-led rather than producer-driven; and that a number of new policy objectives (support for carers and children in need, the development of day, domiciliary and respite care) can be met through a more appropriate deployment of resources" (Harding 1992). But such assumptions also carry several implications relating not least to equity, access, expectations and resources.

The two measures also contain elements of both continuity and change. Like much earlier child care legislation, the 1989 Children Act saw its objective as promoting "the best interests of the child", though, in this case, the legislation specifically sought to achieve "a better balance between the powers of state authorities and families" (Harwin 1990). Again, like a considerable amount of previous legislation, the 1989 Act emphasized the importance of preventive services designed to help families carry out their childrearing responsibilities and lessen the risk of family breakdown. But by the 1989 Act the range of such services has been increased and their scope extended to cover new categories of children.

There is an apparent continuity, too, in the term "community care" that has been an emerging policy objective for adult users of SSDs for the past 30 years. But in that time, although the terminology may have been unchanged, the meaning attached to community care has differed considerably. Three main emphases can be identified, of which that introduced in April 1993 contains the most significant redefinition of the role of SSDs.

The first emphasis, associated with the Health and Welfare White Paper of 1963, saw community care as the creation of an increased range of non-institutional day care and domiciliary services staffed by professional workers in expanding local authority health and welfare departments.

The second, developed especially since the beginning of the 1980s, and very much in keeping with the Conservatives' vision of a reduced role for the state in welfare, emphasized the role of a wide variety of help-giving agents and organizations in providing care. Referring to the role of informal and voluntary care for older people, a government document in 1981 pointed out that "It is the role of public authority to sustain and where necessary to develop – but never to displace – such support and care. Care in the community must increasingly mean care by the community" (Cmnd 8173).

The third and most recent redefinition of community care locates it in the context of an internal market in social care. There are several facets of such a quasi-market. First, is the separation of the roles of purchaser and provider, of the sort that has also been introduced into other welfare sectors. SSDs in general will no longer continue directly to supply services in the way they have done since 1948. And even where they do continue as a provider they are required to develop self-managed units in order to do so. But in the new arrangements, the second feature is a contract based service in which SSDs, once they have identified the community care needs of their area, are required to invite tenders for the supply of services from the private market and voluntary organizations. Where these changes impact directly upon the user – and this is the third important change – is in the appointment of a case manager for each client whose function will be to purchase an appropriate "package of care" on the client's behalf. In doing so, it has been suggested, the user's own opportunity to exercise choice may actually be diminished (Hills 1993).

The origins of such change are not difficult to locate. The report prepared by Sir Roy Griffiths of Sainsbury's in 1988 – *Community care: agenda for action*

(DHSS 1988) laid the foundations for the White Paper *Caring for people: community care in the next decade and beyond* (Cm 849). The idea of service contracting owes much to the American model, while the prototype of care managers with devolved budgets creating packages of care for their clients was initially developed in the Kent Community Care Scheme. The White Paper saw the measures for children and community care setting "a fresh agenda and new challenges for social services authorities for the next decade". Glennerster, by contrast, suggests that the practical reality may be one in which "the claims of the elderly, the new community care responsibilities and the Children Act 1989 will compete seriously in the 1990s" (Glennerster 1992).

Child care and the personal social services

Roy Parker

The nineteenth-century origins

The "modern" history of child care dates from the second half of the nineteenth century. It was during this period that children's societies like Barnardos, the Waifs and Strays and the National Children's Homes were founded, when improvements began to be made in the ways in which children who were in the care of the Poor Law were looked after, and when legislation was first introduced to protect children from cruelty and neglect.

However, none of these changes occurred in a social or political vacuum. The position of children in society had been transformed, by the growth of new technology that steadily reduced the demand for their labour, and later by the expansion of elementary education. Even so, problems of begging, vagrancy, criminality and homelessness among children seemed to multiply. One response was the establishment of industrial schools (the forerunners of the approved schools), another was the reformatories. Nevertheless, it was not until attendance at school was made compulsory in the 1890s that children were considered to have been brought under a new and comprehensive discipline.

Religion played an important part in shaping the early children's services, in particular the revivalist movement that swept the country in the 1860s and which lasted into the early twentieth century. Evangelical causes proliferated, and adherents sought ways in which to help in the saving of souls. The salvation of children became a notable expression of evangelical fervour; but in order for them to be "saved" it was assumed that they had to be separated – and kept separated – from the contaminating influence of evil, debased or feckless parents and from squalor and poverty. They had to be protected from a future of crime, irreligion and pauperism.

The desire to discourage pauperism also had a powerful effect upon Poor Law policies towards children. Separate accommodation began to be provided for them away from the workhouses, in schools, in grouped cottage homes and in foster homes. Emphasis was also placed upon the value of education and training. Children had to be prepared for useful employment. Indeed, the elementary education of Poor Law children was made compulsory nearly 20 years before it was required for all. However, the range of occupations that the children entered was extremely narrow. On leaving the care of the Poor Law most girls went into domestic service and many boys joined the armed services or the merchant navy.

Whereas the voluntary and religious children's societies were anxious to have and retain children in their care in order to protect them from "contaminating forces", the economic imperative of the Poor Law (funded as it was largely from local rates) was to reduce the number of children for whom it was responsible. Both parents and relatives were often encouraged to resume the care of separated children as soon as possible.

Thus, the two principal origins of modern child care were the religious children's societies and a public system based upon a multitude of local boards of guardians. Although the former tends to occupy a more prominent place in the histories, in fact the public sector looked after far more children. However, although different in many respects, both sectors became increasingly affected by a spate of new legislation introduced from 1889 onwards. In that year, for the first time, provision was made for children to be protected against their parents' cruelty, and later from the worst forms of neglect. Until then it was virtually impossible for action to be taken against abusive parents or to remove children from their care.

Although the National Society for the Prevention of Cruelty to Children had been a prime mover in securing the new legislation, other factors played their part, in particular the changing position of women in society. Indeed, the children's cause was carried forward on the wave of a growing women's movement, albeit that that movement manifested itself in various forms, such as the battles for women's suffrage, married women's property rights and a wider choice of employment.

Despite legislative advances, one of the major problems in identifying child neglect or abuse during the nineteenth century was the unexceptional nature of child death. Diphtheria, tuberculosis and measles all took their toll. Infanticide was difficult to detect before the compulsory notification of births in the 1870s. Furthermore, at a time of deep poverty it was difficult to know what was due to wilful neglect and what was not. Child protection made slow progress.

Nonetheless, it was within the legal framework of the 1880s and 1890s that the child care services developed well into the next century. Indeed, it was not until the Children Act of 1989 that there was a far-reaching departure from those legislative origins and from some of the ideas that they reflected. However, despite this continuity significant changes in the socio-economic context of child care were already altering its character and would continue to do so in the inter-war years.

The inter-war years

The 1914–18 war marked the end of an era. The children's organizations suffered major disruption as a result of mass mobilization. There were also thousands of war orphans for whom special arrangements outside the Poor Law had to be made by the state. Most notably, however, the position of women changed. They entered the workforce in large numbers. Partial suffrage was won in 1919 and various campaigns on behalf of children's welfare were launched by a more vigorous women's movement. In addition, because of the scale of the slaughter at the front there were, for several decades, more women than men. The extra unmarried women, who were weakly placed in both the housing and labour markets, provided a cheap supply of living-in staff for homes of all kinds right up to 1960 when the last of this "spinster cohort" retired.

Important though these repercussions were, they were background factors in the evolution of the child care services. Three more direct influences emerged during the years between the wars. The first was the general improvement in the condition of children. In particular, the rate of infant mortality fell for the first time aided by the spread of vaccination and immunization. Children were better nourished (the history of "milk for children" should be noted); they were more regularly examined (the school health service and the maternity and child welfare movement were important here); there was, by now, almost complete compulsory education; housing was becoming less crowded and unhygienic (the provision of council houses dates from the early 1920s and slum clearance from the 1930s), and a sharp reduction in drunkenness (stricter licensing laws were introduced in 1923) was considered to have led to a reduction in both child neglect and cruelty.

However, the effect of these and other factors has to be seen against a background of a falling birth rate (partly attributable to improved methods of family planning) and a falling rate of juvenile delinquency. The size and threat of the "problem of children" began to diminish: at least that was the popular and official view. There was, indeed, a good deal of official optimism about child welfare. Child abuse (less so neglect) was assumed to have virtually disappeared and, after a post-war surge, the number and rate of children in the care of the Poor Law were declining. Partly as a result there was little pressure for change – whether in the public or voluntary sectors.

Nevertheless, a second factor did have a far-reaching impact on the organization of the public system of child care; that was the reform of local government in 1929. Amongst other things it ended the administration of the Poor Law by hundreds of boards of guardians. Instead, the responsibilities for the Poor Law passed to the county councils and the larger metropolitan authorities. The potential benefits were economies of scale; more consistent policies; more effective internal control, and better co-ordination with education and health services. In some places these benefits were realized, elsewhere they were not: not least because of a third crucial factor. That was the question of public expenditure.

After a brief flurry of economic prosperity at the end of the war, unemployment rapidly increased. By the early years of the 1930s it was regarded as a mass phenomenon. Severe measures were introduced to curtail public spending. Just like other services those for children felt the effects. Various schemes were shelved, particularly the improvement of residential facilities; others were reduced. The voluntary children's societies were also affected. Both central and local grants and fees became less common, whilst income from donations and bequests declined.

However, one of the interesting repercussions of the more slender budgets with which child care bodies were obliged to manage was the reduction in the number of children they looked after. On the face of it one might have expected that the turbulence and deprivation caused by widespread unemployment would have led to an increase in the demand for child care services, despite the general improvement in the condition of children that we have noted. That did not happen. This suggests that these services were essentially "supply led" rather than demand- or need-related. The cuts in public spending in the 1980s appear to have had similar results and lead us to much the same conclusion.

The 1939–45 war and after

The complacency that pervaded most of the child care services in the 1920s and 1930s was rudely shattered by the 1939–45 war; in particular by large-scale evacuation. It was as if a stone had been turned to expose the real nature and extent of the problems of child poverty and deprivation. But the separation of children from their parents and the upheaval of being sent to unknown foster homes also brought a new awareness of the emotional problems associated with the disruption of children's lives.

During the war civilian morale was considered to be of crucial importance to its successful outcome. As part of the campaign to sustain that morale great stress was laid on post-war reconstruction. The reform of social policy was a vital ingredient. Beveridge was commissioned to recommend what should be done. One of the keys to his proposals for a comprehensive welfare state was the abolition of the Poor Law.

However, the Poor Law was not only a system for providing relief payments to the destitute, it was also (and increasingly so) a system for providing care for the dependent elderly, the mentally disordered and, especially, for children. If the Poor Law was to be dismantled new arrangements had to be made for public child care. That, together with the sharper awareness of child deprivation, led to the setting up of the Curtis Committee in 1944. It recommended the establishment of separate children's departments in all the major local authorities (Cmd 6922). This, amongst other proposals, became part of the Children Act 1948, an Act that signalled several new departures. First, there was the uncoupling of child care from the social assistance system: cash and care were to be dealt with separately. Secondly, there was the recognition that special training was needed for social workers who dealt with the problems of separated children. Thirdly, there was a clear message that foster care was to be preferred to residential care. Finally, overall responsibility was to be brought together under the wing of the Home Office.

Radical though it appeared to be, the so-called "Children's Charter" of 1948 was in part a consolidation of earlier legislation and it did not cover the work of the juvenile courts in respect to either delinquency or care proceedings. In particular, its critics charged that it failed to deal with the issue of prevention. It was still illegal for the new children's departments to spend money on any child who was not in their care. The government's resistance to lifting that restriction sprang from its fear that were the scale of the required preventive work to be revealed it would also highlight the sources of the problem – in particular housing – and housing was not something that the government could do much about, faced with severe shortages of materials of all kinds in the aftermath of the war. Nonetheless, it is noteworthy that the dominant assumption of the time was that the main problem for the emergent children's departments was child neglect; and, as in earlier periods, that was often difficult to disentangle from child and family poverty. Indeed, throughout the inter-war years and up to the 1970s the issue of child protection was construed almost wholly in terms of neglect rather than abuse, and therefore seen largely as a problem of poor mothering.

Gradually the services for children in care improved, the turbulence of the immediate post-war years subsided and the number of children to be looked after settled to a remarkably steady level. There were no crises or scandals: or at least none that reached the public notice. However, the apparent tranquillity was deceptive. The issue of "prevention" never completely disappeared and by the late 1950s pressure again mounted for a relaxation in the law in order to allow children's departments to spend on preventive measures. That was achieved in the Children and Young Persons Act 1963, an Act that marked a turning point in the history of these services, opening the way as it did to a much wider range of interventions in family life.

New shaping forces

By the 1960s other significant changes were beginning to impinge on the child care services. Four were especially influential. First, the voluntary sector had gone into a post-war decline. Whereas at the time of the Curtis Committee these societies had looked after some 40 per cent of children cared for away from home (albeit many on behalf of the Poor Law), by 1965 that figure had fallen to 14 per cent. Public expenditure on children's services was now concentrated in and on the children's departments rather than being disbursed by way of grants and fees to voluntary bodies. The voluntary children's societies had lost their way; the evangelical zeal and charismatic leadership of the nineteenth century were missing. The idea of "child saving" had begun to assume a more professional character.

However, the emergence of "prevention" provided fresh opportunities for the voluntary sector and initiatives began to take shape around the development of community based services to families rather than the provision of residential or foster homes. Added to which the societies began to specialize, thereby complementing rather than duplicating the public services.

A second change that affected the work of the children's departments in this period was the enlargement of the approved school system. At first, after the war, it was assumed that substantial reductions could be made, but with an upsurge of juvenile delinquency in the latter part of the 1950s the fortunes of the schools were revived. In effect, that relieved the child care system of the need to look after several thousand older boys and girls (but mainly boys). The children they continued to care for were much younger and less difficult; in 1965, for instance, 22 per cent were under school age. This, as we shall see, was to change dramatically.

The third development that emerged in the 1960s and that was to have a major effect on the child care services was ideological. The Labour party was elected to office in 1964. It had a number of plans for the redirection of social policy: one was for the creation of a "family service" that would promote preventive work and minimize the distinction between young offenders and those who were regarded as being in need of care or protection. This not only reflected a conviction about the structural causes of crime but also a wish to shield children from the stigma of criminality and from the penal system. The assumption that there was little difference between the needs of the young delinquent and those of the child destined for care found expression in the Children and Young Persons Act of 1969, although an incoming Conservative government failed to implement its provisions in full.

A fourth trend that was to lead to the complete reform of the personal social services in the early 1970s was also ideological. It derived from ideas about the good management of organizations. The system of fragmented personal social services led, it was believed, to waste, duplication and inefficiency. It was also considered to be ineffective. The new watchwords were amalgamation, co-ordination, unification and integration.

Work was put in train to reform local government and to redesign the health services. The wish to see the personal social services similarly modernized, together with the drive to create a broadly based family service, led to the appointment of the Seebohm Committee in 1965. When it reported in 1968 it did not favour a family service of the kind that had been suggested but proposed instead a more comprehensive unification.

The upheavals of the 1970s

In 1970, following the 1969 Act, responsibility for the approved schools was transferred to the children's departments. At a stroke this added some 8,000 older children to the "in care" population. Later, the approved schools were renamed community homes. In 1972 children's departments themselves were absorbed into the combined social services departments provided for by the Local Authority Social Services Act of 1970. The term "personal social services" had been coined by the Seebohm Committee to describe these new integrated activities. This was significant. The idea of a "family service" had been based upon the need to provide supportive and preventive assistance to families with children. Had this materialized it would have been a rather natural evolution of the existing child care system. As it was the reform was more radical, incorporating services for the elderly, the mentally and physically disabled as well as those for children.

Coming as they did together with the reform of local government the new arrangements were implemented in an atmosphere of upheaval and uncertainty. There was a good deal of local variation in what was done, especially in respect to the interpretation of "generic" social work. Were there to be all-purpose teams or all-purpose individual social workers? If the latter, what was to become of the special knowledge and expertise built up in the former children's departments? As we shall see, whereas the 1970s might be characterized as a period of retreat from specialization, the 1980s saw the pendulum swing in the opposite direction, above all in work with children and their families.

The 1970s were marked by several other changes in what, despite the reorganization, still tended to be called the children's services. The rapid growth in the number in care was one notable feature. This was partly, but not wholly, attributable to the transfer of the approved school children. Yet during this period the number of children coming *into* care was falling. Obviously, children were staying in care longer, and, although much of this reflected a sharp rise in the number being committed to care by the courts for their care or protection, it still suggested that not enough was being done to restore children to their families.

The political consensus was that the apparently relentless upward trend in the number in care had to be halted. More preventive work was encouraged, as was more energetic action to discharge children from care: particularly so from the mid 1970s when reductions in public expenditure had become a central feature of economic policy, and even more so after the Conservative victory in 1979. Alongside the reductions in the number in care that began in 1978 went a renewed policy of promoting foster care in preference to more expensive residential care: the closing and selling of children's homes began to gather momentum.

However, the more stringent economic climate also began to expose long-standing tensions within child care practice and policy. If, as professional, civil rights and financial considerations all indicated, children should be prevented from being separated from their families (and if they were, then restored as soon as possible) the issue of child protection was bound to become more prominent. The death of Maria Colwell, who was killed by her stepfather after having been returned home from care, sounded an unmistakable warning (DHSS 1974). The public inquiry that followed was the first of its kind for 30 years; but now it was followed by a veritable plethora of similar inquiries investigating child tragedies. Those concerning the death of Jasmine Beckford (Blom-Cooper 1985) whilst she was "home on trial" and the events in Cleveland (Butler-Sloss 1988) in which an unprecedented number of children were diagnosed as victims of sexual abuse are probably the best known.

The essential lesson of these inquiries was (and is) that there is a fine line between the protection of a child from unnecessary removal on the one hand and from neglect or abuse on the other. Social workers and the courts have the unenviable task of deciding in which direction a child's best interests lie. That dilemma was made more acute by the "rediscovery" of child abuse and, somewhat later, of sexual abuse. By the end of the 1960s the paediatric profession had renewed its interest in "battered babies" (assisted by new techniques in radiology) and this had spilled over into wider settings. The Department of Health issued guidance on several occasions about the management of cases of "non-accidental injury" (only later termed child abuse) and, in particular, emphasized the need for registers to be kept and professional collaboration to be improved.

The "rediscovery" of child abuse was not an isolated event: it owed much to the convergence of several factors. First, the women's movement had become more active and its influence in the field of child welfare can be seen clearly in, for example, the setting up of two select committees in the mid 1970s: one on violence in marriage (1975) and the other on family violence (1976). Secondly, social services departments gradually became better staffed. The number who were qualified rose by 25 per cent between 1972 and 1974 and by another 50 per cent by 1980. Training raised levels of awareness. More social workers were alert to possible abuse. Thirdly, some statistics about neglect and abuse began to be available, most notably those collected by the NSPCC and first published in 1974. Each year the totals mounted.

Thus, by the end of the 1970s child care was located in new large organizations that were responsible for many more children, both in and out of care, and more of these children were adolescent. The service was having to grapple with an apparent wave of abuse and was confronted by tighter economic constraints. On the other hand there were more and better-trained staff and the upheaval of the early years of the decade was beginning to subside.

Permanence and planning

Alongside the growing concern about child abuse was a strengthening conviction that steps should be taken to ensure that children had stable homes, reliable relationships and committed care. The impetus came from several quarters. One was research findings, especially those of Rowe and Lambert that were published under the title *Children who wait* (Rowe & Lambert 1973). The clear message from that influential study was that children were languishing in care for want of effective planning and that disruptions of their placements were frequent; many could have been restored to their families, whilst others were being denied any prospect of a long-term alternative. At much the same time the idea of "permanency planning" was finding its way across the Atlantic from the United States. In particular, it was associated with the belief that the best form of permanence for many children who were separated from their families was to be found in adoption.

The 1975 Children Act reflected these developments. A number of measures were introduced that made it easier for children to be adopted without the approval of their birth parents and for them to be "released for adoption" without an application for an order having been made. The legislation also enabled local authorities to pay allowances to facilitate the adoption of children in care: and most did.

Nevertheless, inasmuch as "permanency" entailed permanent separation from parents it met with opposition as well as support. It was argued that permanence reinforced the images of incompetent and uncaring parents. It was not more adoption or long-term foster care that was needed but more support for parents struggling to do their best in deplorable circumstances. In particular, opposition to the rationale of "permanency" came from the black community. Permanence for black and mixed race children in care had been achieved almost wholly by placing them with white families. This, it was maintained, was blatantly against their best interests, since a clear sense of racial identity was essential in a racist society.

These and other criticisms of the permanency movement changed its character and led to a more balanced interpretation of the idea. Its influence

179

is now to be seen rather more in the priority attached to participative and soundly based planning than in any one type of solution. Certainly, as we shall see, this is the strong message to be found in the 1989 Children Act. Even so, the underlying conflicts in child care remain, revolving as they do around the central question of "what is in the best interests of the child, now and in the future"?

The 1980s, the Children Act 1989 and beyond

During the 1980s the number of children in care continued to fall (by a third in the decade); more work was undertaken by way of prevention; children's homes continued to be closed (sometimes to be replaced by community based family centres), and concern continued to grow about child abuse, but especially about sexual abuse. In 1988 the Department of Health published national figures for the number of children on the child protection registers, and each year until 1992 the total leapt alarmingly. This not only presented new challenges to social workers (as well as to health care staff and the police) but raised fears that what was happening reflected a more general and deep-seated social malaise. Cherished values and comfortable assumptions seemed to be tumbling.

Hitherto, most concern had been about protecting children in their own homes. Now there was the added disquiet about what they might be suffering in their care placements, especially in residential homes. The "pindown" scandal, which was investigated in 1990 (Levy & Kahan 1991) added to other worrying evidence of children being abused by care staff. Children now seemed to need protection against the protectors.

The 1980s also saw remarkable growth in child care research, in large part as a result of initiatives by the Economic and Social Research Council and by the Department of Health. The essence of these studies was summarized in two important Department of Health publications – *Social work decisions in child care* and *Patterns and outcomes in child placement* (DHSS 1985: DoH 1991). The results revealed many shortcomings and gaps. This, together with heightened media attention to the apparently endless procession of child care scandals and tragedies, intensified disquiet about the standard of the service. One expression of that disquiet is to be found in the report on child care submitted by the House of Commons social services committee in 1984 (HC Social Services Committee 1984). This led to a departmental working party being set up to review child care law, since this was the framework within which the services were operated and controlled. It was one of the most thorough reviews to be undertaken in any field of social welfare for many years.

Its report led to work being put in hand to produce a new, radical and comprehensive Children Bill. The subsequent Act was the most far-reaching piece of children's legislation ever introduced. Its detail and scope are not readily summarized, but several of its cardinal principles should be noted. First, private and public law are brought together: that is, the same considerations apply to domestic disputes that lead to the matrimonial court (private law) as to those procedures that are invoked when the state steps in to protect a child's interests (public law). Secondly, in deciding about the best interests of a child his or her welfare must be the paramount criterion. Thirdly, "partnership" with and between parents must be sought. In practice this means that even if a child is committed to care the parents' rights and duties are not extinguished and the care authorities have to strive to work with them in planning for their children. Likewise, if parents are separated or divorced both continue to have a responsibility towards their child. Fourthly, there is the principle of non-intervention; that is, compulsory intervention to protect children by way of removal is only to be used as a last resort. It must be shown to a court that no other alternative is possible. Fifthly, if a child is taken into care (whether on a compulsory basis or not) the local authority is required to act as a "reasonable parent" in the arrangements it makes and in the care it exercises. Sixthly, local authorities now have a general responsibility for the welfare of *all* children in need in their area and therefore an unambiguous preventive responsibility. Finally, attention must be paid to a child's culture, race, gender, language or disabilities when decisions are made and, where it is reasonable to do so, children's wishes must be taken into account.

Nonetheless, there remain certain strong continuities, if not in law, policy and procedures, then in the underlying problems and issues with which any child care system has to struggle. The six that follow stand out most clearly from the history.

1. There is the abiding question of what *are* a child's best interests and how are they best secured? Are the short-term interests different from the long-term? When are children best protected by separation and when not? Is one child's best interest necessarily the same as another's – even in the case of brothers and sisters?
2. How, without 24-hour a day monitoring, can children be protected from neglect or abuse? In particular, what can we do about violent men?

3. Just how far are poverty, ill-health and disadvantage the precipitating factors in creating the need for a child care system? Indeed, can such a system be expected to succeed without corresponding improvements in the environment in which families and children live? In short, is the child care system dealing with a specially disadvantaged or deviant group or is that group a sad reflection of more extensive social ills? By concentrating on a particular child care system do we obscure the *general* issue of the position of children in society and our collective responsibility towards them?

4. How encompassing should a child care system be? If it concentrates mainly on issues of protection are other functions thereby accorded a lower priority? In particular, is the *promotion* of child welfare through a variety of supports to parents – such as respite care, day care, counselling, better health care or the encouragement of mutual aid – relegated to being a matter of secondary concern? In any case, how will the new responsibility placed upon social services departments to meet the needs of *all* children in their area alter the character of the rather narrowly defined services that exist at present?

5. What is the nature of parental responsibility? More specifically, what should be the balance between the parent and the state and between men and women? In particular, when things go wrong who is to be held accountable?

6. Do we yet have sufficient knowledge and skill (some would say wisdom) to intervene successfully in family life in order to promote as well as protect the wellbeing of children? Will the recent movement towards greater social work specialization in child care lead to better services, and if it does will it be at the cost of a narrowing of their focus?

Suggested reading

Parker (1990) provides a brief history of children's services while Packman (1975) provides a commentary on the post-1945 period. For a broader discussion of certain current issues see Parker (1986), Parton (1985), Bullock et al. (1993) and Dingwall et al. (1988).

Disabled people and the personal social services

Sally Sainsbury

Introduction

Three major themes are important to understanding the development of personal social services for disabled people since the Second World War. First, as in the case of any locally provided service, those for disabled people have been at the mercy of broad policy decisions such as those concerning the economy, the financial and political relationship between central and local government, and the National Health Service. Secondly, while such factors exercise constraint on all personal social services, those for disabled people have been in a weaker position than some others in withstanding the effects, because they have tended to attract less attention. For example, although the 1988 OPCS Surveys of Disability (OPCS 1988) estimated the disabled population to number about six million, this has lacked the political resonance of demographic projections of the numbers of elderly people into the next century, with the attendant anxiety regarding the growth in the "weight of dependency". Disability, unlike juvenile offending, is not seen to pose a threat to personal and communal safety, nor does it attract the horror aroused by the violation of a child's trust in adults represented by abuse cases. Indeed, an important feature of the disability services is the way in which they have tended to be determined by the needs of other groups.

Finally, there has been the significant difficulty of determining what disability is and who should define it. For example, should definition be a matter for professionals and administrators or for disabled people themselves? And is disability an attribute of an individual, or caused by the structure of society? The way in which these questions are answered may evoke very different service responses. A related question is, who is to be included in the disabled population? For example, for most of the post-war period, deaf people, who rely primarily on sign language, have been confidently included in the disabled population by policy-makers. But recently, some members of the deaf community have argued that their difficulties arise not from disability, but because most people do not understand their language, and therefore their position must be seen as analogous to that of members of ethnic minorities. Again, the question of age remains unresolved. It has been customary for local authorities to draw a distinction between elderly and disabled people even though most services available to these groups are allocated

183

according to disability, not age. In contrast, in the two OPCS (Harris 1971, OPCS 1988) surveys of disability, *all* adults have been included, a practice that local authorities themselves have followed in compiling their registers of disabled people.

The post-war development of personal social services for disabled people may be divided into three broad periods: first, that of promotional welfare, from 1948 to 1963; secondly, the period of the establishment of rights to services aimed at achieving choice and control in daily life, from 1964 to 1975; and finally, the period from 1976, during which the issues of the burden of care has dominated policy-making and debate.

1948–63: Promotional welfare

The establishment of the services

Post-war personal social services for disabled people have their origin in Section 29 of the National Assistance Act 1948. As an "Act to terminate the existing poor law", this piece of legislation was of enormous psychological significance. Under the Poor Law minimum services had been provided on a test of means; the new objective was optimum services on a test of need. Expectations were unleashed.

Section 29 of the Act, which established local authority welfare services, gave local authorities the "power to make arrangements for promoting the welfare" of disabled people. In elaborating the meaning of "promotional welfare", the Act is striking in the emphasis given to providing employment services. Crucial to the post-war social policy settlement was full employment. In guaranteeing the right to work, which had been the objective of organized labour since the nineteenth century, government laid on adults below retirement age (other than married women) the *obligation* to work as a necessary prerequisite of the welfare state – an obligation and a right from which disabled people were not exempt. Local authorities were required to reinforce that national system of rehabilitation, training and employment services set up under the Disabled Persons (Employment) Act 1944 as recommended by the Tomlinson Committee in 1943 (Cmd 6415). The wartime shortage of labour, which had made it imperative for injured people to return to "the front", at home or abroad, whether as a civilian or in the armed forces, continued into peacetime, as the country grappled with reconstruction. Local authorities, therefore, were given the power to establish sheltered workshops for those unable to work in open employment, hostel accommodation for those employed in such establishments, and home-working schemes, including training, the provision of materials and the means for selling the products, for people unable to work even in sheltered conditions.

In contrast, other provisions of the Act were brief and vague. Local authorities were given responsibility for providing disabled people with "recreational facilities in their own homes and elsewhere" and "for compiling classified registers" of the blind, partially sighted, deaf, hard of hearing, and "the general classes" of the physically handicapped.

The model for much of the National Assistance Act was the Blind Persons Act 1920, which it replaced. The Act of 1920 had utilized the notion of "promotional welfare" and was intended to remove most blind people from the clutches of pauperism by providing a blind pension, rehabilitation, training and employment, home visiting and the teaching of Braille and Moon in the home. The government encouraged local authority health and welfare departments to use this Act as a template in developing services under the new legislation, and required them to submit their schemes for services to the Minister of Health for approval.

In terms of expenditure, however, the most important of the new duties acquired by the health and welfare departments of the local authorities under the Act was the requirement to provide residential care. It was in this context that the ambiguity of the relationship between age and disability emerged. The Act made no distinction between the elderly and others in need of residential care. In practice, however, although the registers included people across the whole age range, and, indeed, were dominated by those who were elderly, a distinction was drawn by local authorities between accommodation for the elderly (the vast majority in residential care) and that for disabled people below pensionable age. Despite the resources spent on it, residential care accommodated only between 3 and 6 per cent of elderly people, and a tiny minority of younger disabled people. To ensure high quality in care, the National Assistance Act required local authorities to register and inspect residential homes provided by the private and voluntary sectors.

Aneurin Bevan, the Minister of Health, defined promotional welfare in this context in terms of size of institution and relationships between residents and staff: the antithesis of the Poor Law was a small home run as the type of hotel to which the middle and upper classes themselves retired. To achieve the hotel model, people were to pay for residential care. Capacity to pay was to be guaranteed by the state pension, while a nationally determined personal allowance was to prevent destitution once people were in the home.

Elaborating promotional welfare

However, it soon became evident that greater clarification of the nature of promotional welfare was required. In 1951, the Ministry of Health issued a Circular (Ministry of Health 1951) that encouraged local authorities to provide escorts to enable people to go to places of worship and entertainment, to secure access to such places for people in wheelchairs, to provide help in the home and assist people to acquire wireless and library facilities; to provide outings, lectures, games and other recreational facilities, and assist with any transport required for these purposes; and to provide help with adaptations to the home, as well as helping people to take holidays. The Circular, while maintaining and even reinforcing provision for work and training, had the effect of shifting the balance of the Act to give greater weight than had been the case initially to social and recreational services. And it reaffirmed the Act's commitment to the involvement of the voluntary sector, even to the extent of allowing local authorities to use voluntary organizations as their paid agents.

In staffing the new services, local authorities were not allowed to plunder the labour force that already existed to run the blindness services. The duties of the new staff, to be called welfare officers, were broad, ranging from assessing individual needs, home visiting, and encouraging and enabling people to participate in social activities, to liaising with other services, organizing social centres and recreational facilities, and recruiting volunteers to help to implement the Act. For these duties they were to be prepared by a training leading to a "Diploma or Certificate in Social Science or a similar qualification in Social Work of a comparable character". However, because labour was in short supply and places on training courses limited, local authorities were allowed to employ as welfare officers anyone judged to have "a special aptitude for the work", "a broad knowledge of the social services", and "some experience in the field of welfare". It was a concession that ensured that few welfare officers held the recommended formal qualification.

From the outset, the government was clear that those working with deaf people, like those working with blind people, required special training. Welfare officers for deaf people were to be confined to those "fluent in manual language and other methods of communication as an alternative to normal speech". Moreover, it was acknowledged that the needs of deaf people differed from those of the hard of hearing and that social isolation was a problem for both groups. As a consequence, the bedrock of provision for them was to be advice, information, and meeting places.

Developing the services

Broadly, Circular 32/51 provided the basis for the development of services for disabled people until the present. However, only services for blind people were mandatory, those for other groups being permissive until 1960, when few local authorities were without schemes. In that year, the Ministry of Health issued Circular 15/60, (Ministry of Health 1960) that was primarily concerned with the implementation of the Mental Health Act 1959. The Act, largely as a response to anxiety about the cost of the National Health Service, initiated the gradual reduction of beds in long stay hospitals and their replacement by "community care" provided by local authorities. Essentially the Circular extended Section 29 of the National Assistance Act to the "mentally disordered" on a mandatory basis. In the circumstances, it would have been anomalous for services for disabled people to remain permissive, and therefore their services became mandatory as well.

The effect of the Mental Health Act 1959 was to spotlight local authority personal social services generally. Although initially government interpreted community care as any non-hospital care, it came under pressure from academic critics to redefine the term to cover only non-residential care. In the British context, Townsend (Townsend 1962), unlike other theorists such as Goffman and Barton (Goffman 1961, Barton 1959), rejected the irreversibility of the long-term negative effects of institutions on people, and instead, based his objections to institutional care on its denial of access to normal life, which he defined as life with people of all ages and both sexes. Developing the theories that Bowlby (Bowlby 1952) had evolved for children, Townsend argued that, whatever their age, everyone needed "dependable love", and he saw the three-generational extended family as the institution that most effectively met that need. For him, community care meant supplementing, supporting, or substituting for the family.

Townsend's case rested on the failure of hotels for the elderly to become a reality. The demands of post-war reconstruction delayed the demolition of the workhouses in which as many as 35,000 elderly people were still accommodated in 1960, and even in new homes people often continued to share rooms. Many superintendents had worked for the Poor Law authorities and transferred old ideas into the promotional welfare context: it was easier for matron to hold pension books herself and hand out, or withhold, the guaranteed personal allowance than organize residents to pay on an individual basis. Moreover, local authorities varied widely in the way they interpreted their inspection and registration duties. By the 1960s inspection could amount to no more than a cup of tea with matron every five years, or as much as a six monthly two hour examination of the premises.

1964–75: rights, choice and control

The commitment to community care focused attention on services such as home helps, meals on wheels, home chiropody, laundry, aids and adaptions and recreational provision, rather than on sheltered workshops. The main thrust of rehabilitation and employment provision lay not with local authorities but with the government's national employment and training services. Thus, within a decade of the passing of the National Assistance Act, personal social services for disabled people tended to be directed at the "general classes of the physically handicapped" and, because they were associated largely with care and domestic labour, to provide help to women rather than men. Indeed, from the outset, there had been a clear bifurcation on gender lines between local authority services: those associated with employment and disability were allocated overwhelmingly to men, while those associated with "the handicapped" aided disabled women in the home. By the early 1960s, the register of "the general classes" were dominated by women, and especially women above the retirement age (Sainsbury 1970).

Despite the commitment to community care, the balance in expenditure on residential care and day and domiciliary services changed only slowly, and variation between local authorities in non-residential provision was substantial. In the late 1960s, the number of people on the registers of the general classes of the physically handicapped ranged from 1.8 per thousand population in Bromley to 10.1 in Kingston upon Hull, while annual average expenditure per person registered ranged from £1.9s.0d. in Durham County to £28.3s.0d in Exeter (Sainsbury 1970). It was a phenomenon to which academics began to apply the term "territorial injustice" by the end of the 1960s (Davies 1968).

Perhaps of as much importance as community care for the development of services was the emergence of the disability lobby to press for a disablement income, an issue that raised the question of the nature of disability. Many saw disability largely as loss of control in life and of the normal choice range, and argued that a disablement income was essential to restore normality in these respects. At the end of the 1960s and in the early 1970s, younger disabled people in residential homes, particularly those in the voluntary sector, began to agitate for participation in the management of homes to ensure greater choice in and control over the way they spent their lives. The movement, which stopped short of residential accommodation for elderly people, aroused the interest of academics who devised institutional typologies some of which contrasted the "warehouse model" which emphasized the passive reception of care, with the "horticultural model", where the regime was organized to encourage growth in the individual (Miller & Gwynne 1972). Within a decade, "horticultural" experiments were in place based on paid volunteers who, acting as arms and legs for severely disabled people, extended their choice and control, for example, by cooking to the disabled person's instructions, bathing them in accordance with their wishes. Such accommodation was intended as a halfway house where the former residents of warehousing institutions became accustomed to exerting choice and control before moving into their own private accommodation aided by volunteer carers (Dartington et al. 1981).

The movement for a disability income also encouraged interest in access, particularly to public buildings, shops and transport, and gave rise to considerable dissatisfaction with local authority failure to implement the access clauses of the National Assistance Act. Dissatisfaction was fuelled by the development of overseas contacts, particularly with the United States, where the tactics and objectives of the civil rights campaign were adopted by disabled people, and Denmark, which had pioneered a large-scale independent living scheme.

The government response to these pressures was the first OPCS survey of disability (Harris 1971), the immediate outcome of which was a private member's measure, the Chronically Sick and Disabled Persons Act 1970. In the main, the Act strengthened the National Assistance Act, particularly the duties of local authorities to ensure access to public buildings, adapt homes, register people, and provide home helps, and laid on them a new duty: to estimate the number of people in their area as a basis for service planning. Essentially the Act reinforced the existing commitment to day and domiciliary provision, while emphasizing the importance of participation in "normal" activities. It was passed at the end of Harold Wilson's second administration with grudging ministerial support, but provided the disablement lobby with a platform for agitation.

A similar antipathy met the Seebohm Report in 1968, (Cmnd 3703) on which the Local Authority and Social Services Act 1970 was based: a measure that had substantial long-term effects on the administration of personal social services for disabled people. The original object had been to reduce juvenile delinquency by improving services for young offenders and their families: the existing range of services were to be replaced by a single family service offering one door on which to knock and a generic social worker. In practice, however, while many of the relevant services – education welfare, child guidance, the probation and youth services – remained outside the new family service, Seebohm glued together most of the services of the existing children's, health and welfare departments to create the social services department. The immediate impact of the Act was to halt the development of specialisms for the different categories of disabled people that were analogous to those already existing for blind people. Thus, welfare officers skilled in sign language found themselves moved into administration and replaced by generically trained social workers unable to communicate in sign language (Sainsbury 1986).

Moreover, the new departments were preoccupied with implementing the Children and Young Persons Act 1969. And after the publication of the Colwell Report in 1974 (DHSS 1974), the issue of child protection became their major priority. These developments distracted attention as well as resources from the Chronically Sick and Disabled Persons Act (Topliss & Gould 1981), trained social workers were increasingly confined to work with children, and disabled adults of all ages became the responsibility of untrained or assistant social workers and, sometimes, occupational therapists.

However, personal social services for disabled people did benefit from the continued general commitment to community care and government belief in the benign relationship between high public spending and economic performance: local authorities were encouraged to increase their expenditure on all personal social services, including those for disabled people.

Since 1976: the burden of care

For a variety of reasons, the rapid rate of service expansion in the 1970s was shortlived. First, some academics began to question the validity of the concept of need that had been widely used to justify increasing demands for more services, and argued for its replacement with the economic principles of demand and supply (Nevitt 1977). Furthermore, others began to elevate the issue of care and its provenance above the needs and rights of disabled people. For some critics the outcome of post-war social policy had been the creation of a rigid and unresponsive welfare bureaucracy serving the interests of its employees. They looked to the informal networks of family, neighbours and friends to provide the responsive care that people needed: the resources were available in the community if only they could be tapped (Hadley & Hatch 1981). These ideas struck a chord at a time when professional carers were increasingly unionized and their activities hedged about with restrictions. Moreover, they were not unlike those of Bleddyn Davies who, through the Kent Community Care project, sought to substitute community care for residential care, and informal carers for formal carers, in the interests of economy and effectiveness (Challis & Davies 1985).

What bound these factors together was the effect of the oil crisis on the economy and growing doubts about the efficacy of the Keynesian economic principles that had governed economic policy since the war. The Callaghan Government responded in 1976 by reducing the expansion of the social services, although priority groups, including disabled people, were protected and overall the personal social services were allowed a small expansion to respond to the growing numbers of elderly people and the contraction in long-stay hospitals (DHSS 1976). Services for disabled people now developed within a new conceptual framework as emphasis shifted from rights and individual needs to the problems of financing the "burden of care". The change was reinforced by the emergence of a feminist perspective that tended to focus on women as unpaid or low paid providers of care, rather than its recipients (Finch & Groves 1980).

The Conservative victory in 1979 accelerated these changes. Government suspicion of the public sector generally and local authorities in particular, and the decision to tackle Britain's economic problems by cutting public expenditure and, at the same time, increasing the social security bill by allowing unemployment to rise, squeezed the expansion of services for disabled people still further. However, the counter power of the disability lobby continued to exert influence. The government delayed including disability payments in its social security reforms by commissioning a new OPCS survey of disability. The Reports (OPCS 1988) provided ammunition for the disability lobby, resulting in another private member's measure in 1986, which gave disabled people the right to an assessment of their needs by the local authority, and to be involved in that assessment, if necessary through a representative. However, in practice, most local authorities failed to comply with the law, pleading shortage of resources.

The government was forced into a general upheaval of personal social services by the consequences of its relaxation of the social security rules in 1983, which enabled people on social security to enter private residential accommodation, the state paying the difference between a resident's income, less the guaranteed personal allowance, and the price of the accommodation. It was a change that hugely stimulated demand, allowing freedom of choice regarding entry into residential care for the first time. Expenditure on private and voluntary residential care rose dramatically, untrammelled by central or local control. The government was forced to act. First, a ceiling was placed on the fees that it was prepared to meet, and secondly, local authority registration and regulation powers were strengthened by the Registered Homes Act 1984 (Sainsbury 1989). But more was required. The answer was the NHS and Community Care Act 1990, based on the Griffiths Report (DHSS 1988), which promised large-scale reform of the personal social services.

The Act has done much for the benefit of disabled people, who are now guaranteed assessments involving consumers and informal carers. Within local authorities, the separation of their purchaser and provider roles should free those designing packages of care from the constraints on providers. The complaints procedure and inspection units that local authorities must set up, to which their own residential care is to be subject for the first time, should strengthen the voice of disabled people and extend their choice in and control over services.

However, there are also possible disadvantages in the new structure. First, the context of the changes is one of financial constraint, and there continues to be uneasiness about identifying need that cannot be met. Some authorities have stopped expanding their independent living schemes; entry into residential care is based on need not choice; priority for services is given to those on the brink of having to go into a home; in many areas the home help service is being transformed into a home care service that excludes housework; increasingly people are charged for day care, while holidays and other social activities are abandoned, except in cases where there is a respite care element.

Moreover, voluntary organizations of disabled people that combine service provision with advocacy have to split these functions if they wish to become providers under contract to local authorities, and may find that local authority priorities, rather than their own, predominate. Advocacy is likely to attract diminishing resources in the future. Furthermore, while local authorities must involve consumers in community care planning, and thus provide a formal medium through which disabled people may make their voices heard, in practice it is easier for organized groups than individuals to participate effectively, and the voices of some groups tend to be louder than others. As the role of local authorities is weakened generally, it is likely that the NHS rather than social services departments will play an increasingly important role in service development, so that the medical model of disability, with its focus on individual pathology, is likely to be strengthened. Finally, community care itself, as currently interpreted, is inherently passive, despite the rhetoric of consumer participation. Keeping people out of residential accommodation lacks the vibrancy of the vision of participation in all aspects of life and the right and obligation to contribute to society that underlay the National Assistance Act in 1948.

However, there are countervailing pressures that may reduce the negative effects of some of these changes. First, disabled people are increasingly effective advocates of their cause. During the 1980s they began to challenge the political tendency to view disabled people as members of a homogenous group. Some studies began to question the normality of life in private households where large-scale help is required, even where it is sensitively delivered (Owens 1987, Sainsbury 1993). And in the experimental establishments intended to be half way to independent living, some residents have preferred to remain there rather than make the move to life on their own "in the community". Meanwhile, as a disability income to restore the normal range of choice and control failed to materialize, some began to agitate for money rather than services, to secure through the market what they wanted, rather than rely on what local authorities and voluntary agencies were prepared to supply (Morris 1993). Feminists who were themselves disabled challenged the predominance of the male view of disability, and stressed women's particular experience and service needs (Morris 1989). Others began to question the assumption that care provided by relatives is preferable to residential care, and that informal carers are more acceptable than professionals.

A parallel development was the emergence and articulation of the black experience of disability, reflecting different cultural responses to disability, as well as being disabled in the context of racism. It was a situation that predominantly white professionals and semi-professionals working in the area were slow to recognize and understand, while few policy-makers were eager to jettison "colour-blind" provision. The development of advocates for disabled members of ethnic minorities has revealed further complexities. For example, people of different religious backgrounds and regions in the Indian subcontinent have different responses to disability, and their British born children with disability may adopt the attitudes of the majority community rather than those of their parents.

In recent years, some groups with particular conditions have established clear sets of service priorities of their own. Since the later 1970s, deaf people have become increasingly skilled in pressing their claims to be recognized as a community with its own culture defined by language (British Sign Language), which they argue should be recognized as an official language of the UK (Sainsbury 1986). Local authorities began to respond in the late 1970s by reintroducing specialist workers who were skilled signers. But this development was erratic, subject to resource constraints and the unreliability of the availability of training schemes. Moreover, not all deaf people were happy about the social work component of the training which, they argued, assumed a pathological element in the experience of deafness. Furthermore, the success of the deaf community has tended to distract political attention from hearing-impaired people who rely on speech for communication. Although they are numerically more important than deaf people, and growing in number as the population ages, they lack the cohesion provided by language and culture focused on special clubs. The fledgling service of hearing therapists, which is increasingly seen as being the appropriate response to hearing-impaired people relying on speech, has only recently been established, and its training courses are small in scale and underdeveloped. As hearing impairment does not determine entry into residential care, future resourcing of the service is open to doubt.

To some extent, the fissures that have appeared within the disability movement are a tribute to its strength: the resources that have generated internal debate and research have laid bare differences of opinion and interest. These may be exacerbated by the operation of the NHS and Community Care Act, which seeks to target those most "in need": need in this context meaning not the open ended commitment of promotional welfare, but the narrow responsibility of maintaining at home those on the brink of entry into residential care. Furthermore, the atomizing effect of increasing government insistence on markets and consumers, which may benefit some strong individuals and groups within the disability movement, may weaken the lobby's capacity to focus its campaigns effectively. Much will depend on its success in projecting a coherent political strategy. Recent attempts to develop coherence out of the idea that disabled people represent an oppressed class whose difficulties stem from the structure of a society created in the interests of the non-disabled, has itself been the subject of much debate. However, there are countervailing forces that already exist to strengthen the lobby. The international nature of the movement has become marked in recent years. This has acquired greater political importance as ties within the European Community have tightened; good practice elsewhere within the community provides a benchmark for development here. And the lobby is increasingly well placed to look beyond Europe for ideas and objectives in its search for models, such as the large-scale independent living schemes that have emerged in the US and elsewhere, which may be advocated on the British political stage.

However, important as the personal social services have been and are likely to continue to be in the lives of many disabled people, it is important to remember that the experiences of disabled people as a whole, and the strength of the disability lobby, are likely to be more substantially affected by broad shifts in general social policy, such as, for example, a return to a commitment to full employment.

Suggested reading

Morris (1993) presents the case for cash rather than service provision. OPCS (1988) provides an analysis of the characteristics of the disabled population as well as a discussion of definitional problems. Challis & Davies (1985) describe the research and principles that have since come to inform much of current community care policy. Oliver (1989) offers an extended discussion of the disabling nature of society. Finch & Groves (1980) explores the problems of carers. Sainsbury (1993) includes an exploration of the use of and attitudes towards the formal and informal networks of care, and a critique of the Hadley & Hatch (1981) position that interdependent communities exist, are capable of providing most of the care that is required, and that such care, because it is "natural", is superior to, and more acceptable than that provided by formal agencies.

Older people and the personal social services

Robin Means

Introduction

The last two sections have illustrated the marked policy differences in the provision of the personal social services for children and for disabled people. This last section considers elderly people whose "story" is enmeshed within that of disabled people, since they both depend largely upon the same pieces of legislation. Indeed, the tendency to separate them out is questionable since elderly people do not receive personal social services because they are old, but because their later life is coinciding with illness, frailty or disability. No attempt will be made to take the reader through a detailed history of legislative and administrative change since this has been provided by the previous section. Rather, key themes and issues will be drawn out and illustrated with specific examples drawn from the 1940s onwards.

Caring for people: continuity or change?

The mechanism for addressing key issues and themes with regard to the personal social services and elderly people will be to start with the community care reforms initiated by the White Paper *Caring for people* (Cm 849) and the subsequent 1990 Act, and to consider the extent to which these represent a continuity of debates about community care and older people or a radical departure from the past.

The government justified the need for change on several grounds. First, there was concern about the public expenditure implications of an ageing society, especially in terms of the rising social security benefit bill for people in independent residential and nursing home care (Audit Commission 1986). In 1979 such expenditure was only £10 million, but it had reached £459 million per annum by early 1986, the main reason being the rise in number of those in receipt of social security payments from 12,000 to 19,000. Secondly, there was frustration at the repeated failure of health agencies and social services to work effectively together on such issues as the closure of large mental handicap and mental health hospitals and the resettlement of the patients into the community. Thirdly, local authorities were seen as prone to slotting elderly people and others into a limited number of predetermined and unimaginative services that often did not meet their needs. Fourthly, local authorities were perceived as equally inadequate in terms of supporting carers to continue to play the dominant role in helping the majority of those with community care needs to avoid expensive institutional care.

As Sainsbury points out, the chosen direction was not, as many predicted, that local authorities would be stripped of their responsibilities and replaced by new health dominated quangos, but rather that social services authorities should be given the lead agency role for all the main community care groups including elderly people. They were to establish a strategic direction for local provision by producing annual community care plans in consultation with other key agencies and organizations such as health authorities, voluntary groups and user groups. However, this was not the same as encouraging local authorities to be the monopoly or near monopoly provider of community care services. Instead the voluntary and private sectors were seen as gradually taking over the dominant service delivery functions. The role of social services departments would increasingly be confined at the client level to the assessment of need, the designing of care arrangements to meet that need by "care managers" and the provision of funds to finance those arrangements. Local authorities were also being asked to establish a clear separation between their purchasing activities and their remaining provider functions. Overall, local authority social services were being encouraged to become "enablers" with a declining role in direct service provision.

Because of their emphasis upon markets, contracting out and competition, some commentators have condemned the reforms as part of a Thatcherite strategy of marketization of public services that will "guarantee only greater hardship to that section of society that is least capable of bearing it" (Langan 1990). Others have stressed how these reforms reflect broader international trends across policy areas to reject bureaucratic approaches to service delivery and to use developments in information technology to allow decentralized purchasing decisions to take place within devolved budgets (Hoggett 1991).

Certainly, at one level, the reforms reflect how the provision of personal services to elderly people will constantly change as ideas emerge and develop about the strengths and weaknesses of different mechanisms for delivering publicly funded services. And such options will expand as technological change creates new ways of storing information and monitoring budgets. However, in what ways this potential is used will reflect political values. Thus, the community care reforms are based upon a desire to minimize the service delivery role of local authorities but they could have been directed towards a radical decentralization of decision-making and service delivery *within* local authorities.

Optimists about the reforms can argue that they represent an opportunity to break with the past in terms of overcoming a long history of service neglect, when compared to the energy and thought that traditionally has gone into child care services. For example, services for elderly people in the 1940s legislation tended to be institution based, whether provided by the NHS or local government, and they were often starved of funds relative to those available for the acute sick (in the NHS) or for children (in local authorities).

There are many explanations for this neglect but one of the most powerful comes from the political economy perspective on ageing which argues that elderly people "are an ongoing problem in a society where institutions are geared primarily around issues of production and reproduction, where the facilities in the communities which most people retire into are concerned mostly with the serving of the existing labour force and the reproduction of a new one" (Phillipson 1977). It is probably equally important to remember that the "old old" are primarily women and that the services they receive are usually delivered by male dominated professions (Arber & Ginn 1991). Given this duality, the history of service neglect is perhaps not that surprising.

At the same time, the tradition of neglect has sometimes been tempered by "moral panics" about elderly people, either in terms of the shame to society of their poor treatment or in terms of government anxiety about their potential burden upon those of working age because of high public expenditure on their health and welfare needs.

"Moral panics" and the development of services for elderly people

The Second World War and the subsequent reconstruction debate had a major impact upon the shape of personal social services available to elderly people (Means & Smith 1985). These turning points also illustrate the complex ways in which elderly people can shift from being a low priority group for resources to the focus of a "moral panic" about the need for society to show care and concern.

In the early years of the Second World War the state was largely indifferent to the problems of elderly people in coping with the disruptions of war. The focus was upon children and families. Elderly people were initially a low priority for evacuation from urban areas in danger from German bombing raids while many were evicted from hospital beds to help establish the Emergency Medical Service. Once the bombing raids started, elderly people who lost their homes or who could no longer cope were in danger of being placed in public assistance institutions and hence acquiring the taint of pauperism. The government responded by supporting assorted hostel and evacuation schemes designed to ensure that such obvious "war victims" avoided this fate, but these initiatives failed to resolve what was becoming a major social issue.

> The problem of the aged and the chronic sick had been serious enough in peacetime; in war it threatened to become unmanageable. Thousands who had formerly been nursed at home were clamouring for admission to hospitals where families were split up, where homes were damaged or destroyed, and where the nightly trek to the shelters became a part of normal life . . . . (Titmuss 1950)

The response of government to this situation repeatedly showed a concern about civilian morale rather than about the fate of elderly people themselves. Thus, 4000 bedridden and infirm people were forcibly evacuated from

London air raid shelters in the autumn of 1940 because they were seen as a health hazard, a source of lowered morale, and "a serious encumbrance in the presence of an incident" (Cmd 6234).

As the war progressed the concern was less to hide the infirm and "bedridden" from the rest of the population, but rather to be seen to support women workers with caring responsibilities and to protect respectable elderly people who were drifting into public assistance institutions solely because of the disruptions of war. The former concern can be illustrated by describing how the home help service was extended to include elderly people in December 1944. Prior to this the service was restricted to a domestic service for young mothers who had recently given birth. The Ministry of Health became convinced of the need for this extension during the influenza epidemics of the 1943–4 winter. As it explained in a letter to the local authorities: "the Minister of Labour and our own minister are concerned about the hardship which is arising owing to lack of domestic help in private households where there is sickness or where there are aged or infirm persons and the deleterious effects which this may have on service and civilian morale."

The reference to "lack of domestic help", suggests the Ministry of Health may have been less concerned with the difficulties of women aircraft and munitions workers than upper and middle class women who had "lost" their domestic servants to the war effort. The meals on wheels service also emerged in this same period. Here the concern was with the difficulties faced by frail elderly people in queuing for their food rations. For example, one national newspaper complained of how "old people go short of food" while a local paper warned that "many Leeds aged were on the brink of starvation". Such articles called for an extension of meal delivery schemes being pioneered by the Women's (Royal) Voluntary Services [W(R)VS] and local branches of the NOPWC (later Age Concern). A clause was added to the National Assistance Act 1948 that gave local authorities the power to fund voluntary organizations to provide such a service.

However, the most famous example of a newspaper generating a "moral panic" on behalf of elderly people in this period concerns a letter that appeared in the *Manchester Guardian*. This was entitled "A Workhouse Visit" and referred to a visit to "a frail, sensitive refined old woman" living in the following regime:

> But down each side of the ward were ten beds, facing one another. Between each bed and its neighbour was a small locker and a straight-backed, wooden uncushioned chair. On each chair sat an

old woman in workhouse dress, upright, unoccupied. No library books or wireless. Central heating, but no open fire. No easy chairs. No pictures on the walls . . . . There were three exceptions to the upright old women. None was allowed to lie on her bed at any time throughout the day, although breakfast is at 7 a. m., but these three, unable any longer to endure their physical and mental weariness, had crashed forward, face downwards, onto their immaculate bed-spreads and were asleep.

The key point was that this was a "refined" elderly person and not some-one who deserved such poor treatment because of a previous feckless life-style. Rather, this was a war victim trapped within a Poor Law system that had deteriorated since the outbreak of war. Further letters and numerous articles followed the initial letter. A Ministry of Health spokesperson stressed the Department's hostility to such rigid regimes but admitted that the war had interrupted the early stages of substantial improvements. During inter-nal meetings, officials noted that the care of the aged was arousing consider-able public attention, and the Department must not lay itself open to charges of inactivity such as were implied in the Curtis Report in regard to the super-vision of Children's Homes. In this context, the emphasis of the 1948 National Assistance Act upon the development of local authority residential homes is easily understood. As is the strong emphasis upon the hotel concept in which residents would choose to come and hand over 17 shillings, of their 21 shillings pension, as rent.

These examples of policy debates and developments sparked off by the Second World War are illustrative of the two ways in which elderly people can generate "moral panics". They can be defined as a threat to stability because of their numbers and perceived decrepitude or they can be pre-sented as abandoned victims in need of greater public support and sympathy. This mixed pattern has continued. The most obvious example of the former concerns periodic panics about the perceived demographic "time bomb" and its implications for public expenditure. Although containing many sensi-ble proposals, the 1978 discussion document *A happier old age* (DHSS 1978) predicted that by 1986 there would be 24 per cent more people aged over 75 and warned that £10 million, or a third of total public expenditure on the main social programmes, was already going on elderly people. Although the bulk of this was on pensions, the report pointed out that within the health and personal social services the average cost of care and treatment of a per-son aged over 75 was seven times that of a person of working age. At least these figures were presented factually rather than in apocalyptic terms. However, only five years later, the Health Advisory Service in *The rising tide* was issuing dire warnings that the number of people with dementia would rise rapidly because of the growth of the very old and that "the flood is likely to overwhelm the entire health care system" (Health Advisory Service 1983). Such government publications have fuelled a debate about the need to target services only at those most in need, to encourage elderly people to self-provision and for local authorities to become more adept at supporting relatives to maintain their caring roles. These issues are returned to later in the chapter.

"Moral panics" have also continued to appear in terms of periodic scandals about ill-treatment and neglect, usually but not always within large institutions. Perhaps the clearest example of this concerns the establishment of the campaigning group Aid for the Elderly in Government Institutions (AEGIS) which claimed in the mid 1960s that there was widespread abuse of mental geriatric and psycho-geriatric patients by hospital staff. Their book *Sans everything: a case to answer* (Robb 1967) received massive publicity and the government was persuaded to take action through the establishment of the NHS Hospital Advisory Service in 1969. In the last couple of years, elder abuse and elder abandonment have re-emerged as high profile topics with extensive coverage by television programmes such as *Panorama* and professional journals such as *Community Care*, leading to the establishment of a new campaigning group by Age Concern.

The politics of caring and service neglect

However, "moral panics" about particular issues are not a random phenomenon. They are usually based around deep social or state concerns (about law and order, the decline of the family, the rising costs of public expenditure etc.) and are open to promotion and manipulation by pressure groups and other self-interested bodies (Cohen 1973). In the case of elderly people, there has always been deep concern about the costs of "looking after" elderly people and hence the need to ensure that the dominant role in this is continued to be played by the "family".

The true nature of the "family" care of sick and frail elderly people has long been known. In his 1948 study of 600 elderly people in Wolverhampton, Sheldon found that the key roles in the performance of domestic chores and the management of illness were carried out by wives and daughters: "whereas the wives do most of the nursing of the men, the strain when the mother is ill falls on the daughter, who may have to stay at home as much to run the household as to nurse her mother" (Sheldon 1948).

Many commentators in the 1950s claimed such family "care" would be undermined by the creation of the so called "welfare state". Doctors, social workers, local authority associations and voluntary sector pressure groups were all willing to express this view at various times, an attitude especially acute amongst those afraid of bed blockages being caused by relatives refusing to offer a home to elderly patients. Thompson was associated with Birmingham hospital surveys in the 1940s: "It is . . . possible that slackening of the moral fibre of the family and a demand for material comfort and amenity outweighs the charms of mutual affection . . .. The power of the group-maintaining instincts will suffer if the provision of a home, the training of children, and the care of its disabled members are no longer the ambition of a family but the duty of a local or central authority" (Thompson 1949).

The Association of Municipal Corporations in their evidence to the 1954 Phillips Committee on *The economic and financial problems of the provision for old age* (Cmd 9333) complained of "the reluctance of many families to care for their aged relatives" after they entered hospitals which was placing enormous pressure on local authority residential accommodation.

Such a mind set and its support within much of government in the 1950s and 1960s helps to explain the slowness to give local authorities the legal power to provide a full range of domiciliary services (counselling, day care etc.) rather than just residential care and home care. From the early 1950s, the Ministry of Health was claiming that care at home was better than care in institutions and from the early 1960s Townsend in *The last refuge* (1962) and others had exposed the inadequacies of residential care. However, it was not until the creation of combined social services departments in the early 1970s that local authorities had access to general powers to promote the welfare of elderly people. The great fear was that the wider availability of domiciliary care would be used by carers and especially daughters and daughters-in-law to abandon elderly relatives to the state. As a consultant physician argued:

> The feeling that the state ought to solve every inconvenient domestic situation is merely another factor in producing a snowball expansion on demands in the National Health and Welfare Service. Close observation on domestic strains makes one thing very clear. This is that where an old person has a family who have a sound feeling of moral responsibility serious problems do not arise, however much difficulty may be met. (Rudd 1958)

Gradually, overwhelming evidence accumulated that wives, daughters and daughters-in-law together with male spouses continued to provide the majority of care for frail and dependant elderly people. An early 1960s study of 1500 patients discharged from a geriatric unit concluded that "the belief in the decline in filial care of the elderly is unfounded and an as yet unproven modern myth" (Lowther & Williamson 1966). Such conclusions were supported by a series of studies involving Peter Townsend, the largest of which entailed 4000 interviews with elderly people in three different industrialized countries and recommended that rather than being restricted from a fear of undermining the family, domiciliary services needed to be expanded rapidly to support families and help the isolated (Townsend 1963, Shanas et al. 1968).

The gradual acceptance of these findings did lead to a gradual expansion of the powers of local authorities to provide domiciliary services and growing encouragement from central government for a switch of local authority expenditure away from residential care and towards the provision of domiciliary services. There has also been a growing recognition that such domiciliary services should be available to those with nearby carers as well as to those elderly people lacking such informal support. The danger of failing to do this was bluntly put by Moroney:

> By not offering support, existing social policy might actually force many families to give up this function prematurely, given the evidence of the severe strain many families are experiencing. If this were to happen, the family and the state would not be sharing the responsibility through an interdependent relationship and it is conceivable that eventually the social welfare system would be pressurised with demands to provide even greater amounts of care, to become the family for more and more elderly persons. (Moroney 1976)

This is now accepted by central government. One of the six key objectives of the 1989 White Paper on community care was "to ensure that service providers make practical support for carers a high priority" (Cm 849).

At one level this represents a radical shift in professional and government perspectives away from the "moral fibre" discourse of the 1950s and 1960s when the availability of support through government funded services was seen as only likely to reduce a willingness of family members to care for their elderly relatives. At another level, however, one is struck by the continuity of assumptions. It is still assumed that the family ought to care and a failure or refusal to provide physical services (cleaning, shopping, nursing etc.) implies a lack of emotional concern. The advantage of this to governments is that the continuing willingness of women (and male spouses) to perform these roles helps to reduce the need for public expenditure on the personal social services for elderly people.

The health and social care divide

One of the tasks of the 1989 White Paper was to reduce confusion over the respective roles of social services and health. This was attempted by giving social services the lead agency role and by stressing the role of health agencies in the planning process, in joint assessments and in the provision of the health care components of community care packages.

The health and social care divide debate has been continuing throughout the period covered by this chapter. Section 21 of the National Assistance Act 1948 stated that local authority residential care should be available for those "in need of care and attention" and implied that those who were sick would be treated in hospitals, but no clear definition was offered of what was meant by "in need of care and attention". However, as Goodlove and Mann point out: "It seems fairly clear that the authors . . . did not envisage this type of care as being adequate for those suffering from incontinence, serious loss of mobility, or abnormal senile dementia. A 'Part III home' was to be a home rather than a hospital or a nursing home" (Goodlove & Mann 1980). Despite these intentions, the trend over the last fifty years has been towards local authorities taking responsibility for elderly people in these types of situation.

The late 1940s and early 1950s were characterized by arguments between local authorities and hospital boards over the correct placement of individual elderly people, a situation exacerbated by the shortage of beds in both sectors. Hospitals felt local authorities took too narrow a view of "care and attention" and rejected anyone with the slightest health problem. Local authorities felt elderly people who were ill were being dumped on them by health professionals. As one commentator of the time explained, there were a large number of elderly people "stranded in the no-man's land between the Regional Hospital Board and the local welfare department – not ill enough for one, not well enough for the other" (Huws Jones 1952). But hospital beds were more expensive than local authority beds, and so the solution proposed in the key 1957 circular from the Ministry of Health was that the following groups of elderly people were the responsibility of local authorities:

- care of the otherwise active resident in a welfare home during minor illness which may well involve a short period in bed;
- care of the infirm (including the senile) who may need help in dressing, toilet, etc., and may need to live on the ground floor because they cannot manage stairs, and may spend part of the day in bed (or longer periods in bad weather);
- care of those elderly persons in a welfare home who have to take to bed and are not expected to live more than a few weeks (or exceptionally months). (Ministry of Health 1957)

Hospital authorities were also given a list of responsibilities by this circular and these included the "chronic bedfast", the "convalescent sick" and the "senile confused".

At first glance, "the partly sick and partly well" were no longer in no-man's land. They were increasingly being directed to local authority residential homes. However, the circular was riddled with problems of interpretation. Could one always decide if a bedfast resident would die in three months or three years? How clear cut was the distinction between the senile and senile confused? Staff from hospitals and social services were able to use the circular as they bargained over the location of individual elderly people.

Such tensions over the health and social care divide have never been resolved, but the overall trend has been towards social services taking responsibility for more and more dependent elderly people. Reforms brought in by the NHS and Community Care Act exacerbate these trends. Social services authorities now have funding responsibilities for low income elderly people in independent sector nursing homes and health authorities are rapidly withdrawing from the funding of all continuous care beds. This has generated further uncertainty about the health and social care divide. As Henwood points out,

Despite the claim that the responsibilities of the NHS are unchanged, nursing home care is apparently now viewed as social care, not health. Is this contradictory, or are we to accept that there is a real distinction between those needing nursing home care for reasons of ill health and those needing it for other reasons? Sure this is playing *Alice in Wonderland* games with words and semantics. (Henwood 1992)

Nursing care provided by the NHS is free, while social care can be charged for. The responsibility for funding long-term health and social care is thus being shifted covertly onto users and carers by the government. Social services authorities and health authorities are being left to struggle with the consequences of this shift.

Similar health and social care tensions remain unresolved in terms of the contribution of primary health care services to care packages for elderly people. This is difficult enough for care managers from social services when the district nurses relate to a health provider unit or trust, but the situation becomes even more complex when the dimension of GP budget holders are brought in. Such individuals are likely to perceive themselves as purchasers of health care packages that require an appropriate community care response from social services, thus creating a danger of two competing purchasers from two different agencies trying to co-ordinate provision for elderly people.

This has led some commentators to speculate on possible future scenarios. Glennerster, Falkingham and Evandrou have queried whether approved general practices might take on community care powers at least on an experimental basis:

> Social services departments are not necessarily the only or best placed organizations to co-ordinate a package of services for an elderly person. Health centres or the enhanced budget holding general practices could be good alternatives . . . Faced with a competition, local social services departments might be put on their mettle. In some areas general practices might be the most efficient agents to administer services and employ a specialist doctor to combine both the home visits to elderly people that will be required under their new contracts as well as assessments for social care. (Glennerster et al. 1990)

Others have gone one step further because of the perceived need to draw community health and welfare services (including GPs, care managers, home care staff and district nurses) into a simpler and more coherent structure. For example, Henwood et al. have suggested exploring the feasibility of a primary and community care authority based upon Family Health Service Authorities (FHSAs) or, alternatively, the integration of all health and social care purchasing functions within health authorities (Henwood et al. 1991). In other words, the legitimacy of social services and care managers as the lead agents in community care provision for older people remains in some doubt.

Future scenarios: towards a mixed economy of social care?

The whole thrust of the White Paper on community care, the 1990 Act and the subsequent policy guidance is upon the need to stimulate a mixed economy of social care in which the provider role of the independent sector will be greatly strengthened. It is easy to perceive this as a radical departure with the past, but it is important to recognize that it is only partially true. Earlier discussion outlined how central government was reluctant to support a strong local government role in domiciliary service provision for fear of undermining "family" care. One way of justifying this was to emphasize the potential role of voluntary sector organizations. Organizations such as W(R)VS, the British Red Cross and NOPWC (later Age Concern) had developed strong welfare roles during the Second World War and were keen to play a strong part in the reconstruction process. Indeed, they "planted" many of the "moral panic" stories about workhouses and food rationing as part of this strategy to emphasize their potential role, while they, also, lobbied central government in the 1950s against allowing local government increased powers (Means & Smith 1985).

However, local authorities became increasingly frustrated at the failure of voluntary organizations to develop coherent authority-wide services in terms of meals on wheels, day care and visiting/counselling schemes. This created what one commentator called a "wind of discontent in the town halls" (Slack 1960), and led to a growing campaign to increase the legislative powers of local authorities. However, as already noted, these powers were not fully available until the establishment of social services departments in April 1971. Thus, there has always been a mixed economy of welfare in both residential and domiciliary care, and it is misleading to suggest that local authorities have ever been monopoly service providers. In residential care, a voluntary sector has long existed and this was joined by a rapidly expanding private sector from the mid 1980s onwards. In domiciliary care, voluntary organizations have continued to receive grants to provide services from local authorities despite the considerable growth of local authority provision since the early 1970s.

Having said this, the community care reforms still represent a radical development in terms of their emphasis upon creating an explicit market in social care controlled through contracts. Research so far carried out on the reforms suggests that the majority of senior managers are keen to develop a mixed economy and to make services more flexible and responsive to users through developing care management systems (Hoyes & Means 1993, Wistow et al. 1992).

It must be said, though, that such research also indicates that the majority of energy has so far gone on developing community care planning systems and the internal reorganization of departments, and in implementing their new residential care and nursing home assessment and payment responsibilities. There is, as yet, little evidence of a dramatic growth in the use of the independent sector to provide services. In only a few local authorities have the majority of services been contracted out, though many predict that the pace of change in this direction will soon speed up.

My own research with colleagues is supportive of these conclusions, but also illustrative of the very different starting points of individual authorities in terms of attitudes of councillors, the inheritance of services and demographic profile. The "knock on" effect of this for developing a mixed economy in social care can be shown from the following two case studies (Hoyes et al. 1994).

County "A" has a very large elderly population and an enormous independent residential and nursing home sector. It made an early decision to implement a purchaser–provider separation at the level of its 32 district offices for all its functions including child care. Three pilots were established in 1990–91 with a view to these informing a phased county-wide reorganization over a three year period. Care management teams are composed of a wide range of staff (social workers, occupational therapists, home care organizers, etc.) and these teams are perceived as purchasers, with responsibility for a locality or client group. Care management is a service all users receive, with different degrees of professional involvement according to the complexity of their needs and care packages.

By April 1993 care management teams and a purchaser–provider split had been established throughout the county, although delays had been experienced in the delegation of budgetary control to some teams. The county was also planning further structural changes to consolidate and strengthen the purchasing function, and to develop and support the management structure of the inhouse providers. The main effect of this restructuring would be a reduction in the number of districts from 32 to 19, and the establishment of a managerially separate provider division, known as "Community Services – County A".

This authority is very enthusiastic about the mixed economy that it believes will generate more choice for the users of services. However, the large private residential and nursing-home market does not yet extend to other forms of provision such as day services and domiciliary care.

Managers see two sets of issues arising from the division of people away from residential and nursing-home care by providing community based packages. First, there is the risk that the inevitable reduction in the size of the independent residential and nursing home sector will not necessarily see high quality homes survive. To tackle this the department has implemented a system of accreditation using written quality standards over and above the registration requirements. Secondly, there is the need to stimulate a market in other kinds of services. The authority had advertised in the local press and in *Care Weekly* and was opening a process of dialogue with those potential providers who had responded. However, care management teams at the district office would make most purchasing decisions, and the trigger point for market stimulation would be the annual district purchasing plan.

Metropolitan Borough "B". This metropolitan authority retained its traditional service delivery structure with social work teams, home care teams and occupational therapists involved in both assessment and care delivery until April 1993 when a radical purchaser–provider split was introduced into the community care work of the department, with care management teams becoming the "purchasing" arm of the authority. These new teams are composed of a mixture of social workers, home care organizers and occupational therapists. Referrals are allocated by team leaders to one of five priority bands that define the speed of care manager response. Subsequent packages have to be costed (all services now have shadow unit costs) and agreed by the team leader who has to refer upwards if the proposed package is above agreed ceilings. Places in independent residential and nursing homes are bought on a spot purchase basis by care managers, using DSS price guidelines.

This authority has a tradition of local authority provision of services. However, development plans for all services were generated in 1988 and these identified the need for new services and a more diverse range of providers. By the time the fieldwork commenced, the local authority had developed a number of service agreements with the voluntary sector and this included a Crossroads care attendant scheme and day care provision by Age Concern. Movement in this direction has continued, but only modestly, and no major change in this situation is expected in the near future for two main reasons. First, the local authority remains very proud of its own services (especially home care provision) and most members are not willing to consider the contracting out of such services. Secondly, this authority received a low sum from the social security transfer formula and has also faced major expenditure cutbacks as a local authority. This has limited the scope for developing new services outside of existing local authority and voluntary sector provision.

At first glance, both these authorities are tackling the reforms in rather similar ways in terms of their attitudes to developing care management, purchaser–provider splits and the mixed economy. But this is misleading. The cultural shift involved is greater in the metropolitan authority than the county, and the former is developing its mixed economy from a much smaller base. Furthermore, the county received much more additional money from central government than the metropolitan authority in 1993/4 to fund residential and nursing-home care because of the size of this sector locally and this has created the flexibility to shift some of this money into new domiciliary developments. Finally, the radical system of devolved budgets in the county has been made possible by extensive investment over several years in computerized information systems. The metropolitan authority aspires to this model but lacks this infrastructure of past investment to allow care management teams to control real as opposed to shadow budgets within the short, and possibly the medium, term.

There appears little doubt that the provision of social care services to elderly people in the 1990s will be based upon a growth in the mixed economy. However, the two case studies underline that both the speed and the nature of this change will vary considerably from local authority to local authority. Many local authorities will remain an important provider of personal social services to elderly people unless the government decides to take further action to speed up change. Finally, it needs to be remembered that a growth of the mixed economy is not the same as the growth of a more diverse range of providers. The work of Le Grand and Bartlett underlines the economics of scale in the functioning of any market (Le Grand & Bartlett 1993) and it may be that the social care market will become dominated by a limited number of large "players" from the independent sector rather than a diverse range of local and very flexible providers. Whether this happens or not will depend upon how local authorities develop their purchasing roles.

Future scenarios: towards user-centred services?

The last point brings us to the issue of whether the reforms will be developed primarily to control costs (large block contracts with a limited number of large providers) or whether care managers will be encouraged and supported to develop their own purchasing role in which they will put together flexible care packages that draw upon local, often unconventional, providers rather than just relying upon traditional agencies.

The enormous obstacles to such a development need to be recognized. First, it is very difficult to develop a user-centred approach within finite budgets. Local authorities are developing ever more explicit rationing systems in which only those most at risk and most dependent will receive a service. Secondly, this means local authorities are under pressure to minimize the cost of services provided to those who do qualify for help. The focus becomes the cheapest acceptable package rather than an exploration of a wide range of alternatives, some of which might be much more expensive than others. Thirdly, as Allen et al. discovered, elderly service users have low service expectations and are thus the least likely to complain and demand a better and more appropriate response to their needs (Allen et al. 1992). Thus, they are likely still to be put to bed at eight o'clock by a home help or district nurse because that is the latest such a service operates, rather than because that is when they want to go to bed.

The reforms do, however, offer a vision of a more user-centred system of personal social services for elderly people despite the enormous financial problems faced by local authorities. This can best be illustrated by reference to black elders and previous failures to develop appropriate services for them. Elsewhere, with a colleague, I have argued that:

> . . . the changes will have failed if they do not lead to the provision of flexible care packages that are perceived as appropriate and high quality by consumers and their carers. A good test of this will be the experience of clients from minority ethnic groups. Such individuals should receive services appropriate to their needs, not only where they happen to live in local authorities where a significant proportion of the population is from such groups, but also where they represent an isolated household in a largely all-white community. (Hoyes & Means 1993)

However, the performance of social services authorities with regard to black elders has been appalling. Means and Smith in their 1985 study of *The development of welfare services for elderly people* cover the period from the 1940s through to the early 1970s. Not a single reference to race or ethnicity is made, not even in the final chapter that considers future agendas (Means & Smith 1985). Such colour blind attitudes have continued. In *Elderly people from ethnic minorities*, Bowling looked at four different innovative projects that had been set up in different local authorities with the help of central government grants. Overall, he found that all four projects "had to struggle for a role, to struggle for recognition by other agencies and to struggle to gain the confidence of the client group for whom they were working". Bowling argues that these problems flowed from the colour blind nature of existing services which thus failed to attract many clients from minority ethnic groups. This in turn generated complacency; out-of-date information was used to argue that numbers were very low or it was claimed that all their needs were being met in their own community. Hence, there was a "Catch 22" situation in which services could not be developed until a need was demonstrated and it was difficult to demonstrate a need until an appropriate and accessible service was provided (Bowling 1990).

Conclusion

In looking at the development of community care services for elderly people since the Second World War, it is easy to drift into an overly narrow look at detailed policy concerns of the moment such as differential local authority approaches to care management. Hopefully, this section has avoided this temptation through its emphasis upon the importance of broader ongoing debates such as the implications of demographic change and the caring obligations of family members.

This type of perspective enables us to see some of the factors that will drive policy change in the next decade. Above all, government concern about projected increases in the elderly population suggests a growing emphasis upon the need to target expensive care services only at those most "at risk". Those falling within this category, as defined by individual local authorities, may well receive more user-centred services and more choice, but many others will effectively be told that no response can be made to their needs because of resource shortages.

Such concerns also suggest a growing emphasis upon the need for "better off" elderly people to self provision for their own health and social care needs. This is despite extensive evidence that only a minority of elderly people will have the resources to contemplate this sort of strategy within the foreseeable future (Bosanquet & Propper 1991). However, it will be feasible for local authorities to place a growing emphasis upon charging for domiciliary services as a key mechanism for raising revenue. There is evidence that some local authorities are keen to encourage their clients to maximize their take-up of disability benefits (attendance allowance, mobility allowance etc.) so that they can afford to pay more in charges (Means & Lart 1993). A key objective of the community care reforms was to stop the mushrooming of the social security bill for private residential and nursing-home care. It would appear that a new social security tension may be about to emerge as local authorities try to maximize income from the social security system as they struggle to implement the "new" community care.

Suggested reading

Means and Smith (1985) provide a detailed look at the development of personal social services for elderly people from the Second World War through to the early 1970s. Maclean (1989) covers some of the same ground but takes the "story" through to the community care reforms. Material on the impact of the community care reforms upon older people is only just beginning to emerge but Wistow et al. (1992), Hoyes & Means (1993) and Hoyes et al. (1994) provide early insights.

CHAPTER 9
Voluntary action and the state

Marilyn Taylor

Introduction

Voluntary organizations, like the poor, are always with us. For as long as people are free to come together independently to tackle problems or improve conditions for themselves and others, it is likely that they will continue to do so. But, over time, there have been many different views as to the place of this kind of activity in society. How can its energy and resources best contribute to public welfare? Can welfare be left to the spontaneous goodwill of voluntary and community organizations? If not, how are the efforts of these organizations best tied into provision organized through the state or the market and what roles are they best equipped to play?

Voluntary organizations were important providers of a wide range of welfare services in the nineteenth century. Often they were developing provision in areas where the state played little or no role. In others, such as the relief of poverty and the welfare of children, their provisions existed alongside the pervasive role of the New Poor Law.

Early in the twentieth century, Sidney and Beatrice Webb characterized this approach as a "parallel bars" relationship between state and voluntary action, each with its distinctive sphere of operation. However, by the end of the nineteenth century, there was increasing support for the state to play a greater role, while the growth of municipal and central government provided the capacity and structure for it to do so. Developments in the twentieth century thus moved towards the Webbs' second model of an "extension ladder" approach, in which the state would play the central role, providing a national minimum, with the voluntary sector topping it up.

With the advent of the welfare state in the 1940s, it seemed the "extension" would all but disappear. In the eyes of the new Labour government, voluntary provision was patronizing and outdated. But by the 1980s it was the state that was seen to have failed: a radical Conservative government wanted the "active citizen" to take more responsibility and transfer the delivery of welfare to voluntary, or indeed commercial, organizations. In these competing views of welfare, voluntary and public sectors have appeared as rivals for the central position in welfare provision. But others would see this as a misreading of recent history. Instead they argue that the public and voluntary sectors should be seen as interdependent partners in welfare (Gidron et al. 1992).

For students of the voluntary sector, the past 50 years have provided a fascinating opportunity to observe the implications of these different perspectives on welfare. From a situation in the 1940s, where many who were active in the sector must have wondered whether there was a role for the sector to play at all, we have moved in the 1990s to a situation where voluntary organizations are expected to move back to centre stage, albeit with competition from the commercial sector.

This chapter looks at the way in which voluntary organizations have responded to changing welfare policies and at the implications both for organizations within the sector and for the people whom it aims to serve. On the basis of this experience, it asks what policies are likely to allow the sector to play its full part in welfare.

The voluntary sector: definitions and characteristics

The twin pillars of voluntary action that Beveridge identified in his work on *Voluntary action* (1948) – philanthropy and mutual aid – have been a third force in society throughout modern history, alongside the market and the state. The origins of many of the services described and analyzed elsewhere in this book are to be found there: in the educational endowments of the Tudor era; the network of voluntary hospitals that grew during the eighteenth and nineteenth centuries; the friendly societies which were a major source of social insurance for the working classes; the housing initiatives of Octavia Hill, the Peabody Trust and others in the latter half of the nineteenth century.

But what exactly is the voluntary sector? And what part has it played in the provision of welfare?

The Wolfenden report on the future of the sector in 1978 identified four systems of "social helping": the informal, the commercial, the statutory and the voluntary. Voluntary organizations are described by Maria Brenton as formal, constitutionally separate from government, non-profit distributing and of public benefit (Brenton 1985). They are not, as their name would suggest, made up solely of volunteers: Beveridge quotes a study of the sector written in 1945 that claims that, even then, "many of the most active voluntary organizations are staffed entirely by highly trained and fairly well paid professional workers" (Bourdillon 1945). However, some authors require of any organization claiming to be in the sector that it should incorporate some element of voluntarism, including unpaid management committee members (Salamon & Anheier 1992).

Some commentators have stressed the associational or communal form that voluntary and community organizations take (Billis 1993, Butler 1982), as opposed to the bureaucracy of the public sector or the price-driven competitiveness of the commercial firm. While current pressures may pull parts of the sector in the directions of bureaucracy and competitiveness, these authors would insist that the roots of a true voluntary organization must remain in the associational sphere. Others (Evers 1993) argue that, rather than occupying a sphere of its own, the voluntary sector is the point at which informal/personal, market/commercial and government/public systems intersect and it is thus able to integrate different spheres of operation. Such an analysis of the sector makes voluntary organizations essentially ambiguous in nature and hard to define, but highly versatile and responsive to changing circumstances.

However defined, supporters of the sector tend to suggest that there are several positive characteristics that the sector offers to any welfare system. Its flexibility, innovation, and closeness to the consumer in comparison to state welfare (Hadley & Hatch 1981) are frequently cited, although such lists have been criticized as over-romantic (Brenton 1985). There has also been an assumption over the years that voluntary organizations serve the poor (Salamon 1993) and that they are public interest organizations, hence the tax benefits that they enjoy in many countries. Some have claimed that the voluntary sector has a monopoly on values (Jeavons 1992). On the other hand, these organizations have also been criticized as being paternalistic and patchy in their coverage as well as amateurish in the delivery of their services (Salamon 1987).

It is essential for the purposes of this chapter to stress the diversity of the voluntary sector. One of the reasons the sector has always proved so hard to define is the huge variety of organizations contained within it. Beveridge's distinction between philanthropy and mutual aid organizations has been carried forward by Handy (1988), who talks of *mutual support, service delivery* and *campaigning organizations.* To these three categories should be added *intermediary* agencies – umbrella bodies that provide support to other organizations within the sector and charitable trusts and foundations, which dispense money to organizations in the sector. Current policies tend to see the sector as a potential (and alternative) service provider: but this fails to recognize or allow for the fact that, as well as being service providers, voluntary orgnizations have a political role in giving expression to the range of interests within society and a social role in reinforcing common identities and experiences.

In talking of voluntary organizations, therefore, this chapter spans everything from a large household name children's charity to a small support group for single mothers; from a medical research organization turning over millions to a local environmental group campaigning for the preservation of a wildlife site; from a housing association, through large-scale campaigns for homeless people to a tenants' group on a local estate; from the major charities for people with visual or hearing impairments to a local coalition of disabled people lobbying for better provision.

Developments over the past fifty years

The development of the voluntary sector over the period under study can be divided into four overlapping phases.

1. *Redundancy?* Immediately after the war, the introduction of the welfare state meant that the future role of the voluntary sector was uncertain. Some commentators see this as a period when the voluntary sector was "marking time" (Wolfenden 1978) or even "moribund" (Knight 1993).

2. *New roles.* The sector began to gain confidence as the post-war generation came of age in the 1960s, with the arrival of major new campaigning organizations and the influence of social movements in the United States and on the continent. This was the beginning of a new wave of voluntary and community activity that was both complementary to and critical of the welfare state; a wave of activity that gained strength during the 1970s with the growth of self-help and community activity on the ground, and the development and formalization of relationships between the voluntary sector and government.

217

3. *Transition.* At the same time, the limits of state welfare were becoming apparent as the economy faltered and the beneficiaries of the welfare state began to demand better standards and more choice. Calls for more pluralism came both from within the sector and from the "New Right".

The election of a new Conservative government in 1979 provided the opportunity to respond to these criticisms and reduce the role of the state in welfare. Rather than an "extension ladder" these policies envisaged using the voluntary sector as the service delivery "arm" of the state.

4. *Agency.* But it was not until the third term of the Thatcher Government, from 1987 onwards, that new policies began to bite across the board, with major legislation affecting education, health and local government in the late 1980s. This legislation allowed schools, housing estates and parts of the health service to "opt out" and imposed or encouraged the "contracting out" of mainstream services from environmental maintenance to community care.

History is rarely as tidy as this brief summary implies. It is impossible to put precise dates to these different phases of development, or indeed to suggest that they were in any way clear cut. Organizations operating in different fields faced different challenges at different times: the entry of the state into social welfare and leisure, for example, came later than its entry into education and health. There were some areas that were never at any time during this period considered a high priority by government; others where the sector was operating as an agent even prior to the 1940s. It is, however, possible to see different patterns of activity emerging over the period under study in response to government policy, emerging needs, and changing definitions of need.

Redundancy?

As other chapters in this book have shown, the welfare state did not spring out of nowhere. The entry of the state into welfare had been under way since the nineteenth century and voluntary organizations had been adapting to this fact for some long time. Indeed, voluntary organizations were among those campaigning for the state to take greater responsibility. Often the first move towards state responsibility came in the form of funding for voluntary organizations. Friendly societies acted as agents for the state in the social security legislation at the beginning of the twentieth century, a role that Beveridge wished to see continued under the post-war welfare state. The state stepped in with subsidies to universities and voluntary hospitals after the First World War and as it took over the primary responsibility for education, was prepared to support new complementary functions carried out by voluntary organizations in the fields of social welfare, family support and youth work, adult and civic education.

The fact that Beveridge, sometimes dubbed the architect of the welfare state, followed up his work on social security with a treatise on *Voluntary action* (Beveridge 1948) demonstrates his expectations that the voluntary sector would continue to play a role in the post-war era, even against the background of comprehensive state provision. But the legislation of the 1940s, coupled with the election of a Labour government committed to state welfare, must have felt like the writing on the wall for the many voluntary organizations that had been major service providers in the past, especially in the fields of health and social security. Would there be any further need for them?

Worst hit were the friendly societies and hospitals. The former faded into the background, once it became clear that they were not to be used as agents in the way Beveridge had suggested. The hospitals were taken into state ownership along with their endowments, although lobbying ensured that the teaching hospitals kept theirs. A "rump" of some 200 independent hospitals and homes survived, mainly those with a distinctive religious character.

The rising class of new public servants and the politicians of the new Labour government saw little role for the voluntary sector. There were two reasons for this. To the Labour party, charity was an expression of the British class system that they vehemently opposed: "Philanthropy was to us the odious expression of social oligarchy and churchly bourgeois attitudes" (Crossman in Brenton 1985). But, equally important, it did not fit into the new vision of centralized planning on which the new administration had pinned its faith. To Aneurin Bevan, piloting the new National Health Service through its initial stages, the voluntary sector represented nothing more than "a patchwork of local paternalisms" (Aneurin Bevan in Prochaska 1992).

This belief in centralized planning also condemned local co-operative traditions, which were seen as insular and apolitical (Prochaska 1992). This failure to nourish the roots of the Labour movement was to prove shortsighted. For with the benefit of hindsight, a key figure in the Labour party of that time, Richard Crossman, was to comment on the "grievous harm" that the post-war Labour party had done to its mutual aid tradition "which, merging

219

into philanthropy, gave socialism its democratic infrastructure and moral structure" (Crossman in Prochaska 1992). In fact, the co-operative tradition was not wholly lost: working class communities were always more resistant to centralized planning than the post-war Labour party was prepared to realize. But it survived only in the shadows and with little influence until the 1970s revived the importance of local community action.

There were other problems for the voluntary sector. The expanding public sector was a powerful magnet for the highfliers of the post-war era. The voluntary sector could not compete as an employer, although the post-war job market and employment conventions still left many women with energy and ideas to pour into voluntary action. There were also fears that people who had to pay for welfare through taxes would not wish to pay again through charitable donations. A post-war survey showed that 99 per cent of people thought philanthropy would be superfluous with the coming of the welfare state (Beveridge 1948). Many traditional organizations were worried for their future, fearful "that their funds would dry up if the welfare state abolished material need" (Younghusband 1978).

Nonetheless, there were still openings for the voluntary sector, especially in those areas that were not priorities on the welfare state agenda. These included services for elderly people, leisure and youth services: there were no local authority empires in these fields immediately after the war and the manipulation of the youth movement in pre-war Germany left many people wary of state intervention in this field. At a time when calls upon the public purse were high the assets and skills available to the voluntary sector had a lot to recommend them, as did the voluntary effort that they could release. By 1970, the voluntary sector still provided one third of all residential home places for elderly people and the physically handicapped, albeit often on local authority sponsorship.

Local authorities had no legal competence to make non-residential provision but the 1948 National Assistance Act did give them powers to fund voluntary organizations to provide such services (e.g. meals on wheels, lunch clubs, social clubs and so on). The Old People's Welfare Committees and Women's Voluntary Service [W(R)VS] created at the beginning of the war already had national networks that were well placed to exploit these opportunities, and money from wartime relief funds was rechannelled in this direction. A circular in 1950 "urged local authorities to do everything in their power to encourage further voluntary effort to meet the needs of old people". Thus, in this field there was a clear division of labour on the "extension ladder" model:

Central government would be responsible for pensions and supplementary pensions, local authorities would develop residential care, the NHS would offer medical services. Voluntary organizations would be expected to develop visiting schemes and other services for those in hospital and residential care as well as a wide range of domiciliary services for those people who remained in their own homes, especially where they were lonely and isolated. (Means & Smith 1985)

Owen (1964) describes many of the voluntary organizations providing services for the elderly at this time as only quasi-voluntary, in that they were in effect acting as agents for the state. There were some fields, for example services for people with visual or hearing impairments, where charities were getting 100 per cent of their funds from this source (Younghusband 1978). Voluntary activity in these fields was very much along traditional lines and government was in the driving seat. As such, even where the voluntary sector continued to operate as a major provider, it was vulnerable to takeover by the state, once government attention moved on from the major challenges of health and education to conquer new areas of provision (see below). In child care Younghusband (1978) reports that the traditional charities were becoming less and less competitive as local authorities gained experience.

Brenton (1985) asks why the voluntary sector did not take the opportunity to establish social care in particular as their distinctive territory. In the case of elderly care, one reason may have been the refusal of the major organizations involved to co-operate with each other (Means & Smith 1985). Another, for the longer established charities, may have been the struggle to come to terms with the new era and its implications for their activities.

Brenton suggests that to have established themselves as major providers in this sphere voluntary organizations would have required a much greater investment from the state. On the other hand, she argues that the state's failure to provide this support may have been a blessing in disguise. She compares the voluntary sector in the UK favourably with that in other countries where, she feels, the sector has become institutionalized into the establishment as an agent of the state. She argues that the relative neglect by the UK government of the voluntary sector and its determination to invest in public sector provision left voluntary organizations to their own devices. This neglect allowed them to develop a host of new independent roles as watchdogs on state provision and providers of complementary services, thus ensuring "a continuing vitality and independence for the voluntary sector which it might otherwise have lost" (Brenton 1985)

But some commentators who see the voluntary sector in this post-war period as "a dull place, staffed for the most part by people who could not obtain jobs in other sectors" (Knight 1993) overlook a great deal. The very expansion of state welfare created new tasks to be performed, and as the territory occupied by the state grew so did the periphery into which voluntary activity could flow. Indeed, this "moribund" era saw the birth of a whole new range of organizations as well as the strengthening of some whose origins lay in the war years. Apart from the providers already discussed, these included the following now well established organizations formed between the beginning of the war and 1959:

- specialist support for disabled people and self-help networks: the Leonard Cheshire Foundation, the Spastics Society (now Scope), Arthritis Care, the British Epilepsy Association, Mencap, the National Association for Mental Health (later MIND), the Multiple Sclerosis Society, the Muscular Dystrophy Association;
- medical research and promotion: the British Heart Foundation, the National Childbirth Trust, the Mental Health Foundation, the Leukaemia Research Fund;
- environmental organizations: the British Trust for Conservation Volunteers, the World Wildlife Fund, the Civic Trust, the Noise Abatement Society;
- aid for developing countries: Christian Aid, Voluntary Service Overseas, War on Want, the World University Service;
- campaigns: the Anti-Apartheid movement, the Consumers' Association, the Campaign for Nuclear Disarmament;
- umbrella organizations: the National Federation of Community Organizations, the Councils for Voluntary Service;
- advice and counselling: the Albany Trust, the Samaritans, CRUSE, the Marriage Guidance Council and its Catholic and Jewish equivalents.

The spread of the state into new areas provided ready work for advice organizations. The growth of the public sector provided the citizens' advice bureaux, which had been set up just before the war, with a continuing *raison d'être*. In Beveridge's terms, they were explaining public authority to the citizen; helping to protect the citizen against public authority and giving people a sense that there is a helping hand out there. He also saw an important role for the voluntary sector in political education: "Democracy, if it wishes to survive cannot afford to be ignorant" (Beveridge 1948).

Other organizations were freed to broach new frontiers. The King's Fund, for example, released from the need to support basic hospital costs, could move into new arenas, such as training, convalescent provision, dietary matters, experimental schemes (Prochaska 1992). And the more traditional organizations were forced to reassess their roles: a process that began to bear fruit towards the end of the 1950s as they began to break away from conventional provision.

A military retreat is not always surrender. It may be an opportunity to marshal resources in order to advance again. There is a sense in which the retreat of the voluntary sector in the immediate post-war period was a retreat of this kind. Certainly this reassessment was to bear fruit in the years to come:

> Paradoxically, voluntary action was being broadened, sharpened, and enlivened by the very nationalization of welfare that voluntarists had so long opposed. State social reform precipitated change within charitable bodies themselves, bringing many of them into tune with modern conditions. Moreover, state provision was egalitarian and materialistic; it tended to erode those hierarchical values and religious pieties that had brought charity into disrepute in the past. (Prochaska 1992)

In the 1950s, Conservative governments, more sympathetic to charity, had replaced the post-war Labour government and while the growing public sector, its administrators and professionals, were clearly in the driving seat, the continuing relevance of the sector as a "junior partner" was increasingly acknowledged. Indeed, its importance was officially underlined by a new Charities Act that received royal assent in 1960, following the report of the Nathan Committee (Cmd 8710). This Act, the first legislation on charities since the previous century, cleared a lot of dead wood and for the first time extended the power of the Charity Commission beyond endowments. In the early 1960s, the setting up of the Housing Corporation to channel funds to housing associations was further evidence of a growing acceptance by government that the voluntary sector had a valid role to play.

New roles

By the 1960s it was becoming clear that the welfare state was not the answer to all ills and that persistent problems of poverty remained. As the first generation of children raised under the umbrella of the welfare state came to adulthood in the 1960s, new life was breathed into the voluntary sector. New actors and organizations made their voice heard, inspired by the civil rights and feminist movements as well as the air of revolution in Europe and the "spirit of 1968". Over the years they included: Des Wilson of Shelter, campaigning on behalf of the homeless; Ruth Lister of the Child Poverty Action Group; Erin Pizzey of Chiswick Women's Aid; Frank Field of the Child Poverty Action Group and a host of environmentalists.

Initially these voices came mainly from the educated middle classes. They were joined by an army of crusading volunteers, again mainly educated middle class young people, mobilized at home and abroad by organizations like Voluntary Service Overseas, Community Service Volunteers, the Young Volunteer Force Foundation (set up by government) and the Task Forces in London. This move of the middle classes into working class areas, which intensified with the spread of community development, had many echoes of the settlement movement of the previous century. Indeed, settlements themselves were to enjoy a new lease of life with the rise of community based action. The British Association of Settlements and Social Action Centres was launched at the beginning of the 1970s. There were also new or growing needs to be met: the provision of hostels for homeless single people, support for drug users, support for single parent families, terminal care for cancer patients were among those areas where the voluntary sector became a primary source of assistance.

Meanwhile the post-war expansion of voluntary activity in domiciliary care was running out of steam. It was not so easy to get volunteers and voluntary organizations in this field were increasingly going for the easier options of outings and recreation, leaving domiciliary services for the more needy to the public sector. The public sector was colonizing this particular outpost of voluntary activity with the extension of local authority powers in 1968 and the creation of generic social services departments in local authorities in 1971. While the WVS carried on with a lower profile, the National Old People's Welfare Committee broke free of its ties to the National Council for Voluntary Service and, under the new name of Age Concern, followed the example set by the campaigns of the 1960s into the arenas of advocacy and public education.

With the start of the 1970s, the new campaigning spirit spread to other traditional service-providing organizations which, by now, were coming to terms with their new environment. Children's charities that had struggled to come to terms with the new era began to pioneer new specialist and non-

residential services as the state moved to centre stage on income maintenance and social case work. The National Association for Mental Health renamed itself and, as MIND, moved into information and campaigning work.

Sometimes traditional organizations had to die to give way to the newer
generation. Thus, in the late 1960s government had transferred prison welfare and aftercare to the public probation service and out of the demise of
the National Discharged Prisoners' Aid Society rose the National Association for the Care and Resettlement of Offenders: "an outstanding example
of the new voluntary organizations started in the 1960s which could look
questioningly at the present and future, unfettered by past assumptions"
(Younghusband 1978).

Thus:

> The service delivery function of the traditional voluntary body was
> sustained, supplementing public sector provision, but the real devel-
> opment in the voluntary sector came with the emergence of func-
> tions unique to it – those of mutual aid, the provision of information
> and advice and the critical pressure group function. (Brenton 1985)

Younghusband (1978) reports that the post-war difficulties in recruitment
were being overcome with increasing professionalization within the sector
and the new image created by the 1960s generation of organizations. In the
1970s voluntary organizations became "sources of information, centres of
excellence and means of responsible pressure" (Younghusband 1978). This
complementary role was reinforced by the Seebohm report which underlined the importance of voluntary activity but not as a major provider. Any
shift in the balance of provision could "present problems to the local authority which may be led to neglect its own responsibilities and to the voluntary
organization which may be prevented from developing its critical and pio-
neering role" (Cmnd 3703). The relationship between the sectors began to
look less like an extension ladder, and more like a mirror.

The campaigns of the 1960s gave voluntary activity a new respectability
on the left of the political spectrum and established the political education
role that Beveridge had foreseen for it. Spurred by racial tension in the inner
cities at home and by the War on Poverty in the United States, government
itself took a hand in encouraging this new wave of activity. Early initiatives
were the Educational Priority Areas and the National Community Development Programme, set up in emulation of the War on Poverty. The latter in
particular offered support and resources to local voluntary and community

action in a limited number of areas, while the Urban Programme provided resources across a wider base which were to support a much broader range of local activity over a much longer period. A DHSS grant to the Pre-School Play Association in the late 1960s doubled its income and helped it to "spread like wildfire" (Younghusband 1978). Other opportunities for voluntary and community action were provided by a new interest in participation following the Skeffington report on participation in planning (1969) and the Seebohm report on the personal social services (1968). Younghusband (1978) claims that by the 1970s, "practically all voluntary organizations of standing in the social services were grant-aided from public funds".

Encouraged in part by these government initiatives, a third wave of activity developed in the sector: this time involving service users and disadvantaged communities themselves. In a sense the co-operative traditions that had been downplayed by the post-war Labour government were re-emerging, though in different forms. Tenants and claimants were among the first public service users to join together and make their voice heard: in the former case protesting about rising rents and insensitive redevelopment plans or seeking better facilities for children on public housing estates; in the second, setting up welfare rights centres to improve benefit uptake. Later in the decade, women's organizations put play and child care back onto the agenda along with health; and the focus of community organization began to shift from predominantly white tenants' or community-wide organizations to more diverse groupings organized around ethnic or gender identities campaigning for equal rights and against institutionalized discrimination (Thomas 1983, Taylor 1992b).

Central and local governments took steps to create a dialogue with new local organizations. The language of partnership and participation spread across the public sector and investment in community development and voluntary organizations began to rise. While the creation of new social services departments in 1971 had brought more functions into the competence of local government, it also encouraged them to explore and co-ordinate with community resources, as did the earlier Seebohm report, often through employing community development workers. By 1975, there were an estimated 276 full-time community workers in social services departments in England and Wales (Thomas 1983). In Scotland, community development was boosted through a different route, that of community education, with the publication of the Alexander Report on Adult Education in 1975.

Younghusband (1978) argues that the local government reorganization that took place in 1974 forced a reorganization, too, of the voluntary sector's local infrastructure, which provided a range of services to frontline voluntary organizations at local level. More sophisticated and better staffed intermediary bodies were needed to cover larger local authorities and these authorities were able to put funds into their development. The importance of local councils for voluntary service and other local intermediary bodies was to be a major theme of the Wolfenden report later in the decade (Wolfenden 1978).

The importance of the voluntary sector was recognized by central government in the appointment of a co-ordinating junior Minister with special responsibility for the voluntary sector in 1972, followed by the setting up of the Voluntary Services Unit in the Home Office in 1973, with limited powers but with responsibility for co-ordinating central government relationships with the voluntary sector. In the same year funds were put into setting up a Volunteer Centre to promote volunteering nationally, whether within voluntary or statutory organizations. The experience of the National Community Development Programme was not proving a comfortable one for the government: the projects it had set up became a thorn in the Home Office side as community development workers turned into major critics of government policy (Loney 1983). Instead, less high profile short-term initiatives were developed that put resources into community projects.

Government was not the only source of support for the sector. Business too was beginning to show an interest in the community with the formation of the Action Resource Centre to promote business secondments to the sector in 1973 and REACH which put retired business executives in touch with voluntary organizations in 1976. These would be followed in the early 1980s by Business in the Community and a rise in corporate giving as business was exhorted by government to exercise corporate citizenship.

Transition

During the 1970s the economy faltered and the unemployment rate began to rise. Community organizations began to find it more difficult to squeeze significant concessions out of government and found themselves fighting against "public expenditure cuts" and for the Right to Work. One of central government's early responses to the changing economic picture was to prove surprisingly beneficial to the voluntary sector in the short term, although a source of great heartsearching (Addy & Scott 1988). The special employment programmes began with a small Community Industry initiative in 1972, but it was the Job Creation Programme of the mid 1970s that provided

227

voluntary organizations with central government funding to employ people on projects of community benefit for a year. For many small and new organizations (including minority ethnic groups who had very little support until this time) it was their first opportunity to get significant funding and they used the money to appoint staff or to build community premises as a training enterprise.

Over the years from the mid 1970s to the late 1980s, the special employment schemes underwent several metamorphoses. The goals of the initiatives were redefined and the goalposts moved until they became less and less attractive to voluntary and community organizations. They were in any case a mixed blessing. Those organizations who took the money sometimes found themselves with more staff than they knew how to handle, while the logic of the schemes meant that organizations set up for social welfare or community purposes found themselves turning into employment and training agencies. There was considerable criticism from local organizations of fellow organizations who had "sold out" to government paymasters and of national organizations that parachuted into local areas without concern for existing local networks on the basis of funds from this source. It was an experience that still has lessons in the policy environment of today.

If it had been clear by the 1960s that the welfare state was not delivering on all the expectations it had raised, by the end of the 1970s a much deeper disillusionment had set in: "Like philanthropy, government had made a massive contribution to reducing human misery, but it had failed to live up to expectations" (Prochaska 1992). Now the argument was that it was not capable of delivering. One factor in this disillusionment was the economic recession. The conditions that the Labour government had accepted as the price of getting out of economic difficulty had alienated many of its traditional supporters, including the public sector unions. But the welfare state also contained the seeds of its own destruction. As standards began to rise, people began to take what they had for granted and to expect more. Public provision was criticized for becoming too complacent, catering for the providers and professionals rather than the consumers, geared to the lowest common denominator rather than quality services. Critics from the "New Right" focused on the dependency created by public welfare, arguing that it had taken away people's willingness to accept responsibility for themselves and their neighbours. They argued that public services sucked in money with no incentive for efficiency and championed the market as the mechanism best equipped to control welfare expenditure and offer choice (Taylor 1992a, Taylor & Lansley 1992).

Key figures in the voluntary sector were also arguing for change. In 1978, the Wolfenden Report, *The future of voluntary organizations*, funded by two major charitable trusts argued for a greater role for voluntary organizations, an argument that was developed by two of its contributors (Hadley & Hatch 1981). From the National Council of Voluntary Organizations (NCVO) came a call for a "preference-guided society" (Gladstone 1979) where government, in the interests of equity and social justice, would retain a major responsibility for financing welfare but the voluntary sector, which NCVO saw as more sensitive to consumer need, would take over much of the delivery. The "welfare pluralists", as they were known, differed quite fundamentally from the "New Right". They still saw a major role for government in the financing of welfare and they also stressed the importance of political pluralism: they did not see voluntary organizations merely as alternative service providers. Nonetheless, critics were scornful of their failure to consider how a major transfer of funds to the voluntary sector could be effected in a climate of increasing restraint on public expenditure (Brenton 1985).

In many ways, Wolfenden reflected the trends of the 1970s rather than anticipating the 1980s. Government funding to the voluntary sector was on the increase and this chapter has already indicated the ways in which many government departments and local authorities were already encouraging voluntary and community action. But in the event, the report's recommendations were rapidly overtaken by the election of a new Conservative government that had much sympathy for the more radical analysis from the "New Right".

The major planks of the new government's agenda were to give priority to the creation of wealth, to take service delivery away from the state and to encourage the individual, the family and the community to take more responsibility for welfare through informal support and voluntary action. It called for a return to Victorian values and for an "active citizenship": "Those who succeed have obligations above and beyond that of celebrating their own success . . . The responsible individual does not believe that his involvement with others is limited to paying taxes and that's an end to the matter" (Baker 1988). This government saw a central role for the voluntary and informal sectors, for the volunteer and for charitable giving and, on the face of it, also promised to fulfil the aspirations of the welfare pluralists.

In fact, for the first two terms of the Conservative government, policy change was at the level of rhetoric rather than action: although policies to sell council housing, to begin to restrict the powers of government and to limit benefit eligibility were put into motion at this time, as well as the first wave of privatizations.

But the impact of a change in climate was in many ways beneficial to the sector, for it was in the 1980s that "government became the largest single contributor to charitable causes in Britain" (Prochaska 1992). Central and local government funding to the sector doubled in real terms between 1979 and 1987, fuelled particularly by a continued expansion of special employment programmes and the expansion of funding for the housing associations that government wished to see take over from local authorities as the major providers of social housing. Smaller initiatives, like Opportunities for Volunteering and a number of self-help initiatives funded by the Department of Health, joined the special employment schemes as important lifelines for community based organizations as well as encouraging partnership between larger charities and the state.

Local authorities themselves were significant funders of voluntary action. In the metropolitan authorities, which were high spenders on the voluntary sector, many administrations remained in Labour hands and local voluntary organizations found themselves the beneficiaries of the battle between central and local government for the allegiance of the electorate. Metropolitan local authorities were among those funding a different kind of citizenship to that of central government, based on political education and equal opportunities for groups who had long been vulnerable to discrimination. Groups organized around race and gender were joined late in the 1980s by organizations of disabled people, which challenged the disempowering practices of traditional voluntary organizations as well as public sector providers.

Agency

With the third term of Thatcherism the rhetoric of change began to turn into reality. Legislation was introduced to transfer service delivery to the voluntary and private sectors. In some areas compulsory competitive tendering was introduced while, in others, local authorities were first encouraged, and then instructed, to purchase services from voluntary and commercial agencies. The aim was to increase efficiency but also to give more choice to the service user. Local and health authorities were also required to consult with both voluntary sector providers and service users in the planning of services, particularly community care.

For some organizations the new regime offers opportunities. Requirements that local and health authorities consult over a variety of services have given voluntary, community and user organizations more say in service planning. Closer attention to efficiency and good management has encouraged many more organizations to put their operations on a firmer footing. The increasing emphasis on the consumer may also give a higher profile to advocacy services and organizations of service users who gained in number and confidence during the 1980s. For those providing mainstream services, the move to contracts is a chance to clarify and strengthen funding arrangements with government.

But voluntary organizations are not the only players in the new pluralism. The move towards a mixed economy of welfare has created new competitors: private care firms, floated off public services that are now reforming as "not-for-profits" and NHS trusts are in the market for service delivery paid for by the state. With the current emphasis on targeting, private insurance may offer more security for those with enough money to provide for their future care. The introduction of market principles has brought a more competitive ethos into the sector. It is arguable that a sector that lies midway between the market and the state will fare no better in an unbridled market than it did when the state reigned supreme. Certainly, it will be difficult for small organizations to survive in such an environment.

Meanwhile there are fears that funds for anything other than contracted-out services will become increasingly scarce. Local government in particular has been under ever increasing financial restraint, while central government has begun to cut back on programmes of crucial importance to the voluntary sector: most notably the Urban Programme, withdrawn nearly twenty-five years after its introduction. Both central and local government are specifying more closely what they are prepared to fund, and the balance between fees and grants at local authority level is shifting in favour of the former (Taylor et al. 1993, Mabbott 1993).

Some of these problems could be eased if organizations in the sector were prepared to support each other: to create consortia to bid for contracts or to pool fundraising efforts, for example. Larger organizations could consider supporting smaller organizations through subcontracting or sharing expertise. But the competitiveness that comes with the market may run counter to either development.

Ironically, just as the strong network of intermediary bodies is most needed to provide co-ordination and support, their funding is most at risk. Secondary services are not a priority for hardpressed local authorities and, in an individualistic contract culture, support services are increasingly likely to be spot purchased rather than paid for out of a dwindling grant aid budget. The move to unitary local authorities and the reassessment that this involves could leave them and many other voluntary organizations out in the cold (Taylor et al. 1993).

Another theme of the third term Conservative government was "value for money": a drive for economy, efficiency and effectiveness which began earlier in the 1980s in the public sector and came to voluntary organizations through public sector funding. Tolerance of amateurism in the sector was on the wane, although from a government that believed essentially in the "voluntarism" of the sector, there was rather less enthusiasm for an investment in the core funding, management and infrastructure that more professional approaches to management imply.

During the 1980s, there were two "efficiency scrutinies" that affected the sector, the first into the supervision of charities (Woodfield 1987), the second into government funding for the sector (Home Office 1990). While the second endorsed the importance of core funding and investment in the infrastructure, this was not reflected in the Minister's response, which emphasized instead the need for government-funded voluntary organizations to adhere to "accepted" values and to government agendas. This was a quite different message from that communicated by Seebohm in the 1960s. And government has been slow to put into effect the recommendations of the report that stressed the need for government to be more efficient in the way it administers funding.

The government emphasis on efficiency and effectiveness is in tune with the concerns of the sector itself. In the late 1980s the NCVO showed its willingness to put its own house in order by setting up a committee on the management and effectiveness of voluntary organizations. It also lobbied for legislation to implement the recommendations of the Woodfield scrutiny on charities (NCVO 1991). But with the move towards purchase of service, the management services that have been provided by local intermediary bodies are at risk. The Woodfield report eventually led to charity law reform. The Charities Commission had already begun to streamline its administration and in 1992 a new Charity Law squeezed onto the statute book, just ahead of the general election, with an emphasis on improving supervision of charities, giving the Charity Commission more powers and placing new controls on fundraising.

Fundraising had indeed become big business in the 1980s, with the introduction of television appeals and the growth of professional fundraising. But even in this market, charities had powerful competitors. At the beginning of the period under study, fundraising for the NHS, while not proscribed, was frowned upon. Now both hospitals and schools were actively encouraged to raise funds from the public, to the concern of the charities world. One of the most successful appeals of the 1980s was the Great Ormond Street appeal for a National Health Service children's hospital.

And more was being expected of the sector. With the introduction of the Social Fund and restrictions on benefits, for example, people in need were turned away from statutory agencies and told to go to charities or back to their families for support. The boundaries between state and individual responsibility were being redefined.

Voluntary organizations needed to look to other sources of funding. One was trading; sales of goods, related and unrelated to their main mission. But the more voluntary organizations move into trading the more questions are being asked about their charitable and tax exempt status. High street shops are complaining about the competition from charity "thrift shops". As contracting out is extended, private care firms are beginning to ask why they should be competing at a disadvantage.

Donations and volunteering have generally held up over time with a surge in interest from the commercial sector in recent years, although this has been hit by recession. But despite the professionalization of fundraising, there is little to suggest that the average household is giving more now than it did since surveys began in the early 1980s. Indeed, the bumper media appeals of recent years may have already passed their peak. They are raising less now than in the boom years of the late 1980s. And charitable trusts and foundations are a drop in the ocean of the total amounts needed to resource the sector. In all three respects, the UK lags far behind the US, whose policies we seek to emulate. Meanwhile the introduction of the national lottery in 1994, while providing some new money, is seen by some to threaten more traditional forms of individual giving.

Fees remain the principal source of funds and the government a major donor. It is difficult to see how government can withdraw from this central role, although it is tying its giving more and more to the purchase of specified services. The Urban Programme, an important source of funds for local voluntary action, has been withdrawn and employment and training funds are a much less significant source of funds to the sector since the tightening up of the Employment Training Programme in 1988 and the introduction of Training and Enterprise Councils.

Empowerment

What has this history meant for the people at the receiving end of welfare services? One of the remarkable trends of the past 30 years has been the emergence of community and user based activity, revitalizing the mutual aid tradition that was so strong in the working class organizations of the nineteenth century and in the co-operative traditions of the Labour movement. The paternalism of charity, which so disgusted the post-war Labour government, may still be true of some organizations within the sector but has been turned on its head by organizations fighting for their right to speak for themselves, gaining confidence and resources through mutual support and defining their own agendas for change. Their cause has gained strength from the current emphasis on the consumer, although it bears little relationship to the individualist ideology in which this is embedded. But the move to deliver services through voluntary organizations will not of itself bring services closer to the consumer, despite the belief that voluntary organizations are closer to the community. Many voluntary organizations themselves still have some way to go in achieving equal opportunities and user-centred services. And, as smaller and newer organizations, community and user based organizations are poorly equipped to compete in the "contract" or fundraising markets.

Gender

Women have always been central to the voluntary sector. For many years deprived of opportunities on the labour market, the voluntary sector provided them with the opportunity to realize at least some of their aspirations, although men still tended to occupy the positions of most power. To this day, women remain more likely to volunteer than men (Lynn & Davis Smith 1991). The developments of the past 50 years have given more prominence both to women's issues and to women themselves in the sector. The fight for women's equality has been carried though the voluntary sector in organizations seeking more control for women over their health, more representation in parliament, better working conditions, access to child care, protection from domestic violence and from crime.

It has been a struggle to bring women's issues to the top of the agenda. Membership of the traditional women's organizations has been falling for some time, although they have often played an important campaigning role.

In the 1970s, the agenda for community development was often set by men, who retained the official leadership of community organizations even when most of the membership was female:

> Towards the end of the 1970s, many workers were questioning how far they were in fact encouraging women to realise their potential contribution. Feminists criticised the tendency of community workers to focus on issues . . . such as housing and planning, and ignoring issues like play, child care and community care that women in the community identified as priorities and were keen to act upon. (Taylor 1983)

The introduction of women's units in a number of local authorities in the 1970s and 1980s provided support for a wide range of women's activities at local level. But, with the increasing financial pressure on local government, most of these have since closed. One of the most difficult battles to fight has been the belief that the battle for equality is now won.

Nowadays, as government seeks to put the burden of care back into the community, through informal caring, voluntary organizations and private care firms, it is inevitable that women will be the major providers of that care, whether paid or unpaid. For its part, the voluntary sector will have its work cut out to maintain proper compensation and adequate support for women in this role.

Race

As recently as 1978, the Wolfenden report was still talking of voluntary organizations for immigrants, a language that was out of date as soon as it was written. Action on racism, crime and policing and demand for a redistribution of resources to black-managed organizations has put other voluntary organizations on the spot. There are now black-managed organizations in many fields, although mostly at local level. Funds have been earmarked for black organizations under a number of government programmes, including the shortlived fund for local development agencies where black groups were particularly poorly represented. The creation of Race and Equal Opportunities Units in local authorities also released funds for black and minority ethnic groups. And a national management development resource, originally set up under the umbrella of NCVO, became independent in 1991 as Sia.

But it has not been easy for black communities to organize. Community leaders have faced impossible demands both from within the community and from those outside who wish to be seen to consult with black organizations. It has been hard to make the white establishment understand the diversity of the minority ethnic population in the UK, let alone the need for different ethnic groups to organize separately. And the 1980s black voluntary sector experienced the recruitment problems faced by the rest of the sector in the 1950s, as equal opportunities policies opened up promising new opportunities in local government. It has also been difficult for black-managed organizations to make any significant impact on the distribution of resources, especially as predominantly white mainstream organizations have themselves moved to establish their credibility in the equal opportunities arena. The myth that black organizations cannot manage has been hard to shake off. Mistakes, inexperience or conflicts common to many young organizations have come under a much harsher spotlight here than elsewhere in the sector. And current financial restraints are likely to hit the black voluntary sector hard as it contains many of the smaller, newer organizations that are most at risk under current policies. Many are not equipped to bid for substantial contracts and the loss of the Metropolitan Counties, particularly the Greater London Council and the Inner London Education Authority, the closure of Equal Opportunities Units and, more recently, the loss of the Urban Programme have hit particularly hard.

Disability

The voluntary sector has always been a major supplier of services for disabled people, as the "deserving poor". This remained the case after the introduction of the welfare state: specialist charities had the expertise and the infrastructure to provide services for what were almost always minority groups in any one local authority area.

But the specialist charities were always run for – rather than by – disabled people: and in the late 1980s, building on the example of other civil rights campaigns, disabled people began to set up organizations under their own control that challenged the monopoly of the traditional organizations. They also challenged the images of disabled people associated with charitable fundraising, protesting against the increasingly popular television appeals. And they challenged the discrimination that disabled people experience in the UK.

Disabled people's organizations have the same obstacles to overcome as do women's and minority ethnic groups, but some progress has been made. Traditional organizations have been prompted to involve their users more centrally in management; public authorities, caught between the impetus to consumerism from a government keen to encourage business models and the demands of an increasingly militant disability movement, have made some concessions to more user-centred services. Funds are being made available for advocacy services and the duty to consult service users in the formulation of community care plans has given user organizations more status, despite the fact that government's concept of consumerism is essentially concerned with individuals. Campaigns are less likely to portray disabled people as helpless. There is a long way to go, and it is easy to see achievements slip away, especially when economy and efficiency are the benchmarks of good service management. However, it does seem that this is a part of the voluntary sector that is growing.

The future

The 50 years covered in this chapter have seen the voluntary sector move from a position where it was perceived by many as outdated, through a period of expansion into a wide range of new areas and roles complementary to mainstream provision, to a position in the 1990s where it is expected to be a principal provider of welfare either as an agent of the state or out of its own resources.

To extend the imagery of the Webbs, the sector moved from a period after the introduction of the welfare state when it was a rather flimsy extension ladder, to a period when it was a mirror held up to the state. To adopt another metaphor, this was also a period when the state and the voluntary sector operated not as parallel bars but maybe more as concentric circles, with mainstream state provision supported by the activities of voluntary organizations. Now the sector is moving again to a new era when it is expected to be an arm of the state, delivering services under the specifications of central government and regulated by it. For many, this new direction feels as much of a break with the past as the coming of the welfare state must have seemed to the voluntary sector of that time.

The past 50 years have demonstrated the resilience of the voluntary sector and its ability to adapt and play a role whatever the prevailing winds. What shape, then, will the sector be in as we go into the twenty-first century?

For those who become arms of the state, the challenges of this new environment are to become competitive with other suppliers in a new welfare market. But voluntary organizations competing with commercial organizations to operate to a government agenda are likely to adopt more of the characteristics of their public and private sector counterparts. They are likely to face increasing difficulty in justifying their tax-exempt status or maintaining distinctive values that come from their voluntary sector roots; especially if, operating in a market, they are also forced to draw more money in fees from clients. Will there be any point in continuing to call them voluntary organizations?

Those who wish to keep a part of them that is their own will need to adapt to an increasingly competitive fundraising market. This too will place a premium on business skills and marketing. These skills may be admirable as means, but, if they become ends in themselves, they may cause potential donors and volunteers to become disillusioned with the whole notion of charity. A move into the sale of goods as a fundraising device is murky territory as far as charitable status and fair competition is concerned and may lead to a similar loss of trust on the part of donors and volunteers.

For others, the challenge will simply be to survive. People will continue to come together to address their common needs and, if there are no resources from elsewhere, they will draw on their own energies and commitment. But community and user-based organizations have limited resources and, in an increasingly polarized society, they will be making demands on people who are struggling to survive in their everyday life.

Grant aid to these groups has allowed them to set their own agendas and become less dependent on the goodwill of others. Mutuality has been as important as charity in recent years for many people. If grant aid diminishes and welfare again becomes dependent on the donations of time and money of those who can afford it, there is a danger that the voluntary sector will again become the province of the better off in society, with those who have less power dependent on their patronage and goodwill. If so, the hard road to empowerment trodden over recent years will come to nothing. As Frank Prochaska (1992) argues: "If charities were less snobbish and socially divisive than many had been in the 1930s, it was in part because of the rise of the Welfare State, which engendered egalitarian social aspirations".

The experience of the past 50 years has demonstrated the fundamental interdependence between the state and the voluntary sector. But if the sector is to continue as a plural and diverse force in society, it is likely that government is going to have to take a hand, not only as a purchaser of services but as an investor in a sphere of action that releases enormous energies into welfare. This is not to argue against the right of government to specify what it is prepared to fund and to require good management and careful monitoring of those activities in which it invests. But it is to require that government sees itself as having a role in the development of the sector as a vehicle for political as well as service pluralism.

Is this an impossible dream? It would be glorifying the past to suggest that the regime of the 1970s and early 1980s was in any way ideal. There was probably as much bad management, waste and paternalism on both sides of the relationship as in any other era. But what the experience of that time does illustrate is that it is possible for a relationship between government and the voluntary sector to develop where government is prepared to support the sector without needing to control it, and where the sector can act as a mirror to the state as well as its delivery arm.

What is needed for the future, therefore, is a pluralist approach to funding, which supports the sector as pioneer, advocate and campaigner as well as service provider. This requires pluralism in government funding. It requires a continued role for government in promoting an atmosphere in which the private donor is actively encouraged to support a range of activity alongside, rather than instead of, government. It may even require that government itself is plural: the history of the past 50 years suggests that the voluntary sector has fared best when it can diversify its government funding as well as other sources. With the centralization of state power and even the move to unitary government, this is becoming less and less possible.

Suggested reading

Brenton (1985) provides the most thorough account of the development of the voluntary sector up to the early 1980s, analyzing the respective contributions of statutory and voluntary services and arguing for policies that maintain a central role for the State. A more up-to-date overview is provided by Waine (1992).

Wolfenden (1978) is the report of a comprehensive review of the role of the voluntary sector in the social services, laying the basis of the welfare pluralist approach, which is taken further in Gladstone (1979) and Hadley & Hatch (1981).

The edited collection by Ware (1989) sets the current challenges facing charities and charity law in a longer political perspective and goes beyond the relatively well-covered social services field to look at developments in relation to education, overseas aid, medical research and religion.

CHAPTER 10
Markets and the future of welfare

Eamonn Butler

Why change the system?

With forty years' experience of the operation of the post-Beveridge welfare state behind us, there is now a growing belief in the UK that the system as a whole is in need of deep and serious reform.

Increased questioning

Whatever gains it may have brought us, our welfare system is clearly failing to eliminate those giant evils of need, sickness, squalor, ignorance and idleness. Although living standards, housing, and the quality of public education and health might be far better today than Beveridge could dream of, they remain well below what we know is possible.

These advances have been won only at great cost. The UK social security budget is now roughly £80 billion per year, absorbing one third of all public service spending. It is now more than double what it was in 1979 – and is projected to grow much faster than the projected growth in the economy as a whole, reaching £96 billion by the end of the decade, even if unemployment falls and public spending policies remain tight. Politicians do not normally cast doubt on the idea of the welfare state, because too many voters depend on it. But even so, a number of them, left and right, are now openly describing the present system as "financially unsustainable" (Nuki 1993, Field & Owen 1993).

Moreover, social patterns have changed enormously since the 1940s. Can a system that was initiated before the start of the First World War and largely redesigned at the end of the Second really be effective in tackling today's problems?

And today we understand more about the power of incentives. We can well ask whether we might actually be breeding more problems for ourselves. Are we not subsidizing, and so encouraging, the very things we seek to eliminate? By providing money to everyone in disagreeable circumstances, are we simply making such conditions more bearable and so reducing the incentive for self-support? (Howell 1991). Are we tempting people at the margin to adjust their affairs in order to qualify for this support? And is the existence of that option not ethically corrosive: are we encouraging people to shirk their responsibilities, and do we not all know people who are "on the fiddle" (Davies 1993, Pirie 1993b)?

Many of the same incentive questions arise about the delivery of welfare services as well as their take-up. Intuitively, the Beveridge generation supposed that it would be far more efficient to organize our industries centrally: we could end duplication in production, and eliminate the costs of advertising and profit. On top of all this, our central control of the human services such as health and education would allow us to achieve an equality of outcome, so that people's access to essential services could be based on their need, instead of the depth of their pockets.

A few decades' experience of this bold enterprise, however, has revealed the flaws within it. Reluctantly, we are facing the reality that our intuition was wrong. Now we understand the benefits of the profit motive as a spur to better performance; that competition dilutes market power; that having a variety of suppliers and products enables people to choose those particular goods and services that best suit their individual needs; that producers' desire to win and keep customers drives them to innovate and improve.

State industries, by contrast, offered their customers little choice of products, and certainly no escape into the arms of other suppliers. Information about consumer tastes was lost, along with the need to satisfy them. Nationalized industries came to be run more for the convenience of themselves than their customers; operating decisions were made to maximize the political pay-off rather than to use resources efficiently.

State health and education clearly suffered the same problems, although their outright privatization was still unthinkable in the mid 1980s. Thus arose the internal-market reforms, which kept health and education as state services, but unleashed quasi-market forces within them. With those important services well on the way to competition, some policy analysts now wonder whether other human services, such as the assessment and delivery of welfare benefits, pensions and even police services, should be entrusted to single suppliers or whether some measure of variety and quasi-market competition is practicable.

It would have been shocking to ask these questions just a few years ago; but now they are being asked more and more publicly. Nor is it just a short-term panic among ministers trying to grapple with recession and budget deficits; even non-government (or anti-government) bodies such as the Joseph Rowntree Foundation and the Labour Party's Commission on Social Justice have been thinking about these questions too, and thinking about them for the long term (Hills 1993).

Changing the system

So now there is agreement that we should rethink this part of the government apparatus; to look afresh at what the welfare state exists to do, to assess whether its present programmes are actually achieving those objectives, and if not, to devise some better mechanisms to achieve them.

But there is much less agreement about *what sort* of reform would be appropriate. Some say that no enormous structural change is needed, that a little more public spending would cure most of the problems, and that this is affordable.[1] Others believe that the incentive structures of our welfare system are almost wholly perverse and that throwing more money at it will merely amplify the perversity of the outcomes.

Those of us who share the latter beliefs see the problems of the welfare state as being both philosophical and practical. It may be that no solution will be fully satisfactory: certainly, none will work unless it runs with the grain of human nature, and *uses* the power of incentives and of market structures, instead of ignoring or trying to suppress them, as many present-day welfare programmes seek to do.

Philosophical problems

There are several broad strategies that one can adopt in building a state welfare system. Unfortunately none of them is perfect and (as we now know) their side effects can be very perverse and difficult to deal with (Minford 1993).

Universal provision

First, the state can provide essential goods and services to everyone, as it does with health and education. Thus, everyone is assured of at least some access to these services. Indeed, if there is little or no choice of provider, a rough equality of treatment can be imposed. But such monopoly provision kills off the benefits of choice and competition. And most of the output of these state services, by definition, is consumed by the middle class millions rather than the needy few. If a minority of the population were too poor to afford proper food, we would not think of setting up state kitchens to provide a free but nourishing standard menu for us all; so why should we consider providing free state education, or free health care?

Universal benefits

Secondly, we can provide for people's essential needs by paying ourselves universal cash benefits so that everyone can afford at least a range of basic goods and services. We might confine these benefits to people who qualify in some way (just as today all mothers qualify for child benefit); or, if we are being really radical, we might propose paying a general (or "basic income") benefit to everyone, rich and poor.

These universal benefits allow people to purchase the package of goods and services that they (rather than state providers) think best suits their individual needs. But universal benefits also suffer many problems. Again, most of the money is going to people who do not need it. We must impose high levels of taxation if we are to pay for benefits so widely distributed. But the higher the benefits, and the higher the tax to pay for them, the lower is the incentive on people to drag themselves off benefit and into employment: the phenomenon of the poverty trap, or the "why work?" syndrome. But this characterizes much of state welfare today. When we actually look at the taxes people pay and the benefits they receive (the "tax/benefit ratio"), it is clear that the "why work?" question has become bigger and bigger since the 1960s, even during the Thatcher years, although people commonly assumed that benefits were being eroded (Howell 1991).

Negative income tax

A third strategy is to provide benefits (in cash or in kind) only to those who need help, and let the middle classes pay for their own essentials – clothes, food, housing, education, health care and so on. The most thoroughgoing version of this is the "negative income tax", a general benefit that is paid to all those on the lowest incomes, but that tapers off to zero as people's income rises (Omega File 1983). While this tight focus reduces the cost to taxpayers, the loss of benefit when people do try to improve their circumstances is a major disincentive, amounting to a high marginal tax rate on the poor.

Selectivity

A fourth strategy is selectivity, whereby benefits are given on a case-by-case scrutiny. The aim here is to concentrate resources again on the most needy, while denying state support to those who are capable of supporting themselves (wholly or partially) but choose not to because they know they can take advantage of the system. Thus, support is focused while costs are kept down, so incentives remain reasonably positive. But while we might praise charitable bodies for discriminating between beneficiaries on the basis of their apparent motives, it is much harder for state agencies to be so selective – particularly when legislation grants people welfare benefits as of right, regardless of their motives.

Categorization

A fifth suggestion is categorization, in which benefits are restricted to particular groups of people. For example, Beveridge could be fairly sure that when he was helping old people, he was for the most part helping poor people, because most older people were also poor. But with the diverse lifestyles that are common today, such categorization is less and less useful as a means of targeting social benefits.

Any welfare mechanism, in other words, will involve us in an uncomfortable trade-off between objectives, particularly between cost, focus and incentives. So how does the present system work in practice?

Practical problems

When we look at the actual operation of the welfare state in the United Kingdom, these problems can be seen in practical effect.

Poverty trap

Our welfare system imprisons people in squalor, thanks to the poverty trap. People who accept work can find themselves losing a whole raft of social benefits, both cash benefits and in-kind services, making them much worse off as a result. Marginal tax rates of over 100 per cent are hardly part of a market conforming incentive system (Howell 1991).

Complexity

It is complex. Some benefits depend on past National Insurance Contributions; others do not. Some benefits are means tested; others are not. Some are taxed; others are not. Some are cash; others are in kind; some are given as a gift; others as a loan.

Thus, the Department of Social Security administers a truly bewildering array of benefits. The list includes income support, housing benefit, council tax benefit, child benefit, lone-parent benefit, family credit, unemployment benefit, two sorts of retirement pension (and the Christmas bonus), widows' benefit, war pensions, statutory sick pay, sickness benefit, invalidity benefit, severe disablement allowance, maternity benefits, invalid care allowance, disability living and working allowances, the attendance allowance, the social fund, the industrial injuries scheme, and more.

Poor value

Because of its complexity, administrative costs are high. And because of its universality, some of those costs are pointless. Is there not a certain absurdity and inefficiency about a system that takes money out of the pockets of middle class fathers, sends it up to the Benefits Agency, deducts an administrative fee averaging 30p per week, and then pays the residue back to their wives as child benefit?

It was for such reasons that the American economist Milton Friedman once described modern welfare systems as "like throwing dollars at a barn door" in the hope that some will go through the knot-holes. A humorous exaggeration, perhaps: but remember that it costs the Department of Social Security five times as much to pay out a pound's worth of benefit as it costs the Inland Revenue to collect a pound in taxes. Is complexity worth the cost?

Growing cost

And it is a growing cost. Future projections of the cost of the largest state benefit, the retirement pension (which is now costing around £26,000 million) are alarming, with more and more pensioners being supported by a dwindling proportion of working taxpayers. Income support costs another £13,000 million. The cost of unemployment benefit hovers near £8,000 million. Housing benefit stands at about £7,000 million. Child benefit costs nearly £6,000 million. And despite generally improving health, invalidity benefit too is rising to the £6,000 million level.

Politicization

The welfare state is not driven by markets, but by politicians. And political decision-making reflects voting power, not need. Hence the curious persistence of universal benefits, free health and education, and state-run pensions; although they are disguised as programmes to help the poor, their greatest beneficiaries are the middle classes. Since middle class voters far outnumber the rest, why should any politician want it otherwise?

This "public choice" problem explains why the welfare state is so difficult to reform and to rationalize (Yarrow 1993, Buchanan & Tullock 1992, Reisman 1991). Any reform will produce some winners and some losers. But the losers will be vociferous opponents of such reform; while the winners are unlikely to march through the streets in delight. Politicians, naturally enough, opt for the quiet life. However much they recognize the justice of reform, they frequently regard it as "politically impossible".

Inflexibility

In Beveridge's time, women rarely worked, men rarely changed jobs, people normally married and normally worked full time. But today, people change jobs frequently, take voluntary breaks between jobs, often work part instead of full time, work part time in two or more jobs at once, live together without being married, divorce and remarry, have large pensions or savings of their own. In such an age it is often very hard to know who is actually in need of support and who is just taking advantage of it. Is our support really getting to those who need it? Or simply encouraging those who do not?

Moral problems

Because the system is centralized, it is impersonal. The money it disburses is seen as "government" money, so that people regard cheating the system as less wicked than cheating a person, and turn a blind eye to the fiddles of others.

And are we simply subsidizing and so encouraging the things that we are trying to alleviate or reduce? If teenage pregnancies, single parenthood, divorce, unemployment and profligacy are so bad, do we simply increase them by cushioning their effect? And do we meanwhile strangle the opposite values by taxing people who save, people who maintain stable relationships, and people who do everything they can to keep themselves in work?

State provision

Rather than giving people the money they need to manage their own lives, so that they can become effective consumers in the marketplace, a large and costly portion of the welfare state is devoted to actually *providing* services like health and education. And too often, like all monopolists, the state has ended up providing substandard services at above market cost.

If a private business took our cash and then gave us a shoddy service, we would rightly demand our money back. And if we did not get it we would be entitled to sue. But state services have for a long time taken our money, by force, through taxation, and not even told us what services we are entitled to in return. Only now are we starting to demand that specification, and to impose some penalty if the standard is not met, through the Citizen's Charter initiative. At last there are two sides to our contract with government (Cm 1599, Pirie 1991).

But even Charter enthusiasts regard it as only a second-best option. By far the best way to improve value for money in public services is to expose them to the chill wind of competition. A market based welfare system, like a market economy, would aim to capture the benefits of customer choice and competitive supply. It would give people the money (or vouchers) they need to become effective consumers in the marketplace, and allow *them* to make their own decisions about what particular mixture of services would be best for them.

Outline solutions

What, then, are the principles that would guide us to market-conforming reforms of the system? Let us start with the cash benefits.

Empowering self-provision

A welfare system is supposed to redistribute resources from those who are healthy, young and in work, to those who are sick, elderly or unemployed. But our own welfare state handles the problem as if these groups were *different* people, and separates them by a state bureaucracy that administers the money. In fact most of that money, three quarters of the national insurance budget according to John Hills (1993) and others (Falkingham et al. 1993), has nothing to do with welfare redistribution at all. It is simply a lifetime transfer, taken from and made to the same individuals at different points in their lives. In other words, the state is one quarter welfare agency, three quarters savings bank. And because its clients have no choice about how much they will deposit or what rate of return they will receive on their investments, it is not a bank that offers very good terms.

Individual funding

A market orientated welfare system, by contrast, would return those deposits to the control of the customers themselves. It would *empower* people to *save* when they are young, healthy and in work; so that they can *provide* for themselves when they are old, infirm or unemployed.

One way to do this would be to replace much of the existing state benefit structure with a system of personal pension and income replacement funds. People would be expected to contribute into these funds when they could; and they would be entitled to draw benefits from them when necessary.

Such funds could be offered by private-sector bodies, including insurers and friendly societies, and would work along proper insurance and savings principles. The role of the state would be as a welfare agent, topping up the funds of those whose own funds were inadequate to their needs; or paying the premiums of those who for one reason or another could not contribute themselves; or even managing the application of the benefits on behalf of those who were unable to take charge of their own affairs.

Otherwise, there need be no state bureaucracy. People would choose their own fund providers, and competition would tend to bid up the quality and efficiency of that provision. There should be no fraud, because there is no point in cheating your own fund. People would not have to accept off-the-peg welfare any longer: they could select from a variety of plans which, as long as they provided an acceptable minimum of cover, could provide flexible benefits tailored to suit the individual's own lifestyle and preferences.

Welfare and insurance

In any reform of social security, most of what we have to solve is this enormous insurance and savings programme, benefiting primarily the middle classes, but disguised as state welfare. But the fact that most people are perfectly capable of seeing themselves through bad times as well as good, drawing on savings and insurances of their own, suggests that if we sweep away the disincentives of the present system, most of the remainder could do exactly the same.

Yet there will always be people whose needs are correctly categorized as welfare needs, including people who will never be able to provide for themselves. What of them?

Put briefly, *welfare* provides benefits based on needs, regardless of contributions; while *insurance* provides benefits based on contributions, regardless of need. But our welfare state tries to combine the two, resulting in bad welfare and bad insurance (Ferrara 1982).

Some benefits (such as income support or support for the mentally or physically handicapped) are installed principally for welfare motives and operate on welfare principles. Others (such as unemployment and disability benefit) cover inherently insurable risks, and are linked (though not always perfectly) to past contributions. A few (such as the retirement pension) were originally designed along welfare principles (since old people were almost always poor people), although in this case as with most benefits (including the health service) welfare and insurance concepts are combined in the same programme. These two objectives, however, are always in fundamental conflict, and the result is often both bad welfare and bad insurance.

Of course, politicians have much to gain from preserving this confusion. Insurance programmes that benefit their own middle class voters can be sneaked through under the guise of welfare. So any reform is difficult politically. But if we were trying to design a market based welfare state afresh, we would surely try to separate out the welfare and insurance principles: running insurance programmes competitively, along insurance lines; with welfare payments going directly from the state to those who needed them.

Mechanics of reform

As a practical project, then, the reform of the welfare state in order to capture the power of market principles is no easy matter. A radical overhaul might well rationalize the system and lead to a clearly fairer and more efficient outcome; but the piecemeal and reactive way that political decisions are made, in particular the public choice problem, makes it unlikely that any comprehensive reform can be achieved in one jump.

To some extent Norman Fowler, when Secretary of State for Health and Social Security, discovered this with his own radical review of social security spending in the early 1980s. Through the introduction of income support and family credit he made positive moves towards a workable and high incentive negative income tax scheme. But he did much less well at subsuming other benefits within this overall approach: the complaints of the potential losers were too loud for him to endure. And so the system remains something of a patchwork quilt, with holes in some places and over-thick coverage in others.

It seems likely, therefore, that any change will come from the reform (and possibly quite radical reform) of individual programmes rather than the imposition of any "big idea". It could well be a systematic programme, with a vision at the end of it; but the most successful strategy is likely to be one that works through the welfare state, programme by programme, and builds up a comprehensive reform out of small and practical changes (Lilley 1993).

Savings programmes

If we are to be systematic in reviewing the options, it seems sensible to start with the largest programmes.

The basic state pension

With ten million beneficiaries receiving pensions, and almost the whole of the employed workforce contributing towards them, the basic pension is the largest of the cash benefits offered under the welfare state. It is also one of the most difficult to reform: not just because so many people are dependent on it and would be worried about any changes made to the system, but because of the chain letter principle on which it is financed.

The state pension contributions made by taxpayers today are not saved and invested, as they would be in a private pension fund or any other sort of savings plan, but are instead paid out immediately to pensioners today. The future survival of the system depends on each succeeding generation of taxpayers being willing to enter the same chain letter in the hope that their sons and daughters will do the same later. This is an unstable system, particularly in view of the future demography. The ratio of contributors to pensioners, presently more than three to one, is projected to fall to just over two to one within a few decades: not a comforting prospect for those who make up the bulk of the workforce now.

The obvious answer is to move to a funded system, whereby people (or even governments) actually save and invest the money, building up a fund that is large enough to cover future pension obligations and so preventing the possibility that the chain letter will collapse sometime in the future. But it is a huge problem: today's unfunded national insurance pension liabilities are estimated at about £300 billion (Falkingham & Johnson 1993), and are growing at about £15–£20 billion each year. So unless the present generation reneges on their obligations to present-day pensioners, they would face a prodigious burden: paying as now to support their parents, and paying again to build up retirement funds for themselves.

Actuarially, this looks daunting (Nuki 1993). But the higher rates of return that accrue to savers in a funded system, compared to the very modest growth in state pensions, mean that savers in this generation do not have to "pay twice", as one might think. Only a little extra investment would be required.

Financing the gap

The notional rate of return on the state system, balancing what pensioners receive against what they have paid in over the years is about 1 per cent (Butler & Pirie 1983). A private pension investor would expect a return of many times that. So obviously the funded part of any pension would grow much faster than the present state system.

Taxing the funds would lower the effective rate on people's savings, but the revenue it generated would go a long way towards the current pensions bill. Or the government could borrow, passing some of the burden on to future generations of taxpayers.

Given the extra growth of the savings funds, and this cost-easing measure, we could continue to pay current pensions *and* move onto a secure funded basis for the future by paying perhaps an extra 25 per cent on top of our state pension contributions: hardly a case of "paying twice" (Ferrara 1982).

Controlling exit

We would not want to *force* people into a new system that requires them to pay more, whatever the long-term benefits. But any tax inducement for people to opt into funding will eat into government revenues: so how do we continue to pay our current pensioners?

One way might be to keep the tax concession modest. Thus, only a few would think it worthwhile opting out, while most would decide to stay put. By varying the concession up or down, a manageable rate of exit can be achieved. But this would be cumbersome to administer and easy for an incoming administration to reverse.

Another way might be to offer larger tax concessions but to limit the eligible exit group by age. For example, we could allow only older workers to take the tax concession and set up their own funded alternatives, bringing it down the age scale gradually.

State pension entitlement

Or we could reduce our future costs by freezing the state pensions of those who chose to opt out, so that individuals who have made national insurance contributions for only half of their working life (say) would receive only half of the state pension on retirement.

We might even propose that people who choose to opt for funding would lose the whole of their state pension entitlement. This might sound radical, but younger workers could certainly find it attractive: calculating that they had far more to gain by giving up their entitlement to any state pension and investing the cash for themselves.

Wider benefits

Funding, particularly a system of individual private funds, would leave contributors much better off than at present. They would have control over their own savings, and their pensions could not be stolen by politicians.

Personal freedom would also be increased. People might still be required to make some specified provision for their retirement or other contingencies, but they could also be allowed to choose and control how and where they invest, how and when they take their pension, and otherwise to tailor an individual benefit plan that more closely suits their own needs and expectations. They could switch between the diverse plans on offer; and fund providers would have every incentive to maintain attractive packages, to innovate, and keep their products up to date with the latest trends. The reform would take a sizeable flow of resources out of the hands of politicians and officials, and in effect privatize one of the largest elements in the public budget.

The higher retirement benefits would give particular help to the poor, who do rather badly out of the present system, and who, without savings of their own, find it hard to get by on the basic state pension. And because the fund would be a sizeable part of the estate of most individuals, the new system would actually distribute national wealth more equally than occurs today (Field & Owen 1993).

Insurance programmes

Insurable state benefits

Many other state benefits are capable of being administered on pure insurance principles. As with pensions, the state's welfare function would be to up the income replacement funds, or pay the premiums, of those who were unable to do so themselves.

Jobseeker insurance

Unemployment benefit, for example, could be run along insurance principles. It is not a chain letter like state pension, but a straightforward insurance programme: one that is presently run by the government but that could be offered by competing providers.

In the past, commercial insurers were reluctant to contemplate private unemployment insurance because changes in government policy can make a large difference to unemployment levels, and hence to costs. But today a greater confidence has emerged: companies see that, even with an unemployment rate of 13 per cent, the other 87 per cent are still in work and could be paying premiums. Although the incidence is large, it is still quite manageable commercially.

Private jobseeker insurance could be arranged either through the workplace, as part of the employee benefits package, or within individual income replacement funds. Thus, people would simply be required to have some form of unemployment insurance cover, paying some specified minimum benefit, and most would probably select it as part of a standard fund package. They would enjoy the benefits of actuarial soundness and competitive supply.

As in other programmes, the state's welfare role would be to make sure that the premiums of those on very low incomes were paid. This should be done out of taxation, rather than by forcing all employers to provide the benefit; because by keeping down employers' costs we are more likely to generate employment.

Disability insurance

Private companies already offer insurance that provides income replacement during periods of disablement and inability to work; so in principle, invalidity/disability benefit could well be transformed into a private system.

Institutions such as the friendly societies might be particularly well suited to take on the provider role in this case (Yarrow 1993). Friendly societies commonly offer income replacement cover against disability, but they are also keen to do what they can to get people back to work, or to find alternative work that a partly disabled person could perform. Their motive is not just that of keeping costs under control; they have a deeper purpose to help people to help themselves.

Politicians are alarmed by the fact that the numbers of people on invalidity benefit have more than doubled from 600,000 in 1979 to 1,500,000 today – despite the fact that standards of health are generally much better. But the phenomenon seems to have more to do with the way the benefit is assessed and administered, than with personal health. Were private insurers, mutual funds, friendly societies, or even disabled charities themselves to manage the assessment and subsequent review of cases, it is likely that benefits would be paid much more tightly, but much more fairly.

Industrial injuries and sick pay

At present a number of workplace benefits are paid partly through employers and partly by the state through employer reimbursement mechanisms. There has always been a strong case for taking the state out of this process (Pirie 1993a) and making industrial injuries and statutory sick pay employer responsibilities. The November 1993 budget introduced this concept for larger employers, compensating them by lower rates of employer's national insurance contributions; and it seems likely that this principle will be extended quickly in future budgets.

One parent benefit

The state benefit paid to lone parents, particularly single mothers, causes wide political and moral discomfort. One view is that by making it easier for single women to bring up children, we are actually promoting that sort of lifestyle: breaking up families by making divorce less costly, encouraging teenage pregnancies, replacing marriage or remarriage with a life on benefits; and that all this can leave psychological scars on our children (Green 1993). On a wider level, it is said that we undermine the idea of personal responsibility by cushioning the consequences of personal action; and if people are able to shirk responsibility for what they do, the ordinary business of human life becomes impossible.

At the same time, on welfare principles, we would not want to abandon people who, through no fault of their own, are faced with family responsibilities but not the income to deal with them.

255

Self-funded mechanisms

To the extent that most single mothers are divorced or separated, and may well have been in employment in the past, it *is* possible to construct some private sector alternative on a self-funded basis. It could simply be one of the contingencies provided for in a personal benefits fund.

In the case of teenage pregnancies where the individual might never have worked, a personal fund mechanism might still be practicable, with the state paying the initial premiums as a welfare contribution, but with the actual payment of benefit being on insurance lines. Again, we would expect insurance companies and friendly societies to be firmer in the policing of such benefits. The suspicion of politicians today is that many people, particularly the younger women, who are claiming the benefit are not in fact estranged from the father of their child. But only a more local assessment and payment system is likely to be able to deal with this.

Helping parents work

However, by far the best way to promote the welfare of lone parents and their children is to help the parents get back into work. Accordingly, some pressure groups have advocated the introduction of free state childminding services, arguing that the cost would be easily offset by the tax receipts from working mothers and the reduced need to pay out lone parent benefit.

Access to child care is certainly the best solution. But free child care suffers severe cost and incentive obstacles. Other countries where it has been introduced have been astonished by the demand, and the escalating cost. Many mothers find the service so useful that they will go to great lengths to make sure they qualify, whether they are deserving or not.

A better solution would seem to be to allow working mothers to deduct the cost of child care against tax (Pirie 1989). There is a cost in giving concessions to those working mothers who are already rich enough to afford child care without state help; but the numbers seem low enough to be bearable, while the growth in lone parent benefit does not bode well for the future of the present system.

One might look for other piecemeal solutions that conform with market principles. For example, would it be better to set the state benefit higher (or to fix a comparable minimum rate to be paid by any private plan), provided that single parents devoted some or all of it to childminding services that would enable them to work? Again, we might find ourselves helping women who land very well-paid work and who could then easily pay for their own child care; but this "deadweight" cost is plainly preferable to leaving them trapped at home. Or again, should we be helping single parents pool part of their benefit so that they can establish shared childminding schemes?

Welfare programmes

Thus far we have looked at likely future reform of the savings and insurance schemes operated by the state, the bulk of the national insurance bill. What principles would apply when we consider the strictly welfare obligations of the state?

Benefit according to need

Market economists have little faith in any form of universal benefit, which aims to protect the welfare needs of the few by delivering benefits to everyone. By definition, most of the money goes to those who do not really need it. Certainly, universal benefits are easy and cheap to administer, because no checking up is required. But equally, they are very costly if they are to put any reasonable sum into the hands of the neediest recipients. And because they must be costly if they are to do the job, they require much higher taxes to finance them. That in turn puts up marginal tax rates, and deepens the poverty trap.

Focusing our welfare help on those who really need it is clearly preferable, provided once again that we can get over the incentive problem: that people may not risk improving their own circumstances because they would lose the security of receiving regular state benefits.

Selection mechanisms
It does seem reasonable to expect people with their own means, with savings or other assets or good incomes, to take care of themselves. Indeed, we should be encouraging precisely that self-provision. Our welfare help should be concentrated on those who cannot provide for themselves. However, while the existing system uses this principle, it applies it in a very confused way, and with a complexity that generates much hostility. There are in fact several dozen different tests within the present system; each benefit, almost, being subject to a different test.

It would be better to have a single test that would distinguish a person's eligibility for a whole range of benefits, or for some comprehensive benefit along negative income tax lines. This sort of general income support might be less reflective of particular needs than the present battery of specific programmes from housing benefit on down. But equally it would allow people to manage their own budget more as they deemed fit.

Within the present system, any form of means test does embody certain disincentives – a disincentive against saving and an incentive to draw down one's assets in order to qualify for benefit.[2] But much of this is because benefits are seen as simply "other people's money". In a unitized system where individuals were drawing on their own income replacement funds, the direction of the incentives may be quite the opposite.

Another way of reducing the waste inherent in universal benefits would be to use the tax system to "claw back" the benefits given to wealthier people. Thus, every mother might receive child benefit, but wealthier parents would find some (or even all) of it being taxed away. There is still an administrative loss each time the money is taken in taxation, disbursed, then taxed again; but at least some of the waste is recovered.[3] Care is needed, because ingenious families will arrange their affairs so that the spouse receiving the benefits is also the lower earner, enabling them to keep the benefit even though they may be quite well off as a family. But this is possible by linking tax and benefit rules so that those taxed as families receive benefits as families (Walker 1993).

Contracting out

Even within the current tax-funded state welfare system, as with other parts of the public sector, considerable saving and innovation is possible through *contracting out* the administration of some benefits.

Already the market-testing reforms that are being applied to many parts of the civil service, whereby departments and agencies are obliged to check whether other suppliers could do some tasks more cost effectively, indicate that this possibility is squarely on the agenda. Indeed, some local authorities have already taken the initiative, and are now employing outside service companies and advisers to handle assessments, claims, and payment of the various benefits that are under their control.

In the case of national benefits, there may be considerable advantage in widening the net of potential suppliers to non-commercial sources of supply, such as local charities and friendly societies. Being more locally based, they would be less distant when help was actually needed, and better placed than a government agency to assess *who* was genuinely in need of help, and *how* those people could best be helped (Yarrow 1993, Morgan 1986, Evans 1990).

Nor is this a particularly new and radical idea. Friendly societies were given the role of "approved societies" in the 1911 National Insurance Act. Beveridge proposed that they should be "responsible agents" in the administration of sickness benefits, but this recommendation was dropped; and thus began the post-war decline of the friendly societies movement.

State services

The user as controller

Another principle by which we can get positive incentives into the welfare system is to devolve as much of its management down as far as possible towards the service users. An example would be the transfer of the responsibility for social housing away from local authorities and into the management of social landlords such as the housing associations. And one could go further and put most or all of the management power into the hands of the tenants themselves.

The aim is to cut down the chain of command so that decisions can be made quickly and cost effectively: for example, that essential repairs are dealt with speedily, without requisitions having to make their way laboriously up and down some distant management structure. Since service users themselves usually have a better idea of local needs and resources than any distant manager, such self-management can help provide a better and more responsive service at much lower cost.

User management also encourages personal responsibility. Tenant managers in the UK and elsewhere, for example, have been able to turn around the local culture, and to reduce drugs and vandalism far more surely and effectively than their official landlords ever could. And by allowing people to manage their own local services, we give them an important foundation of experience that can help them move out of the social service net and into a world of self-reliance and self-improvement.

In health and education, the same principle is coming through, thanks to the internal market and the Citizen's Charter. More local management in hospital trusts has produced a devolution of budgetary responsibility right down to ward level. When ward sisters are put in charge of their own budgets, for example, they might spend it in quite novel ways, but probably with a better understanding of how it could best be used to help their patients, and spent without waste (Johnson 1994).

Health and education

Those parts of the welfare state that are delivered in the form of actual services are difficult to reform because of their sheer size, and the number of people who are dependent on them and therefore very worried about the possibility of change. The National Health Service, for example, remains Europe's largest employer, and roughly 90 per cent of the UK population are wholly dependent on its provision. The barriers to change are large.

Health insurance and welfare

Health is already privately insurable, and in a market based welfare system we would probably be treating it just like any other insurable benefit. That is, we would require people to have a minimum standard of insurance for their health, just as we presently require them to have a minimum standard of insurance for their cars. If people wanted to pay extra and have a more comprehensive service, they could. And if people could not afford the premiums of the minimum standard of cover, the state would pay on their behalf as a welfare contribution. Thus, the insurance element could operate on sound insurance principles, and the actual service provision could be made by competing suppliers, with all the benefits that competition brings to service users. Meanwhile the welfare element would be clearly separated, its cost identifiable, its operation on proper welfare principles.

Reforming the present system, however, requires much greater creativity than designing a new one from scratch. Many options were discussed at the time of Mrs Thatcher's National Health Service review (Butler & Pirie 1989). In the end, it was decided not to change the whole financial basis of the Service in this radical sort of way, and to keep health care free and tax-financed. Instead more local management was proposed, and a separation of the purchasing and provision functions that would gradually unleash quasi-market forces within the state system.

The reforms need a further push, but the forces they have unleashed will doubtless continue to expand. With purchasers looking to extract the best value for money from their budgets, there is more and more pressure on providers to discover and then improve the cost and quality standard of what they do; and indeed to explore new services and new methods of working, such as more locally based service delivery. Some managers will feel that they should be able to work for private purchasers as well as NHS purchasers; some may set up independently. But certainly, boundaries between the public health care system and the private sector will become more and more hazy as time goes on.

Long-term care

In addition to acute services, national and local government face a rapidly growing demand for day care and nursing-home care, mainly from the increasing numbers of older people (Nuttall 1993, Laing 1993).

Long-term care is again insurable, and some insurance companies are now offering it. But given the existence of free state care and our high rates of taxation, few people regard the cost of the product as worth the benefit. But if we used the tax system to encourage people to provide for their own long-term care in retirement, perhaps simply integrating it into the current pensions tax reliefs (Butler 1992), the rising cost to the taxpayer could be trimmed while people could enjoy more secure and better quality provision in a competitive market.

Education finance

In education it is perhaps even harder to set market principles to work, although a start has been made on establishing an internal market by allowing schools to opt out of the present hierarchical decision-making system and receive their funding according to the number of pupils they can attract. Again, the broad incentives have been turned in the right direction, making schools concentrate on the quality of what they are actually doing, and convincing parents that they do a good job.

While the need for healthcare is a risk that we all face, education is rather different. At least some people, those who are quite sure that they are not going to have any children, will never need it. So it is harder to justify forcing everyone into some sort of insurance plan. Yet there are some general benefits of having a literate and numerate population.

The traditional market orientated response has been the education voucher. Here, all parents are given a voucher that is equal to the cost of a state education. If they choose to spend more, they can take the voucher to a private school too: the state will pay the voucher's worth to the school, and the parent can top up that payment to the full cost of the school's fees. The same principle would work even if education were wholly private: the state voucher would ensure every family's access to a basic education, but those who could pay more would be free so to do.

261

Despite the presence of several voucher enthusiasts in Mrs Thatcher's Government, however, the voucher never arrived. It has many political difficulties: parents have to understand how it works, state schools have to turn themselves into competitive voucher-catching institutions overnight, experimental trials are difficult to organize without losing the whole concept of the voucher as a way to promote the widest possible choice (Omega File 1983).

The present internal-market structure, however, is close. With local management, open enrolment, and the state money following the child, there is a virtual voucher at least within the state funded system. The next steps are presumably to expand the number of schools opting into this new mechanism, and then to expand the funding principles to allow parents to patronize independent schools as well as state schools.

Again, the boundary between the public and the private sectors will become hazier. And quality control techniques such as the Citizen's Charter will continue the trend. Before too long, and perhaps without realizing it, we could see state services being provided in a much more competitive way – indeed, perhaps with the state being no longer much involved in the provision, but being much clearer in making sure that those services are accessible to those with a welfare need for them (Cm 1730).

Conclusion

There are many ways in which one can introduce market principles and positive economic incentives into the welfare state. One can opt for a radical set of changes, which handle most national insurance benefits as genuine insurance risks, and which give individuals charge of their own contributions and benefits through the establishment of unitized income replacement funds.

Alternatively, one can keep the tax-funded system of state benefits, but recast some of the existing structures so that the economic incentives are made to work in a more useful direction.

One can tackle the problem benefit by benefit, or in terms of a package of related benefits, or in terms of the system as a whole. One can make the change optional and voluntary, or introduce an element of compulsion. One can make changes right away, or introduce them over many years.

As in all attempts to reform the welfare state, politics rather than commonsense will decide what can and cannot be done. But if we are to reform the system, we should be starting with an understanding of the enormous power of personal economic incentives – for good and ill – and a vision of how to use them positively in the defeat of poverty. Armed with that, one can then move systematically through the whole range of social benefits, one by one, working out in each case the best option that is consistent with the principles we have identified.

With 40 years' experience behind us, we can now see that the state is not actually very *good* at providing welfare. It is certainly very bad as an insurance company. The time has come to prise the welfare state out of politics, to liberate those who are trapped into dependence on the government whether they need and want it or not, to empower people to make their own provision for the contingencies they face through their lifetimes. If we devolve the decisions to the people, and confine the state to its proper role as a welfare agent – then we will have a much better defence against those giant evils of want, disease, ignorance, squalor and idleness, and might just create a social insurance system that Beveridge himself would have been proud of.

Notes

1. John Hills argues that social spending will not rise much beyond today's 25 per cent of GDP, unless state pensions are realigned to rise along with incomes rather than prices, in which case another 5 per cent of GDP would be required. But this itself is an enormous amount; over £30 billion (equal to a rise in standard rate income tax from 20p to 45p in the pound or an increase of VAT to 30 per cent).
2. This is particularly true of families that are trying to enable an elderly relative qualify for long-term care services, where gifts and disposal of assets to family members are easily practicable options.
3. The same principle can be applied to "category" benefits such as disability benefit, as proposed in the November 1993 Budget.

Suggested reading

The Beveridge Report (Cmd 6404) is instructive for the author's clear grasp of the incentive problem that could (and eventually did) arise.

For income maintenance programmes and varied proposals for their future see Howell (1991), Hills (1993), Falkingham & Johnson (1993), Field & Owen (1993). The future potential of friendly societies is discussed in Evans

(1990) and Yarrow (1993), while the future funding of long-term care is discussed in Laing (1993). The introduction of quasi-markets into various services of the welfare state is discussed in Le Grand & Bartlett (1993).

CHAPTER 11

Social policy and the active society

Malcolm Wicks

If we are to approach the year 2000 with confidence, let alone summon up the courage to enter a new millennium, much will depend on social policy. To pursue the dream of building the good society as the alternative to the inequality and immorality of capitalism is the challenge for the Left. It is a particular test for the Labour party as it seeks to win the next general election after four successive defeats.

Supporters of the welfare state have undoubtedly been on the defensive since the advent of Thatcherism, and have been uncertain of their ground for a much longer time. Economic troubles confronting both the Wilson and Callaghan Governments in the 1960s and 1970s, together with a failure to develop a coherent social strategy, produced anxieties and uncertainties about the welfare state long before Mrs Thatcher became Conservative leader in 1975 (Wicks 1987).

Looked at objectively, Thatcherism in its early years had an attractive story to tell, as illustrated by this quotation from a keynote document during its Opposition years.

> The Conservative approach entails living within our means, paying our way in the world, mastering inflation, reviving the wealth creating part of the economy and encouraging all those on whom it depends. This approach means less bureaucracy and less legislation, lower taxes and borrowing, higher profits leading to more investment and more employment, and reward for enterprise and hard work. (Conservative Party 1976)

It was essentially a story of unfettered capitalism which, without waste and over-government, would see the unleashing of enterprise and hence, in the slightly longer term, more industry, more entrepreneurship, more jobs and more affluence for all. It was an attractive story, in part because there would be no victims, except perhaps wastrels and scroungers. For, while there would rightly be an attack on waste, no one in real need would be harmed. In fact, the National Health Service would be safe "only with us" and economic growth encouraged by monetarism would allow both lower taxes and protected services.

Certainly, when viewed from the vantage point of the mid to late 1970s, the contrast with the faded prospectus of Labour could not be starker. Here was vision and audacity, certainly a clear strategy. Moreover, a few specific policy pledges, most notably the "right to buy" policy for council tenants illustrated this attractive alternative to the top down welfarism of a statist, paternalistic Labour party.

The reality, of course, has been very different. You only have to look around. Is Britain a land flowing with milk and honey? Are our people proud of the society created by our masters this last 15 years? Moreover, in terms of specifics, the Tories' prospectus has simply failed. For most households, taxation has increased. While the political spotlight has been on lower income tax, overall the tax burden has increased for the average household, thanks to a doubling of VAT, increased National Insurance contributions and, of course, the Poll Tax. This tax illustrated not only the unfairness of Tory fiscal policy, but also the sheer dogmatism of Thatcherism. It was her undoing and with her went the Poll Tax itself.

Moreover, that inevitable accompaniment of monetarism, mass unemployment, is seen increasingly as the social and economic distortion that it is: driving up public expenditure not only in obvious areas such as social security and training, but also in other fields such as law and order. And one significant result of the abandonment of the post-war commitment to full employment has been the growth of the very "dependency culture" that Thatcherism was pledged to destroy.

Thus, we have the modern Conservative paradox: the refusal to intervene through economic instruments to encourage jobs led inevitably to forced intervention to support the incomes of growing numbers dependent on state social security. Less public policy was equated with more public spending. Consider the evidence: in 1992/3 5.3 million people received Income Support, compared to just three million in the late 1970s. Today a staggering 28 per cent of families with children draw either Income Support or Family

Credit in the most dependent culture Britain has witnessed since the Second World War.

"Majorism" does not exist, except as a minor variation on yesterday's tune. Yet because there is no vision, no strategy, no purpose, and because economic recession and huge public debt demands its own agenda, we are left with the extreme, and most vicious, end of rag-bag Thatcherism.

Moreover the development of health "trusts" (at a time of unprecedented public distrust of governmental objectives towards the NHS), opt-outs of grant maintained schools, and the cutting of unemployment and invalidity benefits indicate a greater thrust to the right than that witnessed under Mrs Thatcher herself.

If now however the arguments for welfare are to be stated with confidence, very much more is required than either an effective critique of Tory social politics or an advocacy of a return to the position of 1979. Much will depend of course on the development of specific policies in a formidable array of fields. There is no shortage of questions. How to move from the reality of community neglect to the goal of community care? What family policy is needed given rapid social change? What package of child care and nursery education should be developed to meet the needs of the under-fives? How do we bring training, jobs and economic prosperity to the inner city and out-of-town estate? These important questions can be matched in social security, health, education, housing and many other areas.

But these are secondary to some wider considerations. For the Left now needs a coherent foundation and structure on which to build a true welfare society. This task calls for confidence and critical self-appraisal in equal measure.

Labour's approach to social policy bears the inevitable hallmark of the party's history. The Labour party was created from several political movements that were growing stronger at the end of the nineteenth century. Some were relatively new, while the trade unions already had long histories. The Labour Representation Committee was born at the very dawn of the century, in February 1900. Inevitably the party, when it came into formal being in 1906, drew on its experience of contemporary and economic circumstance. Not surprisingly, much of this was about the condition of labour. High proportions of the workforce, and even more of trade union organized labour, worked in the large-scale industries: millions in the coal mines, the shipyards, in steel and other heavy industries. The labour force was predominantly male, working in masculine trades. Although significant numbers of women worked in the labour market, most worked at home, often in difficult circumstances with many children to care for and feed.

People's housing was predominantly owned by private landlords, accounting for some 90 per cent of dwellings in 1900. The vast majority of children left school at tender ages. There was no health service worth the name and only the most primitive welfare state. Lloyd George's pensions were only introduced in 1908 and the first step towards national insurance was taken in 1911.

In these conditions the Labour party was born, its constitution constructed. Early policy related to the conditions of the day and those that predominated in the early decades of the twentieth century. The battle for trade union rights was central. And faced with exploitation, dangerous conditions and inefficiency, the public ownership of the "means of production, distribution and exchange" was a pre-eminent objective. To achieve decent housing for a working class electorate that all too often knew only the private tenement, municipal housing was developed. And, with the unity that was forged in the heat of the Second World War, the coalition government and then Attlee's Labour administration created the modern welfare state. Its heroic aim was to vanquish the common enemy – the five giant evils, identified by William Beveridge in his report as idleness, want, disease, ignorance and squalor.

These policies were collectivist ones that required large-scale, institutional means for their implementation – the trade union, the nationalized industry, council housing, the town hall, the welfare state and the Labour party itself. Faced with big forces that exploited working people, working people needed big institutions to defend them. It was more Morrison than Morris.

This approach wore the badge of its era and has many victories to its name. Slum clearance was one, alongside improving health standards, the school medical service, workers' protection, national insurance, family allowances and so much more besides. But policies and means born at the turn of the twentieth century offer no clear guidelines to see Britain into the twenty-first century.

At its best – and it is often at its best – Labour's cry is a strong one against injustice. At worst, however, the Labour voice can become an echo of yesterday's Britain: a nation of massed workers in the great industries, a society of tenants, when the relative poverty of the majority contrasted starkly with the riches of the few, and when a majority working class looked to the council, the trade union and the party for change.

Today that Britain now represents the minority. But in the midst of recession and mass unemployment, with homelessness increasing and beggars on the streets of our capital city, this can easily be forgotten, not least by MPs who weekly in their constituencies and advice surgeries see those human reminders of yesteryear. Economic injustice has focused attention on a past – Beveridge's five giant evils – and discouraged a look into the future.

Yet in 1996, or whenever the election comes, the electorate as a whole will have different characteristics. The vast majority – eight or nine out of ten – will not be out of work. Most of those in employment will probably have rising living standards. Electors will be ambitious for themselves and their families in terms of economic wellbeing, housing, health, careers and education. It may be keeping its head down in recession but Galbraith's *Culture of contentment* (Galbraith 1993) is out there to confront, challenge and cajole.

This chapter therefore tackles some fundamental matters for the Left in determining its modern approach to social policy. It starts with values and highlights citizenship. It then seeks to place policy within the context of change by asking how people live and work. Some broad objectives are then outlined. A final task is to consider means: holding the mirror at top–down statism – the traditional face of Labour "welfarism".

Values: a citizenship of rights and responsibilities

> Liberty without equality is a name of noble sound and squalid result.
> (Hobhouse 1911)

Labour requires a new framework to guide its thinking and its policy into the new century. Elsewhere, in *A new agenda*, five Labour MPs set out our analysis and made out the case for an agenda that involves both a reaffirmation of ends and a radical revision of the means for achieving them. This section draws on that analysis (Campbell et al. 1993).

As described below, such an agenda will be framed against a context of change. But we do not start our argument and analysis with a clean sheet nor within a moral vacuum. Rather it is built on values that derive from a rich and dynamic British, European, and indeed, international radicalism, much of it socialist.

Democratic socialism should be the cornerstone. What, however, is "democratic socialism"? It is inspired by no one tradition, philosophical school or set of beliefs. Rather it derives inspiration, ideas and experience from a range of historical strands. Christianity, the Levellers, the Chartist campaign for parliamentary democracy, trade unionism, feminism, Marxism, and other radical and liberal ideas, campaigns and ideals which have all influenced socialist thought and action.

Given the mixed origins of democratic socialism, it may lack the theoretical coherence of, say, Marxism or other comprehensive ideologies and is consequently a constant frustration to political analysts. However, drawing as it does on the concerns and beliefs of ordinary people, it is practical, robust and enriched by the strengths of many viewpoints. Above all else it is non-sectarian. The description "broad church" is often used cynically, but it is a truth, and a strength not a weakness.

Crosland, in *The future of socialism* (1956) reviewed the traditions of British socialism. He concluded in part that there are some fundamental differences between different schools of socialist thought and that the doctrines are often mutually inconsistent.

> Thus, Fabian collectivism and Welfare Statism require a view of the State diametrically opposed to the Marxist view. The syndicalist tradition is anti-collectivist. The Marxist tradition is anti-reformist. Owenism differs fundamentally from Marxism and syndicalism on the class war. Morrisite Communes and Socialist Guilds are incompatible with nationalization: and so on.

Crosland however noted that "the single one element common to all the schools of thought has been the basic aspirations, the underlying moral values. It follows that these embody the only logically and historically permissible meaning of the word 'socialism' ".

Equality

What then are the ideals – "the underlying moral values" – that inspire democratic socialism? A good starting point is the definition provided by William Morris, writing in 1894:

> . . . what I mean by Socialism is a condition of society in which there should be neither rich nor poor, neither master nor master's man, neither idle nor overworked, neither brain-sick brainworkers, nor heart-sick handworkers, in a world, in which all men would be living in equality of condition, and would manage their affairs unwastefully, and with the full consciousness that harm to one would mean harm to all – the realization at last of the meaning of the word "*COMMONWEALTH*". (Briggs 1962)

Central to Morris's definition and to democratic socialism is a passionate belief in equality: the belief that all citizens should be born with equal rights, that they should give, and receive, respect to their fellow men and women, that they should contribute their best to society and take on a fair share of responsibility according to their abilities and receive a fair and equal share in the distribution of resources.

To believe in equality is to reject fundamentally the view that access to decent housing, good health services or education should be decided on the accident of birth, race, gender, inheritance of wealth or current income. It follows that a fundamental guideline for contemporary policy must be redistribution as a means of equalizing individual life chances. This belief does not entail levelling down, but, on the contrary, equal access to the best life chances.

To outline so starkly what Tawney once called "a strategy for equality" may indicate an innocent idealism altogether out of kilter with the mood of the 1990s, with its wretched "me first" cynicism. The challenge however is to match aspiration with determination.

Liberty

But what of liberty? One of the great ironies of modern politics is the ability of the conservatives, of whatever party, to portray themselves as the champions of liberty and, furthermore, to contrast liberty with equality, arguing that the two are incompatible and that equality will inevitably deny liberty and freedom. And what great freedoms does the modern conservative care most about: the freedom to enable babies to live and not to die because of adverse social conditions; the freedom of the young to get jobs, whatever their class or colour; the freedom for old people to live out their lives in decent housing, and not to die from the cold when bitter weather strikes? Of course not. Nothing could be further from their minds: indeed their own actions, when in government, further deny such fundamental freedoms. Rather they define "liberty" and "freedom" so narrowly that they become mere labels to justify their own privileges and bloated life styles. Can it be coincidence that such terms are employed by the rich most passionately and consistently to defend their "rights" to buy privileged education and medical care for themselves and their families, heedless of the consequences for the rest of society?

This has always been the case. Throughout our history, and stretching back at least 200 years, the Conservatives and other defenders of the status

271

quo have opposed reform measure after reform measure, be they concerned with factory conditions, taxation, education or health, on the grounds that they somehow infringe liberty and freedom. In the 1945 general election campaign Churchill, in his first radio broadcast, charged that a socialist policy was abhorrent to British ideas of freedom. Attlee replied in the strongest terms:

> I entirely agree that people should have the greatest freedom compatible with the freedom of others. There was a time when employers were free to work little children for 16 hours a day. I remember when employers were free to employ sweated women workers on finishing trousers at a halfpenny a pair. There was a time when people were free to neglect sanitation so that thousands died of preventable diseases. For years every attempt to remedy these crying evils were blocked by the same plea of freedom for the individual. It was in fact freedom for the rich and slavery for the poor.

The time-honoured Tory tradition continues: the misappropriation of the most inspiring words in the English vocabulary in defence of the most obscene privilege.

We see it, at present, in the contrast between the government's tacit support for those company directors that award themselves huge salary increases, while promoting legislation to abolish wages' councils. In the vindictive vocabulary of contemporary conservatism "liberty" is dragged screaming from the dignity of the dictionary, to serve as a conscript concept – to support the attack on trade union rights and the "right" to work longer hours for less pay in unsafe conditions.

In contrast, and it could not be a greater one, to us true liberty is a key building block in creating the new society. Liberty has implications for a social, economic, political and international agenda. Liberty is crucial for true citizenship, entailing that balance between rights and responsibilities, entitlements and duties that enhance dignity.

Community

Early radicals, most notably supporters of the French Revolution, added "fraternity" to form a trinity – liberty, equality *and* fraternity. Today we would use the term community. But that is no search through the political thesaurus to find, for its own sake, a more modern term. Rather we feel that today it is the very absence of "community" that lies at the heart of our social malaise.

The 1980s, that have dragged on so wretchedly into the present decade, were – are – the years of the individual. From on high we were commanded: "There is no such thing as society." We should not be surprised that people acted accordingly, whether it was the young thug who seized what he wanted, the company director who paid himself thousands of pounds more a *week* (despite the often lamentable performance of his company) or the politician who sought to enhance individual over collectivist values.

Rising crime rates, mugging and brutality, hooliganism, the rundown of the inner city, and City fraud are all inevitable consequences of a culture that applauds the selfish, the greedy and the grabbers. The egos and vanities, the wealth and the power of the few are enhanced and, because we are told that we cannot afford decency, indecency thrives. Poverty increases, dependency develops and, at the extreme, for want of good policy, community neglect masquerades as community care, and the destitute dwell in shop-doorways. Honest citizens find themselves daily – and literally, not only metaphorically – passing by on the other side.

Radicals reject that ignoble "individualism" that is jungle Conservatism. Rather we respect the individual as a social being and one that is interdependent on *family*, *community* and *society*. For us the focus is not on just one of these concepts, but on all. Moreover, we believe in the *equal* rights (and responsibilities) of *all* individuals. For us the good society is one that recognizes the needs, and seeks to utilize the skills, of all citizens for the community as a whole.

Today, community is under pressure and, in some areas, has been all but destroyed. For too many citizens it is a sad fact: there is no such thing as community. There are too many examples: the elderly woman in the high-rise block afraid to venture out after dark; parents who are afraid to let their young children play alone; the estate weighed down by deprivation and despair where unemployment is the norm; the person with mental illness wandering the streets of our capital city. All testify to this grim reality.

Public policies do not help. Housing policies mean that both local authorities and housing associations are unable to house that mix of citizens of different backgrounds and family circumstances that make for true communities. As a result increasing numbers of new tenants come from the most impoverished and insecure backgrounds. Politicians and commentators then find to their horror that majorities of tenants on some estates are single parents, unemployed and dependent on state welfare. This is presumably a puzzle to Tory MPs who have voted for cutbacks to housing investment, and support those economic policies that drive up unemployment and those social policies that abhor child care and decent training.

Planning and often policies that place no value on communities are also to blame. If, in our small towns and suburbs, it is the post office and pharmacist that close and only the video shop and take-away pizza that flourish, then we are in trouble. Planners in far away central offices, calculating how to make prescriptions and pensions more cost-effective, reveal their accountants' mentality, preoccupied with the price of everything, but not the value of local identity and neighbourhood.

We recognize that there is no easy, or short-term, search for community. It is an elusive concept and involves no easy turning back of the clock of our social history. We do believe however in community and seek to support those policies that enhance it. Good practice in schools, social service departments, police forces and health and community services is apparent and must be built upon.

There is nothing wrong with the accoutrements of personal affluence, but if the numbers of personal stereos, Nintendos, mobile phones and cars grow in number, while public transport, health services and schools decline in quality then we are in trouble. We do not wish to see a "society" where crime increases, detection rates remain low and home security gadgetry has to increase; where more opt for private health and education for want of an effective public alternative, and where the roads are clogged up, despite more road schemes, because no one has backed decent public transport alternatives.

Citizenship

This section has outlined the basic values – equality, liberty, community – that we believe represent democratic socialism. To guide our thinking and policy development through the choppy seas of change there is no one theme that predominates. However, people are searching for some certainties, some moral foundations, as they reject the menacing Tory values of the last 15 years. Individuals search not just for affluence, important though that is. Rather they seek a more general state of wellbeing that has an ethical dimension. That is why community strikes a chord and why there is renewed concern about the family.

A unifying concept and one that offers guidance to public policy is *citizenship*. The key work is that of T. H. Marshall (1950):

> Citizenship is a status bestowed on those who are full members of a community. All who possess the status are equal with respect to the rights and duties with which the status is endowed. There is no universal principle that determines what those rights and duties shall be, but societies in which citizenship is a developing institution create an image of an ideal citizenship against which achievements can be measured and towards which aspirations can be directed.

As the quotation indicates, the concept of citizenship is an evolving one, representing a goal for a civilized society that has certainly not yet been attained.

Marshall distinguished three elements of citizenship, civil, political and social. By the last he meant "the whole range from the right of a modicum of economic welfare and security to the right to share to the full in the social heritage and to live the life of a civilised being according to the standards prevailing in the society".

The concept of citizenship is crucial, raising as it does a key question for a democracy, namely what are the fundamental rights *and* responsibilities of citizens? The question of the balance between these two is the key test. Often, the debate is approached more narrowly: too narrowly. Depending on political persuasion, the emphasis is placed solely on responsibility *or* rights. Some argue that citizens should take on greater responsibilities – for the misdemeanours of their children; for the care of their elders; filling labour market gaps; for crime prevention; and for much else besides – but refrain from mentioning what rights citizens should expect in relation to some of these things. Others are equally narrow. They demand further rights – to child care, to a decent income, to jobs etc. – but do not address the question of their own responsibilities in society.

It is therefore the issue of rights and responsibilities – the balance between them, and the implications for the state and other institutions – that offers one of the most fruitful ways of advancing the debates that have been started in recent times. To focus on one without the other, *either* one without the other, is crass, too narrow, merely partisan. But a focus on *both* rights and responsibilities provides a useful entrée into some of the key policy questions that Britain faces.

Some of the key questions are as follows:

- What are the fundamental rights and responsibilities of citizenship, as we approach a new century?
- How have these changed in the wake of social and economic developments around family life and employment?
- What costs, as Titmuss asked, relate to these changes and should they be allowed to lie where they fall?
- What are the caring responsibilities of modern families, given changes relating to the dependence of children, and increasing needs given ageing within the extended family?
- Which responsibilities should become legal obligations?
- What are the rights of families, in relation to, among other things, income support, child care and the care of elderly relatives?

Social change: how people live and work

Three crucial institutions – the family, work and the welfare state – are all experiencing rapid change: their futures are uncertain. Compared with say the UK in the late 1940s, or the 1950s, there is great uncertainty about their future course.

Many critical social policy questions depend on how these three institutions interact. Whether we are concerned about family incomes, social security, policies towards one parent families, or care of young and old, policy judgements depend on family, work and welfare state futures. These three things are important too because they concern the relations between men and women in modern societies and modern economies. While essentially a private matter, such relations have profound public policy consequences.

Family futures

Given current trends, and what we can reasonably predict, how will family life develop up to the early years of the next century? This review is based closely on an earlier analysis (Kiernan & Wicks 1990).

Smaller and older

The ageing of the population has implications for both family structures and family responsibilities. Ageing extends the family across three, four or more generations, while influencing significantly the distribution of care. But care

276

flows in both directions: elders care for their grandchildren, while grown-up children look after their frail parents.

There is both an ageing of the population and an ageing of the elderly population itself. The largest increase between 1991 and 2025 is among those aged 85 and over. There will be a 56 per cent increase here, from 900,000 to 1.4 million.

Household and family size

Households will become smaller in the future, continuing a trend that is already apparent. By the year 2001, average household size will be 2.42, against 2.57 in 1987 and 3.09 in 1961. The number of one person households increases from 5.3 million to 7.1 million. Most will be among the elderly population, but the numbers are also growing among younger groups, as more younger people choose to live as singles, postponing cohabitation and marriage, and as a consequence of divorce.

Fertility rates into the next century will remain low, although, on current trends, higher than in much of Europe, east and west. The average number of children per family is, and will continue to oscillate, about 1.8. The EU average is just 1.6. In Italy it is a very low 1.3, in Spain, also 1.3, and in Germany, 1.5.

Family diversity

As in the 1980s and early 1990s, the trend will be towards family diversity, albeit even more so.

- By the twenty-first century most couples who marry will live together before marriage.
- Partly as a consequence, average age at first marriage (which increased by two years in the decade up to 1991, and which is currently 25.5 years for women and 27.5 for men) will rise: young people will continue to avoid marriage at young ages.
- The numbers and proportions of those who do not marry will rise.
- Many cohabiting couples will have children. Up to the next century these families will be less stable than married couple ones, and more deprived, but these differences may lessen over time (McRae 1993).
- A growing minority of couples will marry after they have had their first or even second child, following the Swedish pattern.
- Most men and women, however, certainly in the early years of the twenty-first century, will marry: probably somewhere in the region of seven or eight out of ten people.

- Marriage, as now, will be a risky enterprise, somewhere between one third and two fifths of new marriages will end in divorce.
- A fifth to a quarter of all children will have parents who divorce and others will have cohabiting parents who split up.
- Significant proportions of children will therefore spend some of their childhood in a one parent household. These children will, in general, be poorer and less well-housed than others.
- Remarriage rates will decline, giving way to greater cohabitation in second, and subsequent, relationships.
- The number of step-families – *de jure* and *de facto* – will continue to grow.
- Many children will experience a complexity of family arrangements during their childhoods. The proportion of children having the conventional family lifecycle – parents married at the time they are born and continuing married until they are grown up – could fall as low as 50 per cent.

Work and the family

Alongside changing family patterns, important employment trends affecting family life, and hence social policy considerations, also need to be recognized. Here some key trends can be summarized.

- *Female employment.* By 1990 71 per cent of married woman were employed, compared to just 10 per cent in 1931.
- *Dual worker families.* In 1990 60 per cent of families had both parents in employment.
- *Part-time work.* By 1992 there were almost six million part-time employees, but while 45 per cent of female employees were part-time, this was true for just 6 per cent of men.
- *Domestic work.* Despite women's employment, work inside the family remains unequal, while child care is also still the mother's responsibility.
- *Ageing and caring.* Demographic trends mean shifts in the patterns of care and the consequent work.
- *Later entry and earlier exit.* Young people are entering the labour market at later ages, due to more schooling and training, increasing higher education, plus unemployment. And workers are retiring earlier, either voluntarily or through redundancy.
- *Collapse of full employment.* Unemployment reached one million at the end of 1975, two million six years later and it hit three million later in the 1980s and in the early 1990s: four million on a true count.

Social policy objectives

Earlier in this chapter the fundamental values that provide the foundations for a modern welfare state were outlined: equality, liberty and community. Citizenship, it was argued, provides a unifying concept. The balance between the rights and responsibilities of the citizen is an important perspective in a number of key social policy arenas.

For socialists and radicals this "back to basics" strategy needs to be developed for a new era, demographic, social and economic, altogether different from that which prevailed either when the Labour party was born or when modern social policies were crafted. Clear policy objectives are therefore necessary, within which specific programmes can be devised. The prime objective is the development of the "active society", to borrow a term from the OECD: "the basic thrust of the 'ACTIVE Society' is to foster economic opportunity and activity for everyone in order to combat poverty, dependency and social exclusion."

The contrast with the mass unemployment, inequality, poverty and marginalization and dependency of the 1990s could not be greater. To create the "active society" involves a battle with formidable foes: discrimination based on race, gender and age; and the cancer of cynicism and pessimism. It also involves mobilizing a formidable array of public policy instruments, many of them outside the conventional field of social policy. But the student of social policy should spend more time looking at economic policy and employment and rather less at the minutiae of Income Support and the mechanics of the Social Fund.

How do we move towards the active society? First and foremost by reinstating the goal of full employment as a key objective of economic strategy. So let us remind ourselves of the words of William Beveridge on unemployment, or idleness, not out of sentimentality but because they ring true as a testing text for the 1990s and beyond: "Idleness is the largest and fiercest of the five Giants and the most important to attack. If the Giant Idleness can be destroyed, all the other aims of reconstruction come within reach. If not, out of reach in any serious sense and their formal achievement is futile" (Cmd 6404).

"Full employment", however, is not the same as that achieved in the 1940s and 1950s. Today it must apply to men and women; it is unlikely to involve the same job for life; it will involve education and training at different career stages; and it should be balanced with family commitments. It must also entail high quality, well paid work, and not any job for its own sake. The achievement of the full employment objective depends on developments that lie outside the scope of this chapter: Britain and Europe's ability to compete effectively with emerging economies, within the Pacific rim, Eastern Europe and Latin America.

This is a very different vision to that of the Conservative government that seeks to compete by driving down wages and working conditions, abolishing workers' rights and the wages' councils, and rejecting Europe's Social Chapter.

The road to full employment will be more difficult than that travelled in the post-war period. But if the goal cannot be achieved then, as Beveridge warned, the prospects for reconstructing our community are bleak. Poverty will grow, social security resources will be squandered and other objectives, including good health and education, will be less realizable.

If work is central to the creation of the active society then it is important to question conventional definitions of work. What is the nature of work in modern society, how do we define it, what work do we most value, what forms of work will grow in importance in the future if welfare is to be maximized, and what are the implications of our answers to these questions for public policy?

These issues will grow in importance in the 1990s and certainly in the early decades of the next century. Why are the questions important? Let us look at some official definitions. According to *Social Trends*, "the civilian labour force includes people aged 16 and over who are either in employment . . . or unemployed". The "work force" is the "work force in employment plus the unemployed". These definitions exclude so much of the most important work undertaken in society. In particular, of course, it excludes much female "economic activity". It certainly excludes most of the tasks involved in childrearing, household activities such as cooking, washing, ironing, etc, and it excludes most of the care of elderly people and others with disabilities.

These vital things are also excluded from other crucial definitions – definitions that are key political and economic indicators – such as gross domestic product. According to the Treasury, GDP is "the value of the goods and services produced by United Kingdom residents, including taxes on the expenditure of both home produced and imported goods and services and the effect of subsidies". But the services that are produced and included under this heading are only the ones in the formal economy.

What does this mean? The perspective of the Martian is helpful. Let us imagine her looking down on our society, observing two households. In one lives a person engaged in welfare work: a social worker perhaps or a home help organizer. This worker leaves home in the morning and is responsible for the welfare of many people. It is a stressful job, but it is remunerated. It is important work, but there are holidays and there are training days and, on retirement, a pension. It is a job that is recognized by society and has some status. She is certainly recognized in the official arithmetic of labour force, GDP, and public expenditure.

Next door another carer lives. But she provides care within her own extended family to one or more relatives living with her (or nearby). The Martian observes that the work is equally stressful, and that sometimes more hours are expended on the care than in the first household. But, and the Martian is puzzled by this, the second carer is not paid, she gets no holidays, and no training and ultimately no pension. (She has no social working qualifications but copes OK!) She also gets little recognition, although increasingly politicians and pundits pat her on the back and applaud the vital work. Social scientists even study her efforts. But she is not part of the "labour force" and, curiously, she is of no formal value to society as she is not counted in official definitions of the nation's product or wealth.

It is not the purpose here to consider the specific policy implications of this line of analysis. In the past the argument has been trivialized: demands for "wages for housework" can easily be lampooned, or, when taken seriously, become an argument of those who, regardless of key social, demographic and economic developments, would somehow wish to return to an age of clear gender divisions in society and its economy.

My guess however would be that increasingly these kinds of questions will move from the academic to the practically important. As women's employment patterns become more like those of men the question of "who cares" in society – for very young, for frail and for old – will become vital and politically important, as many of the traditional carers become fully active in the formal labour market, in the formal labour force and as part of GDP. (In practice, of course, an informal [or "black"] economy occupies precious space between the formal and the household or domestic economy.)

The borderlines between what happens within the family and what happens within the economy, between the social and the economic, and between formal and informal care are difficult to determine but cannot go unchallenged. The debate will only start properly – there is already of course a growing literature – when we challenge the implicit assumption that some of the most important work in society effectively, because of masculine official arithmetic and official definitions, "counts for nothing", to borrow Marilyn Waring's words (Waring 1988). In several countries attempts have been made to measure the unpaid household work that is undertaken. Some have related this to official measures of GDP.

Recently, the Australian Bureau of Statistics undertook a study, based on a time-use survey. It covered about 1000 private dwellings in Sydney. Any assessment is confronted by difficulties, conceptual, methodological, etc., but some "experimental estimates" were reached. For Australia as a whole, "[the] estimated value of unpaid housework for 1986/87 ranged from $137.3 billion for the individual function replacement cost approach using award wage rates to $162.8 billion for the opportunity cost approach using average wage rates". As a percentage of GDP this represented, according to the opportunity cost approach, 62 per cent, and, for the individual function replacement cost approach, 57 per cent. Other studies have estimated unpaid household production as 60 per cent of GNP for the USA (1976); 44 per cent of GNP in France (1975); and 32 per cent of GNP for Finland (1980).

These estimates cover household work in general. Sociologically, they are significant. In policy terms it is the caring tasks that are most interesting. Our estimate, at the Family Policy Studies Centre, was that Britain's 6.8 million carers provided care that could be valued at between £23 and almost £38 billion (Wicks 1994).

The achievement of the active society depends critically on economic policy and employment and on wider recognition of "work" than is conventionally allowed for. However, the pursuit of the active society has still wider implications. It is only in the context of the active community that full citizenship can flourish. It is only when people gain access to jobs and hence independent wellbeing that the dependency culture is shattered, only then that individuals can tackle with confidence their responsibilities in the economy, the community and the family.

The active society will be a force for greater equality, liberty and true community. It is a powerful battering ram against the gates of inequality and social provision. It is, in essence, a key to social solidarity and the integrated society.

In the 1990s such forces for integration need all the help they can receive. During the twentieth century interdependence and community developed and were maintained in many different ways – industrially, through trade unions, the fellowship of work and the communities that resulted; in society through what we term "the welfare state".

What are the modern equivalents? They are hard to see when the symbols of the age – owner occupation, the private pension, the motor car and the personal computer – stand more for individualism than for community.

Thatcherism was, in part, an attack on forces for integration. The politics that boasted "there is no such thing as society" was responsible for attacks on key societal institutions: the welfare state itself, the education system, the BBC, public service and the trade unions.

Social policy can become again a powerful force for integration and solidarity. Consequently we need to consider how different, and often very specific, policy proposals impact on the wider community and the public interest. An important illustration of how this can easily be forgotten is the renewed debate about the relative merits of "universalism" as opposed to selectivity or "targeting" within social security. Recently the advocates of targeting have been in the ascendant. Why, its advocates demand, have universal benefits, when by definition they go to the rich as well as to the poor? Why not target benefits more efficiently on those who "really need them"? There are many important specifics to consider in this debate, not least the impact of selective benefits on incentives and the poverty trap, the take-up problem etc. But the wider implications of targeting can easily be forgotten. The attack on access to universal benefits, such as pensions and Child Benefit, is more fundamentally an attack on the concept of a welfare society as a badge of citizenship.

"Selective" implies a particular society: a fundamentally unequal society, but a society of alleged equal opportunity, with the poor on the outside, excluded from mainstream society, different from ordinary citizens. Means testing is about doing good to these poor, but according to strict, defined rules. As Richard Titmuss used to remark: "poor people's services are invariably poor services".

Universalism, by contrast, is not about poverty first – and last – but about citizenship. It is about the range of risks that all citizens face during their lives; about the good society intervening to produce greater equity. It recognizes that if, as a general principle, we construct social policies for all citizens, then all citizens have an interest. They are utilized by all on a regular basis and can be defended by all. They are forces for unity and solidarity. Means testing by contrast is a force for division, resentment and poor policy. One of the tragedies of the Tory years is that we have to fight again the battles of yesteryear, in defence of decencies we once felt had been achieved for all time. Today, dressed up as "targeting", the means test rears its ugly head again. But, despite its modern nomenclature, it is essentially the difference between designer jeans and denim – no difference, the same fabric.

Willing the means: a democratic social policy

While from the perspective of the Left, and indeed from a wider constituency concerned about fairness and justice, the "New Right" scenario for welfare is easily confronted, those aspects of it that have some appeal to public opinion need to be recognized and understood. These concern the critique of the welfare state as overbearing and bureaucratic, uniform and grey. Moreover, this critique from the Right has an uncanny resemblance to the attack on aspects of welfarism that has come from the Left, but to appreciate this point we need to go back a little.

Central to democratic socialism is the belief that it is mainly through parliament that inequalities can be attacked and social justice achieved. Indeed, Bevan argued that: "the issue therefore in a capitalist democracy resolves itself into this: either poverty will use democracy to win the struggle against property, or property, in fear of poverty, will destroy democracy" (Bevan 1961).

However, the recent history of the welfare state shows that the role of the state is problematic. State interventions in housing, education, health and incomes have substantially changed the conditions of society and have therefore been beneficent. But such state intervention has not always contributed to the enhancement of freedom, and the perception of the state has suffered accordingly. Certainly, many council tenants, NHS patients and social security recipients do not regard their relations with the state as wholly positive (to put it mildly). In too many areas, and in too many individual cases, the state (and sometimes the professionals and officials who represent it) is viewed as harsh, unsympathetic, intolerant, prejudiced and unhelpful.

A major explanation for popular wariness about the state's role in many areas of social policy is the way in which welfare is delivered, through large state bureaucracies, some organized centrally, some locally. All too often they seem remote from the needs of clients and customers, even when delivered by supposedly "local" government. (The recent development and growth of unelected quangos to deliver health, housing and education only exacerbates this problem.)

The growth and administration of welfare organizations can be understood in the context of radical and socialist theory within Britain. The British Labour party came into being with a profound belief in the power of central government, local authorities and other public bodies to do good, to promote human welfare and to eradicate inequalities. This involved recruiting large forces of well-trained staff, developing bureaucracies and drawing up rules and regulations. All this was necessary, indeed desirable, if building homes, running schools and ministering to the sick were to be undertaken competently. This was the socialism of Sidney and Beatrice Webb and Herbert Morrison that spawned a hundred Fabian tracts and gave impetus to the London County Council and many other municipalities. It was the socialism that was, in no small measure, responsible for many significant achievements.

Faith in this approach faltered in the 1960s and 1970s and there developed a growing uncertainty and anxiety about the relationship between the citizen and the state, and an awareness too of other potential conflicts: professionalization versus participation, efficiency versus democracy, and bureaucracy versus accountability.

Some of the critique of state services has been exaggerated, and knowingly exaggerated by the enemies of collectivism. Moreover we should be wary of the strange ideological alliances that developed between New Right enemies of the welfare state and some libertarians and "power to the people" advocates. The ideological climate that favoured Mrs Thatcher's victory in 1979 was, albeit in only a small part, created by some who should have known better. As David Donnison has argued: "Those on the far Right and the far Left who are hostile to the state as such may pull down the institutions around which humane and unifying loyalties can be mobilized – loyalties we destroy at our peril" (Donnison 1983).

The lesson from all this is that while faith in basic values remains steady, socialists must rethink methods and avoid the mistake of confusing ends with means. The policy instruments that seemed right in the early decades of this century are certainly not necessarily right as we approach the twenty-first century. Modern social policy needs to draw on an alternative radical tradition which found expression in the Labour movement. Indeed, Halsey (1978) has asked how "the movement which had invented the social forms of modern participatory democracy and practised them in Union Branch and Co-op meeting, thereby laying a Tocquevillian foundation for democracy, was ironically fated to develop through its political party the threats of a bureaucratic state".

Yet today that radical tradition is expressed through many modern campaigns, organizations and community groups that emphasize the power and rights of the individual to organize human affairs on a small and democratic scale, through industrial and housing co-operatives, well-women clinics, voluntary organizations and playgroups.

In some respects, the Labour party is not easily placed to understand some of these questions because, being the party of labour, it is better at receiving and implementing the wishes of the staff of welfare bureaucracies than it is at recognizing the anxieties of consumers who are, in any case, unorganized. Yet, without adequate and close control, welfare bureaucracies, health authorities, social service departments or education agencies can grow because of the ambitions and aspirations of senior staff in ways that do not inevitably increase the sum total of human welfare.

The challenge for radicals is to draw on the Left's democratic tradition and to think through the lessons for social policy futures. The stakes are certainly high: if the "New Right" are allowed to continue their hijack of "choice" and "freedom" as part of a vocabulary designed to dismantle the welfare state, they will be powerful weapons in the campaign for inequality. If however they become key concepts in the development of social policy they will be revitalizing ingredients in the renewed search for greater equality.

But what would a "democratic" welfare state look like? This is not such an easy question to pursue as some of the rhetoric of "participation" and "decentralization" might suggest. It involves fundamental questions of power and, in the past, some have too readily assumed that solutions would be easily found.

Lenin in *The state and revolution* pronounced that: "under socialism all will govern in turn and will soon become accustomed to no-one governing". As Anthony Wright (1984), who quotes this passage notes: "We know the rest of that particular story." Today, "the generation of 1968 has completed the long march through institutions". For them, perhaps, Lennon, rather than Lenin, captures the mood, yet "power to the people" is easy to sing along to: more difficult to achieve. We must not, for instance, adopt too readily solutions that depend on, or assume, that ordinary people want participatory systems that eat too much into leisure time. As George Bernard Shaw noted, the trouble with socialism is that it requires too many meetings. Political activists may find fulfilment through a seemingly endless series of meetings in draughty halls, but that is their problem.

Moreover, it should not be taken for granted that voluntary action is necessarily superior to statutory action. Sometimes it may be, but it can be equally remote, less reliable and it is often less accountable.

Social policy must involve, in part, the spreading of power and the decentralization and democratization of services and systems of administration. We must rethink the relationship between the citizen and the state, be wary of providing benefits without also conferring clearly understood rights, and be suspicious of developing services that are not run by democratically elected or accountable bodies. Above all else we must measure progress, not by the growth of bureaucracies or the increasing strength of professional staffs, but by output, both the number and quality of services provided and the increase in standards, self-esteem, power and liberty of ordinary people.

This requires a rigorous democratic agenda. At its heart will be a renaissance of local government, but this does not involve reinventing the municipal status quo pre-Thatcher. There is a strong case, for example, to integrate the NHS administrative structure, now increasingly expensive and unaccountable, within a reinvigorated local government. For education, local education authorities should be concerned with setting frameworks, monitoring performance and providing support and co-ordination. They should not be concerned with the day to day responsibility for the management of schools, which is best left to teachers, supported by governors, parents and senior students. The democratic agenda should also involve participation in housing and social services.

Welfare state futures

Since becoming an MP in 1992, I have held regular advice surgeries. All too often, I witness one future there. It is a future we must reject. The unemployed, the poor, those in debt, the wretchedly housed and the homeless come to seek assistance. All depend on the welfare state, indeed depend too much, through powerlessness and poverty. They seek modest things: a slightly larger council flat, a loan from the Social Fund, a letter to the Social Services Department or, sometimes, more effective service from the NHS – the life-saving heart bypass surgery, soon, not in the next financial year.

If this is the "welfare state" we are in deep trouble. And, of course, we are. It is not the task of the Labour party to defend that dependency state. Indicators of true welfare are not greater social security spending, more loans from the social security office or higher housing benefits. A true indicator is the fulfilment of individual independence, built in part on good employment and, in part, on a foundation of social rights.

It is time to liberate the concept of "social security" from the leg irons of conventional usage. How do we create a socially secure society? What are the contemporary forces that make for insecurity and how do we combat them? If we can tackle these questions, then we can use precious resources to provide decent pensions and benefits to those who require them through retirement, sickness, disability or family commitment.

The future witnessed weekly in my advice surgery is that devised by this Conservative government these last, long 15 years. It is their political attempt, partly successful, to move towards a residual welfare state: reserved for the poor, guarded by the means test, under the shroud of stigma. If their historic mission finally succeeds it has impacts not only on the weak, but on all citizens.

The forces that created the post-war welfare state were many and varied, several from radical and socialist movements. It was the historic role of the Labour government in 1945 to serve as midwife to modern social policy. In the mid 1990s, Labour's task is still more important and certainly more complex. It is to defend, create and inspire. To defend the good that remains of the welfare state. To create a new vision and strategy. And to inspire a new generation to construct the new welfare community, the just society. It is a formidable task, an exciting challenge. A good and decent one to take up as we approach a new century, a new millennium.

Suggested reading

Richard Titmuss (1968) and (1974): two crucial texts from the founder of British social policy studies. While written during an earlier generation, his thoughts, themes and philosophy ring out as powerful guidelines for the troubled 1990s. David Donnison (1991): a powerful and stimulating statement from one of Britain's leading social scientists. George & Miller (1994) present a prospective analysis of British social welfare while Campbell et al. (1993) provide a policy outline for the future, which includes both a reaffirmation of ends and a radical revision of the means for achieving them.

CHAPTER 12
Accountability and empowerment in welfare services

John Stewart

The necessities of public accountability

Those who exercise public power should be answerable to those on whose behalf they exercise it. In the welfare system power is exercised by institutions and by those who work within them. Taxes are raised to provide resources; resources are allocated between different activities; services are rationed according to the resources available; the form and nature of the services is determined. The cumulative effect of these decisions has critical effects on the life and welfare of the members of the society who depend upon the welfare system. The exercise of those powers can only be justified by public accountability.

There are different forms of accountability, apart from public accountability. Indeed, public accountability depends upon the existence of other forms of accountability:

- management accountability is the accountability of managers to their superiors in the organization;
- professional accountability is the accountability of professionals to the standards of their profession as enforced by professional associations;
- contractual accountability which is playing an increasing role in the welfare system is accountability to the terms of the contract;
- client (or as some would now have it customer) accountability is direct accountability to the individuals who receive the service.

In the public domain, where public power is exercised and expenditure incurred, these different forms of accountability have been developed within public institutions set within the framework of public accountability.

Public accountability requires two differing elements if it is to be fully developed. The first is that those who control public institutions should be required *to give an account* to the public of their exercise of power. The second is that there should be a means of the public *holding them to account*. Both are necessary for the full development of accountability. To give an account is of only limited value if there is no means of acting upon it. Holding to account will not be adequately based unless there is a full and open account to which there is public access, so that a judgement can be made.

Traditionally in the welfare services, as for public services generally, the giving of accounts has been ensured by debate and discussion in parliament and local councils. Holding to account has been secured by the accountability of ministers to the House of Commons and by the accountability of the House of Commons and of councils to the electorate.

Whether these forms of public accountability were adequate given the growth in the scale of public service and in the extent of publication can be doubted. The open government necessary for giving an account is lacking particularly in central government, and the work of parliament and its select committees is necessarily limited thereby. The doctrine of ministerial responsibility has been under strain. The division of responsibility between central and local government was a means of spreading the burden of public accountability, but the low turnouts in local elections indicated a weakness in accountability at local level.

The crisis in public accountability

In addition to existing weaknesses, public accountability has been weakened by two changes. The first change has been the increasing centralization of responsibilities for local decisions. The clearest example is the capping of local government expenditure, which covers wide areas of welfare spending such as education and social services. This means that local authorities no longer have the right to set local taxes at a level above the cap. At present that cap takes some account of past expenditure, but over time it is likely that every local authority will be capped at the standard spending assessment which is the government's formula-based assessment of their need to spend. Since, with increasing central government constraint on local government expenditure, nearly every local authority would be forced to spend at the standard spending assessment – the only exceptions being the few local authorities spending below that level – central government will in effect be determining the level of local taxation in every local authority. The only role of the local tax would then be to confuse people as to where accountability lay. For accountability for local expenditure increasingly lies with central government.

In other fields too central government has assumed responsibility at national level. One example is the national curriculum, with the related arrangements for national testing. In effect the Secretary of State for Education has assumed responsibilities from schools and local authorities. This chapter is not concerned with the merits of this change, but with its consequence in increasing the burden of public accountability on ministers.

The second major change in the institutional framework of welfare services has been the replacement of control by and accountability of local elected councillors by appointed members. This has been through:

- the transfer of local government responsibilities to boards with members appointed directly or indirectly by central government ministers;
- the transfer of local government responsibilities to boards with self-appointed members;
- the removal of local government representatives from boards to which they were previously appointed.

The result of these changes building on previous structures means that the health services are run by regional and district health authorities, family health services authorities and health service trusts – all of them controlled by appointed boards. Training and Enterprise Councils, largely self-appointed, exercise major responsibilities for training programmes. Further education colleges now have their own governing bodies and are responsible for their finances to the Further Education Funding Council, itself an appointed body – as grant maintained schools will be responsible to another funding council. Self-appointed housing associations play an increasing role in the provision of social housing. Housing action trusts and urban development corporations have taken over responsibilities from local authorities in specified areas of certain towns and cities. Now police authorities are constituted, separated from local authorities, with councillors appointed but also with five appointed members and three magistrates constituting just under half the board.

The cumulative effect of these developments, building on the already existing structure of largely appointed health authorities, is that these bodies will constitute a major part of the system of local governance, exercising powers and responsible for expenditure, equivalent in scale to that exercised by local authorities. These bodies exercise substantial powers at local level,

They will make choices on local priorities within their sphere of operation – indeed they are constituted for that purpose, yet they are in no way accountable to local people.

They may choose to give accounts to local people, although for many of these bodies the requirements of public accountability in giving accounts are significantly less rigorous than those on local authorities. Neither their members nor their officers are subject to surcharge. They are not required to appoint monitoring officers for financial and legal propriety. Some of them meet in private and on none are the requirements for open meetings and access to information as wide-ranging as on local authorities.

But even if the obligation to give accounts was fully developed for these bodies, there is no means by which local people can hold them to account. There will be problems that arise:
- financial mismanagement may take place in regional health authorities;
- a grant maintained school can run into difficulties;
- a training and enterprise council can become bankrupt;
- an urban development corporation may pay little attention to the views of local people;
- a health authority may ignore the dominant view expressed in local consultation.

These may happen – indeed all of them have happened – but there is no means by which local people can hold these authorities to account.

The only means by which these bodies can be held to account is the long line of accountability to ministers, themselves accountable to the House of Commons which is accountable to the electorate. In so far as these bodies make local decisions effecting local people such an approach to accountability is inappropriate. The overall effect is, in any case, to add to the burden of accountability on ministers. The doctrine of ministerial responsibility is under strain. Ministers – of any party – have not shown a readiness to accept responsibility for activities directly under their own control. It is hardly realistic in those circumstances to assume that ministerial responsibility resolves the problem of public accountability. Through the growth of appointed boards and the assumption of responsibility for local authority decisions by central government a crisis in public accountability for welfare and other services is building up. The whole burden of public accountability cannot be borne by ministers nor by the Cabinet.

The counter-arguments

It will be argued that the development of contractual accountability can resolve the issue. Increasingly, as for example, in the health service between the district health authority as purchaser and hospitals and trusts as providers, organizational and inter-organizational relations are governed by the purchaser through the contract. Accountability is then accountability by the provider to the contract. Whether that meets the requirements of public accountability even for the contractor may be doubted. The excuse when a problem arises that "we have carried out the contract – so we are not to blame" can be an evasion of accountability rather than its celebration.

But for the district health authority (DHA) as purchaser, the existence of contracts highlights the issue of accountability. It raises the issue of who the district health authority is responsible to for determining the requirements for which it is contracting. The Audit Commission (1993) has said that each district health authority should "debate and clarify its underlying values so that its purchasing plans reflect agreed strategic priorities. This process will be contentious and difficult, and it is doubtful whether the NHS is professionally, managerially or politically ready for it. But in the long run such clarity will be essential if real headway is to be made with the broad aims". The health service reform makes clear that the role of the district health authority is to set "its" local priorities. That exposes the issue of public accountability, and with the lack of local accountability challenges the legitimacy of the DHA in making decisions on behalf of local people – a lack of legitimacy that undermines the role of the appointed boards.

Market accountability can also be argued to be a substitute for public accountability, rendering it unnecessary because outcomes are determined by the hidden hand of the market. It is doubtful whether that would ever be regarded as adequate for welfare services that have been provided in the public domain because market outcomes were regarded as inequitable and/or against the public interest. But, in any event, what is being introduced into welfare services is not the market of market theory in which, in a situation of perfect competition, customers choose the services they want at the price they are willing to pay. What are being introduced are not markets, but quasi-markets consisting of a series of disaggregated market mechanisms. They are more often producer markets in which the consumer has little choice. Services are provided free at the point of delivery. Such quasi-markets do not behave in accordance with market theory, according to which the spontaneous operation of the market leads to optimum efficiency. The outcome of quasi-markets cannot be assumed to lead to optimum efficiency or even to the outcome sought by those who designed them. Such markets have to be regulated and managed to ensure outcomes are in accord with public policy. So the issue of accountability is unresolved because there has to be accountability for the design and the management of such quasi-markets and therefore of their outcome. The spontaneity of the market of market theory may lead to the accountability of the market but quasi-markets that are designed, regulated and managed leave the issue of public accountability unresolved.

William Waldegrave (1993) in his Public Finance Foundation lecture entitled *The reality of reform and accountability in today's public service* has argued that:

> . . . services are not necessarily made responsive to the public simply by giving citizens a democratic voice, and a distant and diffuse one at that, in their make-up. They *can* be made responsive by giving the public choices or by instituting mechanisms which build in publicly approved standards and redress when they are not attained.

He later says that:

> . . . the government have not in any way altered or undermined the basic structure of public service accountability to Parliament and hence to individual citizens. But we have made it useable. We have strengthened those formal lines of accountability by making our public services directly accountable to their customers.

This argument begins by assuming that the requirements of democratic accountability are adequately met by accountability of ministers to Parliament. This ignores the point made in this paper that that line of accountability has never previously been asked to bear the whole burden of public accountability and is now being asked to bear a burden that is totally unrealistic.

There appears to be an assumption that consumer responsiveness is an alternative to accountability to elected bodies. Local authorities have shown in recent years a concern for consumer responsiveness which goes alongside their accountability to the electorate. Responsiveness and public accountability are not alternatives: they can be and are combined. But, and this is the key point, consumer responsiveness is no substitute for public accountability. As we have seen the appointed boards are allocating resources, setting priorities, determining the nature and level of services, which set the framework within which services are provided and within which consumer responsiveness develops. Accountability to the individual customer cannot replace public accountability, because the individual customer will not always receive the service they seek. Services are rationed; priorities are established; conflicts between different "customers" have to be resolved. For these decisions customer accountability is not enough – not all customers can be satisfied. There has to be public accountability for these collective decisions and where those are choices made locally, Parliamentary accountability is not only overburdened, it is inappropriate.

Rebuilding public accountability

The growth of government by appointment raises issues of public accountability that are not resolved by contractual accountability, market accountability or accountability to consumers, although there may be roles for each of these. In so far as there are weaknesses in the procedures by which these bodies give accounts of their activities or by which they are checked, legislation could be introduced to place on these bodies at least the same requirements as are placed on local authorities for reporting procedures, open meeting, access to information, monitoring officers, and external audit. Such changes could be achieved without fundamentally altering the institutional structure.

However, as has been argued earlier in this chapter, public accountability involves more than giving an account. If the issue of how these appointed boards can be held to account by local people remains unresolved the crisis in public accountability has not been met. One approach would be to make these bodies (e.g. health authorities) subject to direct election. There are then issues about the fragmentation of government at local level that would have to be faced, as a proliferation of elected bodies constitute the government of local communities.

The other alternative would be to base public accountability on the local authorities. This could be achieved in a variety of ways, from the local authority assuming direct responsibility for the services provided by these bodies, through assuming responsibility for setting contracts for services (e.g. assuming in health the responsibility of the district health authority), to assuming responsibility for appointing such boards and ensuring that the boards are accountable to the authority. All such approaches are possible now that local authorities have learnt, partly under the pressure of government legislation, to operate in a wide variety of ways apart from direct provision.

If, in one way or another, public accountability at local level is to be based on local authorities, it raises the issue of the adequacy of the public accountability of local authorities – an issue relevant in its own right to this book, because of the wide range of welfare services provided by local authorities. Public accountability has too often been regarded by local authorities as adequately fulfilled by the election of the council and by the responsibility of officers to that council and its committees – even though the turnout at the elections averages only between 40 and 50 per cent.

Public accountability as a moral principle

If public accountability is the basis on which the exercise of public power is justified, it is hard to accept that it is achieved by periodic election alone. Although such elections provide the basis on which public accountability can be built, the role of public accountability in providing the legitimacy for public action demands a continuing relationship. Public accountability should be regarded as a moral principle expressing a sense of stewardship in those who act on behalf of the public: as a principle it has to be expressed not merely in elections, but in a continuing relationship between an authority and its citizens.

Margaret Simey (1988) has expressed this in her account of her experience as chair of the Police Authority in Merseyside,

> Accountability is not about control but about responsibility for the way in which control is exercised. The distinction is a fine one but it is of fundamental importance. In other words, accountability is not an administrative tool but a moral principle. Of those to whom responsibility is given, an account of their stewardship shall be required. It is a principle whose purpose is to govern the relationship between those who delegate authority and those who exercise it.

She saw that this should govern not merely the relationship between the Police Authority and the Chief Constable but between her and her fellow councillors and "those who in turn delegated authority to us and to whom we ourselves must be accountable".

Once public accountability is recognized as a moral principle, based on stewardship requiring a continuing relationship, then the nature of giving an account is transformed. It is no longer a one way process in which the citizen is informed but a relationship through which those who govern and are governed inform each other in a process of learning: a process that can effectively merge being held to account and giving an account.

Translating principle into action

The principle has to be translated into action and here there is a need for innovation in approaches to building an active citizenship – which is what is implied. There is a need for as much attention and as much energy and drive to be given to this task as has been given in recent years in the welfare services to management innovation and in previous periods to professional development.

Possible lines of advance are:
- the development of referenda as a means of citizen choice, including citizen initiatives putting forward proposals – the argument for referenda lying not merely in the vote but in the public discussion they generate;
- citizen charters that are not about the public as customers but the public as citizens with the right to know, to explanation, to be listened to, to be heard and to be replied to;
- the development of the role of citizen as members of juries to explore policy dilemmas – in which experiments have taken place in Germany and other countries (Grunow 1991);
- the creation of community forums, both for communities of place and of interest, in which public issues and concerns can be expressed and responded to;
- building on the role of the elected representative so that being a representative becomes a part of a relationship of active representation.

Only if local authorities can give a continuing meaning to accountability can they provide the basis for resolving the crisis in public accountability, which is not merely about the growth of appointed boards and the growing burden on the overstrained doctrine of ministerial responsibility. It is about the inadequacy of traditional models of public accountability both at central government and at local level. What has been suggested is the development of public accountability as an active relationship and the building up of local government both to reduce the burden on ministerial responsibility and

297

because, particularly in environmental and welfare services, the active relationship required is more easily established at local level.

Beyond accountability towards empowerment

To build up local government is not sufficient unless it pursues the active relationship suggested. Indeed, that active relationship can and should go beyond accountability towards empowerment. As it has been argued that central government should be ready to pass power to local authorities, so should local authorities be ready to pass responsibilities to citizens where those responsibilities can be exercised directly, resolving in the responsibility of the citizens themselves the issue of public accountability. In that way empowerment becomes part of the strategy for meeting the crisis in public accountability. Empowerment differs from the approaches suggested to public accountability. The issue of public accountability arises when power is exercised on behalf of others, albeit, as was suggested, in an active relationship with those on whose behalf it was exercised. Empowerment means that power is exercised directly by the public, so that the issue of public accountability is dissolved.

Empowerment has to be sharply distinguished from the emphasis given by local authorities and health authorities and by the Citizen's Charter on getting close to the customer. This has led to public authorities seeking to make their services more responsive to the public, carrying out surveys, instituting customer care programmes. William Waldegrave might have had more basis for his argument that the Citizen's Charter movement had resolved the issue of public accountability if he had shown that the changes had empowered the public, rather than made the services more responsive. The Citizen's Charter is not about empowering the public. Even in the area of customer choice, there has been little development. Most of the changes in, for example, the development of the internal market have been about increasing producer choice. Even in education where there has been an emphasis on parental choice, there has been little extension of choice in practice and a significant reduction in choice over the curriculum. These developments are important in building up the quality of public services and making them more responsive to the public. They do not, however, pass power to the public.

Empowering the public as opposed to responding to the public requires further steps. To give the public more power removes issues from the provider of welfare services:

- to give choice to individual members of the public means that the provider does not determine the choice;
- to give the public the right in a referendum not merely to express views but to determine the issue, means that the public and not the authority decides;
- to set up a community forum not merely to discuss issues but to determine how, for example, resources are used, means that the authority has shared or even given up control of the allocation of resources provided within a framework of policy and within the resources available, which necessarily limits the choices available.

Empowering the public may reduce the burden of public accountability: it does not remove the issue, because there are limits to the extent to which it can be carried. Empowerment takes place within a framework of collective choice for which the issue of public accountability has to be faced.

Who is to be empowered?

Any serious thinking about empowerment must involve not just clarifying what is meant by the term but asking who is to be empowered. It is not sufficient to speak in general terms of empowering the public because a distinction can be drawn between:

- the public as customer;
- the public as citizen;
- the public as community.

The public as customer focuses attention on the individual user of a service, although it has to be recognized that in many public services there is more than one customer. Empowering the public as customer involves extending the choices available to them or at least, by making clear the service to which they are entitled, giving them the means of securing redress as well as providing equality and ease of access. It does need to be recognized, though, that this may escalate the demand for services and thus the requirement to ration them.

The public as citizen focuses attention on the individual as part of the process of government itself. Citizens may or may not be users of a service but irrespective of whether they are users of a service they are entitled as citizens to a share in decision-making on issues in the public domain. It is not only the users but also the citizens who can be empowered.

299

Empowering the public as citizen involves being clear about rights (for example, the right to vote, the right to know, the right to explanation, the right to be heard and the right to be listened to), and about how they can be enhanced. These are basic rights necessary for discourse and decision in the public domain. Empowering these rights as citizen involves treating these rights as basic conditions whose full potential is yet to be realized. And, of course, beyond civil rights, the citizen has economic and social rights, for without these a citizen may lack the basis to play a full part in society.

The public as community provides a focus beyond the individual, whether as user or as citizen, and on the collective concerns of those who live within an area. In every community there can be shared interests, views and concerns, which may, however, only be identified through processes of debate and discussion. Communities can be regarded both as collective customers for services, such as clean air provided not to individuals but generally, and as the citizenry, whose collective action seeks to shape services, mould the environment, and mark out the way of life that distinguishes individual cities, towns and villages. Empowering the public as community involves giving them the right to participate in and, whenever possible, determine issues affecting the community through direct control and through such institutions as neighbourhood forums or community councils. Empowering the public as community involves the creation of new democratic frameworks that may be concerned with the full range of activities that can be undertaken by the local authorities on behalf of their community.

The dilemmas of empowerment

Reconsideration of empowerment needs to go beyond intellectual discourse. One of the major challenges for the coming decade will be to find ways of carrying forward all three strands of empowerment. However, this will not be simple as there are major dilemmas:

- empowering one customer can be disempowering another, if their interests are in conflict;
- empowering the citizen can lead to decisions that disempower particular customers;
- empowering the citizenry as the community will lead to decisions that are opposed by some individual citizens;
- empowering the present can disempower future generations.

The dilemmas can be illustrated by the following examples:

- a decision on a planning application satisfies one customer but dissatisfies another;
- a patient on a waiting list for an operation is delayed an appointment because another patient has greater priority;
- a local authority evicts certain tenants for racial harassment.

In short, actions that empower some may disempower others. To have regard only for the customer or citizen or the community at large is not enough. It is all too easy to make simple mistakes. One is to assume that the local authority can empower the public as citizen and community through periodic elections alone. A second is to assume that because some citizens or customers are empowered, all are empowered. Too often an authority assumes that in access for all, all have equal access. Yet there is a disparity in power of which an authority should be aware and which can only be overcome by purposive action grounded in understanding.

A third mistake is to assume that because a local authority or other public authority is (or is assumed to be) an expression of the public as citizens or as community, there is no need to empower the public as customers. Because a service is provided to meet a public purpose does not mean that individual customers should not be given choice within the limits set by public purpose. Equally, because the standards of service may be determined by the public purpose and debate does not mean that they should not be expressed as rights for the customer.

In simple terms, there is a need for a balance between the interests of customer, citizen and community both in the short term and the long term, just as there is a need for a balance between different groups. The nature of that balance will vary from service to service and from activity to activity depending on the nature of public purpose and the type of activity. What is clear is that achieving that balance will require redressing an imbalance created by disparities of power.

Conclusion

The argument of this chapter has been that there is a growing crisis of public accountability in the welfare services because the traditional model of public accountability is under strain. Changes in recent years have meant than an increased burden is being placed on an already overstrained doctrine of ministerial responsibility by the removal of functions from local government and by the growth in appointed or self-appointed boards that lack their own

301

basis in public accountability. It is argued that these trends need reversing but that more is required to turn public accountability into an active and continuous relationship. Such development could be associated with empowering the public whether as customer, as citizen or as community, although because empowerment necessarily takes place within wider frameworks of collective choice the issue of public accountability remains. Empowerment would help to create the active relationship on which public accountability should rest.

Suggested reading

The context is discussed in Simey (1988) and Waldegrave (1993). The system of accountability in five major public services is set out in Day & Klein (1987).

CHAPTER 13
Quality in welfare services

Lucy Gaster

Fad or necessity?

A recent survey of local authorities in England and Wales (Local Government Management Board 1993) found that a third of local authorities had formed a corporate policy for quality and a further 40 per cent were in the process of doing so. By December 1992, 28 charters had been published under the government's Citizen's Charter initiative. In 1991, when the first module on service quality was introduced on a new master's programme at the School for Advanced Urban Studies at the University of Bristol, it was hard to find suitable material about quality from the welfare sector. By the end of 1993 it was almost impossible to avoid the word in any publication, whether about the public, private or voluntary sector. Wastepaper baskets up and down the country were full of "standards", "charters", "service quality contracts" and "promises" from banks, public transport, local authorities and health authorities.

Does this proliferation of written material mean that the delivery of services has really changed? If so, how has it changed, and how were the decisions made as to the direction of change? Are quality policies simply a veneer, aiming for the glossiness of some parts of the private sector, in keeping with the times? Translated to the welfare services, are they perhaps a survival policy, part of an attempt to stem a tide of policies that may leave purely residual services high and dry? More positively, does the recent emphasis on quality perhaps signify renewed faith that welfare services are a key to the country's future? Do they provide the opportunity to bring them up to the top standards to which all citizens have an inalienable right? Finally, does all this talk of quality mean, first, that quality in welfare services did not exist before; and, secondly, that once thought of, there are some simple "recipes" for putting it into practice?

Not all these questions can be answered here, but my aim in this chapter is to show that, despite the cynicism and sloganizing that are beginning to dog the quality debate, and despite the very real problems and issues that arise when considering what we mean by "quality" in the welfare sector, service quality *is* to be taken seriously.

In this chapter, I look at four aspects of quality. First, there is the question of what kind of quality? The relevance of concepts derived from private sector experience, and the public sector origins and theoretical frameworks are described. This provides a context for thinking about why quality is on the welfare sector agenda at all, and whether it will stay there. Next, some different ways of defining quality and the "quality chain" are examined in some detail: these both provide the springboard for questions of implementation and measurement (not considered here) and are a trigger for thinking about the future: this is done in the final section.

What kind of "quality"?

Private sector quality: can it be left to the "customer"?

"Service quality" as it is interpreted in this chapter is not necessarily the same as that in the minds of central government ministers or of the many purveyors of private sector practices in the public, welfare sector. That kind of quality is essentially managerial. It is aimed at increased efficiency (not, of course, a bad thing, but not synonymous with quality). It is measured by customer satisfaction and market share, by the winning of contracts and by profit levels. It tends to emphasize the need for standardization and "zero defects" – appropriate enough for manufactured goods, but totally inappropriate in a service culture where sensitivity and responsiveness and a willingness to experiment and improve are the key requirements. It is, in sum, an approach that depends on the premise that the operational environment is that of the market.

This private sector approach to quality – developed by "gurus" such as Deming (1986), Juran (1979), Crosby (1986) and Peters & Waterman (1982) in the United States, by Oakland (1989) in the UK, and largely based on statements of faith rather than systematic research, has some benefits to

304

offer welfare services. It emphasizes the importance of the "customer", and it helps towards an understanding that services need to be properly designed, with an attention to detail that has often been missing in the public services. It is not, however, enough in itself. This is because the market option, and the world of competition, is not appropriate to or effective in the provision of most welfare services.

Welfare quality, like many other aspects of welfare, needs to incorporate some expression of active involvement – empowerment, even – of consumers and citizens. It requires negotiation and a clear understanding that some aspects of quality will almost certainly need to be traded against others, whether because of resource or legal constraints, or because the interests of different sets of consumers and producers do not coincide. It needs to acknowledge that even if only current users (if they can be defined) are involved – and the net in fact needs to be spread far more widely – they rarely have the power of choice supposedly available in a free market.

For welfare quality needs, above all, to acknowledge that welfare services are public goods and that quality involves more than just the immediate consumer. They are complex services, involving an array of different organizations that include not just the statutory sector, powerful though it is as the main fund holder, but also large and small voluntary organizations, community organizations, the private sector and the public at large. All have a part to play, in a way that simply is not applicable to the workings of the private market.

Consumer choice

In a market, quality is measured through levels of satisfaction and market share. Effective market mechanisms therefore require individual consumers to be able to exercise choice. Without rehearsing the arguments in detail (see Le Grand 1993), this requires three things: a range of services from which to choose; enough information on which to base informed choices; and the power to choose freely between known options. Not all these conditions apply in the private sector: monopolies and oligopolies restrict choice, as of course does poverty; and private companies are generally pretty selective about the information they make publicly available. In the welfare sector, for different reasons, the conditions for real consumer choice apply even more rarely.

First, most direct consumers of public welfare (or even proxy consumers such as GPs or social workers) do not have access to data on which to base informed choices. Despite a statutory duty to provide far more information than the private sector ever does, the speed of change, complexity of the services and circumstances of service use (crisis, vulnerability etc.) would mean that a *Which?* of welfare, even a local one, would be an extraordinarily difficult project.

Secondly, welfare consumers generally have neither the power of the purse, nor the confidence to confront professional judgements, nor the option of walking away from the services once inside the welfare structure. In addition, some services are compulsory, with enforcement required by legislation for the safety of individuals and society.

Thirdly, the range of choice available in practice to individual consumers is likely to be restricted: block contracts limit the total number of suppliers, while "spot contracts" create fluctuating demand, potentially driving smaller producers out of the "market" altogether.

On top of this, the type of performance requirements included in contracts and the need to be financially viable create pressures on welfare providers to "cream-skim" (that is, take the easiest and most profitable cases). Some parts of the "market" – the chronically sick, single parents, people from black and ethnic minorities, even people who smoke – could be (and are) denied a service altogether.

In these circumstances, quality cannot simply be judged either from "satisfaction" levels or by the number of users. Even where real choices do exist and people can stop using particular services if they want to, the mere possibility of "exit" does not help managers to know in what respects the existing service quality needs to be improved. Traditional market research can help, as long as the right questions are asked. However, as the private sector is also finding, direct communication and dialogue with consumers is likely to provide much more useful answers.

In purely practical terms, and leaving aside considerations of ethics and equity arising from the fact that welfare services are *public* services, market mechanisms are unsuitable and inappropriate as the starting point for quality.

Welfare service quality

However, even the use of "voice" as the route to quality is not straightforward. In the welfare market, the long chain of purchaser–provider–subcontractor–assessor of needs makes for a wide gap between the user, consumer and citizen on the one hand, and those with power to make decisions on the other. These gaps are compounded by the lack of accountability of many of the bodies now responsible for the procurement and provision of welfare services (see Chapter 12). There is no obligation to involve local people, as voters or as service users.

If individuals, in the role of consumer or local citizen, are relatively power-less to affect the quality of welfare services, a different, more participative approach is needed. This applies not just to service delivery and measure-ment, but to the sphere of policy-making too. Quality as it is experienced derives from how the service is defined. There is no sense in democratically involving the public or anyone else (staff, for example) in the quality of deliv-ery if they have had no opportunity to say what they think is important and necessary – the service objectives, priorities and standards – in the first place.

Neither the right of (accountable) organizations responsible for services to have the final say, nor the need for leadership and commitment at "the top" is in dispute. However, the interdependent actions of a wide range of "stakeholders" and "interests" affect the overall service quality: their involve-ment is also essential (see Sanderson 1992). The role both of frontline staff and of the public, as consumers and as citizens, is highly significant. The position of individual consumers and of some groups of consumers and non-consumers is relatively weak. This needs to be recognized and responded to, through policies to improve consultation and participation with local people. Positive action may need to be taken to ensure that the voice of the least powerful is heard and their rights addressed.

Public choice and pluralism

The current charter-based approach to service quality, which depends for its success on complaints and league tables, could be seen as an illustration of "public choice" theories. Such theories assume that both consumers and producers act rationally in their own best interests: self-interest is the funda-mental basis of decisions. However, it is a confused argument. Public serv-ants may in practice work in ways that serve their own interests (alongside other more altruistic forms of behaviour), but the emphasis on the role of the "customer" in these charters means that in practice providers must act in the interests of others.

Public choice theory emphasizes the role of the individual. It does not explain why, in the public sector and particularly in local government, the councils that started in the mid 1980s to emphasize quality tended to be

Labour authorities with a collectivist orientation. These quality and public service initiatives were often led by newly elected councillors uncontaminated by traditional local government cultures and practices. They were anxious to reassert the democratic role of local government, bringing to the debate a concern for the rights and needs of society as a whole. This included not only current service users, but also the local community, and excluded users and citizens. At the same time, they saw that public services as currently provided were often simply not good enough or consistent enough to meet even the minimum demands of actual, current users ("customers"). Such quality policies grew from a mixture of pragmatism and political ideology.

This approach to quality implies that several parties, all with more or less equal rights (though not equal power), are automatically involved in issues of quality. It is not down to the individual or professional, in the role either of producer or consumer, to determine the nature of quality in welfare services, or how it is to be achieved: collective effort is required. If a theoretical framework is needed for the consideration of quality, the multiplicity of groups with different interests suggests that a pluralist analysis is more appropriate. It is this that informs the rest of this chapter.

Quality on the agenda – past and future

While much of the rest of this chapter will be concerned with definitions, we first need to consider whether quality really is an issue for the 1990s and, if so, why? In order to look at the future, we need first to look at the past.

At a rather general level, it can be argued that welfare services should have certain properties that ensure that they meet the needs of both society and of individuals and their families. Many of these properties can be expressed in quantitative terms, and that is how, during the life of the welfare state, it has largely been done. If new needs were identified, extra provision was made. An incremental process led to the *ad hoc* building up of a variety of services, whose justification for their existence, and the way that they were provided, was largely determined by generally well-intentioned producers with little idea of what consumers really wanted or needed.

At the organizational level, similar processes took place. In strongly hierarchical organizations, even strict procedures could not entirely bridge the gaps between the formulation of policy and their actual implementation. Such gaps were reinforced through the formal and informal discretion available to professionals and other frontline staff (Lipsky 1980). They tended to implement services as they "knew best". The result was great variation between services, with very little monitoring for consistency, equity or effectiveness – a curious contrast with the "New Right"'s critique of the welfare state, founded as it is on the assumption of factory-like homogeneity of public services.

Pressures for a change in attitudes and practice came from two main sources. First, the squeeze on resources for the public sector – "the party is over" – came as early as 1976. New demands could no longer be met by an "add-on" approach. By 1979, with the advent of Thatcher's Conservative administration and the ideological bias against the public provision of services, the scene was set where, increasingly, the whole welfare sector was in a position of having to fight for every penny, and to justify its very existence. This meant that such services had to be far more explicit about what they did and what they were there to do, to be clearer than ever before that quantity was not enough: quality was now of the essence.

At the same time, the producer dominated approach to service provision began to give way to an understanding that consumers and the public were not in existence just to take what was on offer. Underlined by the low turnouts in local elections, public services such as those provided by local government needed greater public support if they were to survive. Services had to be of good enough quality for local communities to make the effort to preserve, protect and campaign for them. In the early 1980s, few public services were eligible for such support, being bureaucratic, remote and often inefficient and patronizing.

Programmes began to be introduced in the late 1980s to address these factors. In the National Health Service, the emphasis was on the quality process. Ideas about quality control, quality assurance and, eventually, total quality management (TQM) became in turn the slogans of the day. However, like many top–down management initiatives (these were mostly introduced and fostered, through financial incentives, by what is now the Department of Health), it is difficult to be sure of the efficacy of these programmes – have they helped change staff behaviour, has the public benefited? Some aspects of the "hotel services" may have marginally improved in some hospitals (patient surveys tended to concentrate on this aspect of the health services); nursing-led procedures for quality assurance in the disposal of needles and other processes were developed (Dalley 1991); the respective roles of "managers" and "professionals" in managing quality began to be questioned (Ellis 1988). What was missing, it would seem, was any philosophy to back what appeared to be the latest management fad.

309

If a philosophy existed, it came more clearly from local government, where local citizens' charters, beginning in York and Harlow in 1989, symbolized an attempt to express a new relationship with the public. The instrument here was not the adoption of quality processes, but a statement of what the service was intended to do – its *outputs and outcomes* – together with the provision of means of redress (complaints systems) if it did not come up to scratch.

It was this approach, informed by a rather different, more individualistic ideology, that underlay the Citizen's Charter initiative adopted by John Major's Government in 1991 (Cm 1599). The main weakness of the national "charter" approach is that, without an involvement of consumers and citizens in the setting of the standards, without an assessment of need and without programmes of implementation to ensure that the standards are met, their credibility in the minds of the public is distinctly limited. Hence the overloading of the wastepaper baskets referred to earlier. The public needs to be convinced that these charters really mean something: past evidence of how services have been provided do not inspire confidence in the present efforts.

This is not to dismiss what has been achieved through the charter approach to quality. There may be a lot of confusion about objectives, but the pressure to be clear what is the nature of the service, and to communicate – even negotiate – with consumers and the public, has provided a potentially invaluable starting point for really thinking about quality.

Much legislation of the past decade has produced many problems for both consumers and producers of welfare services. However, as far as quality is concerned, the new laws have undoubtedly had the incidental and important benefit of forcing, willy-nilly, a much clearer and more explicit definition of services. In some cases, such as the 1990 NHS and Community Care legislation and the 1989 Local Government and Housing Act, there has also been a specific requirement to consider the views of "users" and tenants. This has led to a greater awareness of the need to define "the customer". The very word "customer" is, for the reasons already given, inappropriate for most of the welfare services. But to think about who it is who uses, or who has a right to use and to speak about, the whole range of services, the consideration of *citizen* rights as well as consumer rights, is beginning to put pressure on welfare professionals to be less precious about their "professionalism". And in those organizations with values of equity and equality, the voice of those who have in the past been excluded from exercising their citizen and consumer rights may now also be heard.

At the same time, new management practices and structures – the delegation of budgets and the decentralization of services, more teamwork and multidisciplinary project work – have begun to lead to better understanding of the interaction between the organization and the community (the "frontline"). The role of frontline staff begins to be more clearly recognized and valued, the chains of command begin to be shortened, the possibility emerges of aligning responsibility with control nearer the point of service delivery. This provides an infrastructure for a more responsive service relating to local and different needs. The concept of "tight-loose" organizations, with clear central policy frameworks and resources and devolved responsibility for action begins to take shape.

This means that the foundations for fully fledged quality programmes are beginning to be laid. This, if the welfare sector is to survive, is a helpful, indeed essential start.

Defining quality

As all the texts – and common sense – emphasize, defining quality is not easy. Despite the apparent ease with which national "standards" are being developed, there are considerable limitations to them. Quality, particularly service quality, is not an objective, technical "fact", but a series of dimensions and characteristics whose importance will vary for different people at different times.

It is only necessary to think of one's last visit to a hospital or doctor to realize this. At the beginning, especially if one is in pain, the need for pure relief is uppermost. As time goes on, the relationship with the medical staff – do you feel free to ask questions? do the answers appear to be honest? – is likely to become more significant. If one is frightened or staying for a long time, the soothing or harsh nature of the environment, the suitability of the diet, visiting times for relatives, all start to become more prominent. Once the treatment is complete, you may reflect on whether the choice of treatment was itself suitable, whether any choices were even offered, whether enough information about the treatment process and after-effects was given. At the time, gratitude was possibly the dominant feeling. Later on, it becomes possible to be constructively critical.

So the subjective view of the consumer will vary enormously, according to circumstances. Measuring quality through "satisfaction" levels has, therefore, limited value. It can be helpful, but a more practical way of defining quality is needed as well.

A detailed definition of quality appropriate for all welfare services would be hopelessly cumbersome and bureaucratic. Some kind of framework is needed. This falls into three parts. First, we need to distinguish between ideal and attainable quality, and between attainable and minimum quality. Secondly, the gaps between what the consumer expects or hopes for, and what the organization can offer – and the resulting levels of "satisfaction" – have to be narrowed down. Thirdly, the actual characteristics of each service that make up its definable quality need to be classified in terms that can be understood and debated by all the stakeholders.

The very process of defining quality of welfare services helps to identify issues that, on present trends, are likely to arise in the future. This section therefore goes into some detail about the three approaches outlined above.

Ideal, attainable and minimum standards

Quality can be high, low, or anything in between. Therefore, it is important to be clear which is intended within a quality improvement programme. Can a service be "good enough", or is "quality" more than that? If so, can intermediate, "attainable" levels of quality be targeted on the road to achieving "ideal" quality? Can the danger of working to the lowest common denominator be avoided?

Despite limitations of resources, staff capacity or other constraints (the pressure of new legislation, for example), it is a useful exercise to try to define the "ideal" quality of a particular service. This may seem academic, but the advantage is that it makes explicit, in a way that a more "realistic" discussion might not, the underlying values and long-term strategic objectives seen from a range of perspectives. It is particularly important to include members of the public at this stage, in the form of actual, potential or past consumers and as members of the local community, so as to avoid cosy producer and professional dominated definitions.

However, there must be a second stage to this process, which is to think about what is achievable within a given timescale. This "attainable" standard will be shaped in accordance with shorter term priorities. An aid to this phase is an organizational analysis that identifies existing practice and areas for immediate improvement or consolidation. A distinction might be made at this stage between those areas of activity within the quality group's control, and those that depend on the co-operation of others, including the public.

Finally, there is the question of minimum standards, the level below which the service quality must not drop. For an organization that has not thought very much about quality before, this may have to be the starting point. For example, some areas of "good practice" will certainly already be in place. Rather than seeing them as a kind of threat that appears to challenge other, perhaps easier, ways of doing things, these examples can be used positively to construct a basic standard to which all can work. Sometimes the "good practice" may come from other organizations carrying out similar functions (a "benchmarking" process). There is a danger here: if traditional (mainly quantitative) performance indicators are solely derived from this minimum level of quality, the tendency is for it to become the norm (Carter 1991). New kinds of qualitative performance indicator are needed that encourage constructive consumer feedback, and that encourage higher levels of performance, leading to greater job satisfaction. Such performance indicators would focus on teams rather than individuals (quality is almost never an individual matter alone) and be part of an "enabling" rather than a restrictive, non risk taking and hierarchical organizational culture.

The issue of which kind of standard is being sought – minimum, attainable or ideal – becomes particularly important in the context of the contract culture, as we shall see.

Expectations and satisfaction

Consumer satisfaction is not acceptable as a sole way of defining quality in the welfare sector. Some problems with this have already been identified, arising from the very imperfect market of welfare provision, from the fact that welfare involves more than just the consumer, and from the unequal relationship between service providers and consumers. Nevertheless, the notion of public satisfaction can be useful if it is *combined* (through a process of negotiation) with the views and requirements of other stakeholders and interests (not excluding staff) to make up the overall quality standard of each of the services that constitute the welfare sector. But if this is to be done, the concept of satisfaction itself needs to be analyzed.

How do individuals – satisfaction is a very individualistic notion – judge whether a service is satisfactory or not? The answer depends on two key factors: the stage of the service when satisfaction is being measured; and the initial expectations of the service.

313

Take timing first. If you are asked, even anonymously, what you think of the service while you are still receiving it, you may give a different answer from one that would be given, say, six months after the service was complete. Later on, the power relationships are different and you are more certain about the outcome: at an early stage you are dependent on the service providers, unwilling to cause any possible antagonism and unsure of the probable outcome. The answers to a "satisfaction" survey at either of these stages will be very different.

Secondly, levels of "satisfaction" are affected by initial expectations and actual experience. Although past experience of many welfare services has led to low expectations of welfare services in general, it is easy to dismiss survey findings showing low levels of satisfaction on the grounds that public expectations were unrealistically high. Conversely, service providers are sometimes afraid that asking questions about satisfaction levels will itself raise expectations that cannot be met. They claim that if you ask consumers what they want, they will simply want more. In the constrained financial circumstances in which most welfare services operate the result could be more complaints and greater dissatisfaction, even when the service is improving.

In practice, both satisfaction and expectations tend to be adjusted according to actual experience. If consumers know what to expect and have some faith in the good intentions of the service providers, better understanding develops, even if the ideal result cannot be achieved because of resource or other constraints. Feedback based on realistic expectations helps to pinpoint areas for potential improvement. Also, clear mutual expectations and reasonable levels of satisfaction may in themselves improve the quality of the service in the form of more effective communication, a key element in all face-to-face services.

It is easier to be satisfied with some services than with others. Public libraries always come top in satisfaction surveys of local government. Personal welfare services, whose results tend to be unpredictable and which raise far higher levels of personal anxiety, are likely to come lower in the league tables. This does not, of course, necessarily mean that they are of low quality. It does underline the need to be cautious about the results of surveys.

Three dimensions of quality

The concept of negotiation has been at the heart of much of the discussion in this chapter. Standards can be at different levels: what levels? Satisfaction can be differentially interpreted: how can common ground be established? Resources may be far short of what is needed for the "ideal" service: how can the "essential" ingredients for quality be agreed? Consumers may have very different interests from each other, while residents, citizens, voluntary organizations and a whole range of other interested parties may have conflicting views as to what they mean by "quality": can a common language be developed that enables these issues to be thrashed out constructively and practically?

There are no simple answers, as I have said, but recognizing some of these dilemmas and contradictions should help to avoid the pitfall of simplistic, short-term solutions. A quality project is a long-term project, probably taking a minimum of three to five years to become established as a "normal" way of thinking, once the initial commitment has been made. It depends heavily on explicit or implied values and, if it is not to drop from view as soon as the next management or political "flavour of the month" arrives, it needs to be linked clearly with long-term strategic objectives.

This inevitably means that quality will be defined differently in different organizations and over time. Starting points will differ, as will intended outcomes. However, some of the quality processes, involving organizational structures, cultures and change, may be similar, and this will help organizations learn from each other, rather than starting from the beginning each time.

Several writers – Donabedian (1980), Stewart & Walsh (1989), Parasuraman et al. (1988) – have come up with the notion that quality can be seen in three basic dimensions: the "technical" quality, or fitness for purpose (what Bouckaert & Pollitt (1994) call the "objective" quality); the non-technical quality reflecting the service relationship; and the environmental quality, or "service surround", which is the context for the other two.

Having worked with these concepts for several years now, they seem remarkably robust. They are helpful at a practical level, to make sure that all angles are covered; and they are helpful at an analytical level, identifying, for example, the actual focus of different quality programmes such as quality assurance or quality control. Finally, they show that definitions of quality that emphasize standardization – non-variance and "zero defects", "conformance to specification" and "fitness for use" or for "purpose" – though highly relevant to manufactured goods, are not by themselves enough when it comes to services.

What do these three dimensions consist of? The simplest way of answering that question is to divide the quality characteristics of any service into

315

those that describe what the service is actually meant to do; those that relate to how it is to be done; and those that describe the physical circumstances that can enable the first two groups of quality characteristics to be put to maximum effect.

To resume the medical example, if an injection is given in such a grumpy or rushed way that the patient is made to feel like a "non-person", they are unlikely to feel able to ask questions or to return if something is apparently going wrong; if they have been kept waiting for hours in unpleasant, unwelcoming surroundings without any explanation for delays, they will not be in a mood to listen to advice, however pleasantly and honestly delivered. In either case, the effectiveness of the actual medical treatment could well be diminished, if not cancelled out. If communication is poor, the wrong diagnosis may be made, or different treatment options may not be considered. All these aspects need, therefore, to be included in a definition of the quality standard being aimed at, and all three dimensions are interdependent, even though their relative significance will be different in different services. Thinking about one dimension without consideration for the other aspects is likely to reduce the overall quality.

Thus, when it comes to implementation, if the focus is only on the "non-technical" or environmental aspects of a service, programmes of "customer care" may be introduced which, while useful in improving personal interaction, do not tackle underlying issues relating to the objectives and nature of the service. Expensive quality assurance programmes may be introduced which, with their emphasis on procedures, actually increase bureaucracy without ensuring that the product is one that consumers (and here I do not just mean fund holding health and social care "purchasers") in fact want or need.

Possibly most important of all, the identification of these three strands in defining quality gives a kick-start to the process of negotiation on which the eventual definition – and standards – must be based. It is sometimes quite difficult to disentangle the "technical" from the "interpersonal" aspects, especially in personal services where most of the service is interpersonal. However, thinking about services in this way makes it possible for all concerned to understand more clearly the essential nature – the technical quality – of a *particular* service, while perhaps setting broader standards for how all services provided by a single organization should be delivered. Similarly, broad policies can be developed for the quality of the physical environment, including not only buildings and signposting, but also the queuing and telephone response systems that are part of the infrastructure on which each service is built.

Once the key characteristics under each dimension are identified (and each party to the discussion is likely to have a different view as to what is important) the need for "trade-offs" can be considered. This process – the shift from the "ideal" to the "attainable" – would take into account such criteria as statutory and financial requirements, the needs of different groups, the capacity of the organization to deliver, and the values such as efficiency or equality that will give some characteristics priority over others.

For example, is it better to have a quick throughput, with very short waiting times and short waiting lists, or might consumers be willing to wait longer if they feel that full consideration will be given to their problems when they are seen? Can external pressures such as government performance indicators be weighed against internal and public requirements, balancing the need to achieve outcomes as well as throughputs, developing a preventative or developmental rather than a firefighting approach, thinking short-term *and* long-term?

Many of these questions could be debated under the heading of the "non-technical" dimension of quality – an aspect that is likely to be missed in the climate of contracts, which emphasize the short-term and the technical aspects of service delivery.

The quality chain

Attention has so far focused on the idea of negotiating definitions of quality, building on the collective role of consumers and citizens. However, when thinking about how services are designed (or, if not consciously designed, how they operate in practice), it is useful to consider the different stages of production required to achieve the service as it reaches individual consumers. This is the "service chain" or "quality chain".

Very few services are under the complete control of one individual or team alone. Almost all depend, in part or in whole, on the actions of others. Mapping and linking the different actions together, including the stages of service planning and design, helps to identify the key elements of a service as well as possible weak links. At each stage, there is a both a producer and a consumer, traditionally located within a single organization, but increasingly, in the fragmented world of welfare, dispersed among a variety of organizations.

This mapping process can have two results. It helps identify who should be party to the process of negotiating the overall quality of a service. It may also throw up questions of who has responsibility at each stage, and whether that responsibility is matched by appropriate levels of control. In a "blame" culture it is easy to shrug off responsibility, as Catherine McDonald (1992) showed in her study of a county social services department's approach to quality. Councillors, senior managers and team leaders were all variously identified as "weak links" in the chain of implementation. At the same time, several of the managers interviewed felt that a crucial block was the attitude of frontline workers. They needed, it was thought, to be "liberated", to be given "permission" to deliver a quality service. This pattern, in a hierarchical and departmental culture such as this appeared to be, would not be uncommon.

In this chapter, processes of implementing policies to improve quality are not being discussed. However, in any implementation scheme, the connections between the different elements in the service chain, and the development of a culture that supports the process of strengthening weak links and making connections between them (rather than passing the blame literally down the line) are key elements for quality organizations to consider.

Some key issues for the future

Basic principles

Most of this chapter has been devoted to examining why quality is important to the welfare services and what the concept of quality might mean in practice. The exact definition and the quality standards that are derived from that will vary from service to service. It is likely that in all cases there will be considerable emphasis on such factors as reliability, sensitivity, viability and maximal choice. Factors such as efficiency, equality and equity would also be included by some, though my preference is to see these as related but separate factors (Gaster 1994).

While there is certainly no "right way" to define, introduce, implement, monitor and evaluate quality, certain issues will be important and of continuing concern. These include the following:

- Definitions need to be multidimensional and to differentiate between longer-term "ideal" standards and shorter-term "attainable" standards. They should not depend solely on consumer satisfaction, but this should be taken into account.
- A new way of thinking needs to be evolved, where values are explicit,

objectives clear, and each element in the service chain is committed, supported, involved and rewarded in improving services. This requires a new culture and possibly new structures. Hierarchical and bureaucratic methods of working are inappropriate, while professionals need to reassess their roles. Different skills – of negotiation, networking, teamworking and "enabling" in its broadest sense – may become more important than some of the traditional skills that have contributed towards a producer dominated culture in the past.

– This way of thinking has much in common with "total quality management" (in so far as it can be clearly defined), but in addition stresses the importance of involving key participants and interests, including unions, professional organizations, the voluntary sector, and above all, consumers, citizens and frontline staff.

– Following from this, quality is a process of negotiation, requiring clarity as to what is or is not negotiable, and recognizing that neat consensus will not necessarily be achieved.

– Issues of accountability and participation are crucial to service quality in welfare services.

– Devolved decision-making within clear policy frameworks is likely to provide great potential for improving personal services where the quality is largely in the actual interaction between provider and consumer.

– In so far as quality is a function of public satisfaction, it is important to recognize that as quality improves, expectations will rise: satisfaction levels will probably never quite catch up. A high level of complaints can actually be a good thing, not a sign of failure, since they may demonstrate public confidence in getting a response, compared with past assumptions that "they won't take any notice".

Is it possible?

It will be apparent from the discussion at the beginning of the chapter that the aim of improving the quality of welfare services, vital though it is for their survival, could easily be hijacked by other agendas. Already, quality is becoming synonymous with value for money and especially with saving money in the eyes of government ministers (for example when awarding Chartermarks under the Citizen's Charter initiative). Much of the language and the processes imported from the manufacturing private sector and from the market economy is inappropriate – or limited in value – for welfare

319

services. These have collective and community responsibilities and relationships with consumers (not "customers") that, to counteract the disempowerment of many if not most actual and potential consumers of these services, require active processes of consultation and participation.

While this approach to quality may seem eminently logical and appropriate, four factors may inhibit the successful implementation of local quality programmes in the future. These are:
 – the imposition of national standards;
 – the impact of contracts;
 – the fragmentation of services;
 – the costs of quality.

The idea of "standards" is intimately bound up with quality. However, national standards could not only produce standardized approaches to service that, by definition, undermine *local* flexibility and responsiveness. They could also, backed as they often are by national performance indicators, result in a minimalist approach that is actually the opposite of what quality should be about.

So, whatever national guidelines exist – in the name of regulation or deregulation as the case may be – it should be possible to develop local interpretations. These would be based on the views and needs of key local interests and links in the quality chain. The imposition of externally defined standards can be reassuring up to a point. But since such standards will always be subject to local interpretation and implementation they could, if they by-pass staff and ignore the needs of consumers and local communities, even be counter-productive to the search for quality.

Secondly, the nature of contracts and their specification leads to similar concerns. Very few stakeholders/interests are generally involved in the construction or monitoring of contracts. The interests most likely to be squeezed out, however good the intentions, are the consumers, especially those most often excluded from the policy process because of discrimination, poverty or ignorance. Contract negotiation is simply too complicated and, as research has found (Smith et al. 1993), the arguments and discussions between the "big boys" of social services and health departments almost automatically put other groups off the agenda. An extra complication arises if voluntary organizations, for example, are seen (or conveniently labelled) as having a "commercial interest" as a potential provider of services.

In addition, the legalistic nature of contracts and the culture of enforcement rather than co-operation are, despite any "quality clauses" that might be included, likely to lead to rigid interpretations and contract specification of ever increasing amounts of detail. Consequently, levels of discretion and flexibility just where they are most needed – at the point of service delivery – are decreased. This, too, militates against a concept of quality that understands and responds to different needs.

Thirdly, there is the issue of "fragmentation". This relates most specifically to the "service chain" described earlier. When the chain spreads across several organizations with different values, service objectives and recruitment policies, not only is it difficult to maintain reasonable levels of service consistency and to provide clear channels of redress; it is also difficult for service producers to know where responsibility lies and how different organizations can effectively co-ordinate their actions in the best interests of the consumer. This is of course an issue that affects not only the quality debate, but also issues of accountability and empowerment. However, it is when getting into the details of service design, and identifying the ever widening range of stakeholders and interests, that the complexity and manageability of the whole process comes most clearly into question.

Last but not least, there is the issue of cost. This is partly connected with contracts, in so far as purchasers are increasingly demanding proof of existence of some kind of standard quality assurance system and providers are feeling that their competitive edge will be enhanced by being externally certificated (for example, through the British Standard 5750). Development and maintenance costs of such systems are high, and could easily altogether rule out some organizations, particularly the smaller voluntary and community based agencies.

Systematic approaches to developing a quality "culture" are essential, but standardized approaches are not. The welfare sector desperately needs diversity and, by building on existing strengths, organizations can develop quality systems without sacrificing their own individuality. Requiring BS 5750 or its equivalent is fine and easy for the client or purchaser organizations. It can be a heavy price for the contractors or provider organizations to pay, without (because of the emphasis on processes, not outputs or outcomes) necessarily benefiting the consumer.

Some organizations are, not surprisingly, frightened at the apparent costs of quality. This is partly for the reasons stated above, partly because, among all the other priorities and constraints, devising and implementing a quality programme can appear to be the last straw. Certainly there is an investment price, one that few industries these days do not think it worth spending: but there are also benefits. Acquiring a "competitive edge" is one such benefit. Providing a better service, to the satisfaction of workers, consumers and paymasters (councillors, boards and government in the first place, ultimately the public as taxpayers) is another.

Conclusion

High quality is essential for survival of welfare services. It is both inappropriate and impossible to take a mechanistic approach – quality is not a matter of aiming for standardization, "statistical process control", "zero defects". Flexibility and responsiveness are the keys to welfare quality based on a real understanding of needs and requirements. Quality standards have to be negotiated. Like any negotiation, this means that some aspects of quality have to be "traded off" against one another. It is no longer up to the producer to work on the basis of unstated assumptions of what is "good" for consumers. Quality policies can be used to reduce uncertainty and increase reliability, but they must also encourage innovation and responsiveness. This means that risk taking needs to be encouraged, but within clearer confines and with greater public understanding and political and managerial support.

Organizations can learn from each other, but there are no ready-made solutions: everyone has to think through for themselves, as individuals and in groups, what quality they want to achieve, what they can achieve, how they can put it into effect, how they can assess and review their service quality, and how they can account for it.

Finally, quality is value-based. In the welfare services, it needs to be clearly linked with their initial purpose and *raison d'être*. It needs to be an integral, normal way of working at individual, team, department and preferably organizational levels. It is not an "add-on" or a quick fix – three to five year timescales are probably needed just to get it established. Even longer will be necessary to make it a normal way of life. Meanwhile, there is an array of forces which, while ostensibly increasing pressure for improved quality, may in practice militate against it. Over-specified contracts, unco-ordinated, fragmented services, and the inflexibility of nationally imposed standards can lead to rigidity, complexity and cynicism. So it will be a struggle to keep the idea of "quality" going. Nevertheless, if welfare services wish to survive and prosper, that is just what they will have to do.

Suggested reading

Sanderson (1992), Bouckaert & Pollitt (1994) and Gaster (1994) review quality in public services from different angles. Between them, they look at policy implication; definitions and measurements (through series of case studies across Europe); and the components of quality policy and management in UK public services.

Lipsky (1980) is a highly readable exposition of the position of frontline workers and the constraints that affect policy implementation in practice. Gaster & Taylor (1993) provide an up to date picture, based on case study research, of the way "participative democracy" is developing in local government. Thomas et al. (1993) is a series of papers that analyzes the background and future scenarios for key aspects of two welfare services, social services and housing.

Bibliography

Abel-Smith, B. 1958. Whose welfare state? In *Conviction*, N. McKenzie (ed.), 55–73. London: McGibbon.

Abel-Smith, B. & P. Townsend 1965. *The poor and the poorest*. London: Bell.

Addison, P. 1987. The road from 1945. In *Ruling performance*, P. Hennessy & A. Seldon (eds), 5–27. Oxford: Basil Blackwell.

— 1993. *Churchill on the home front*. London: Pimlico.

Addy, T. & D. Scott 1988. *Fatal impacts? The MSC and voluntary action*. Manchester, England: William Temple Foundation.

Ahmad, W. 1993. *"Race" and health in contemporary Britain*. Milton Keynes, England: Open University Press.

Alcock, P. 1992. Social insurance in crisis? *Benefits* **5**, 6–9.

— 1993. *Understanding poverty*. London: Macmillan.

Alexander, R. 1984. *Primary teaching*. London: Cassell.

— 1992. *Policy and practice in primary education*. London: Routledge.

Allen, I., D. Hogg, S. Peace 1992. *Elderly people: choice, participation and satisfaction*. London: Policy Studies Institute.

Allsop, J. 1989. Health. In *The new politics of welfare*, M. McCarthy (ed.), 53–81. London: Macmillan.

Allsop, J. & A. May 1993. Between the devil and the deep blue sea: managing the NHS in the wake of the 1990 . t. *Critical Social Policy* **38**, 5–23.

Amin, K. & C. Oppenheim 1992. *Poverty in black and white: deprivation and ethnic minorities*. London: CPAG, The Runnymede Trust.

Arber, S. 1990. Revealing women's health: reanalysing the general household survey. In *Women's health counts*, H. Roberts (ed.), 63–92. London: Routledge.

Arber, S. & N. Gilbert 1989. Men: the forgotten carers. *Sociology* **23**(1), 111–18.

Arber, S. & J. Ginn 1991. *Gender and later life*. London: Sage.

Audit Commission 1986. *Making a reality of community care*. London: HMSO.

— 1989. *Urban regeneration and economic development: the local government dimension*. London: HMSO.

— 1993a. *Their health, your business: the new role of the District Health Authority*. London: HMSO.

— 1993b. *Practices make perfect: the role of the Family Health Services Authority*. London: HMSO.

Avis, J. 1981. Social and technical relations: the case of further education. *British Journal of Sociology of Education* **2**(2), 145–61.

Bacon, R. & W. Eltis 1976. *Britain's economic problems: too few producers*. London: Macmillan.

Baker, K. 1988. Speech to the Bow Group Annual Dinner, London, 27 April.

Balarajan, R. & S. Raleigh 1993. *Ethnicity and health: a guide for the NHS*. London: Department of Health.

Baldwin, J. 1990. *The politics of social solidarity: class bases of the European welfare state 1875–1975*. Cambridge: Cambridge University Press.

Ball, S. J. 1990. *Politics and policy making in education: explorations in policy sociology*. London: Routledge.

Banting, K. 1979. *Poverty, politics and policy*. London: Macmillan.

Barker, R. S. 1972. *Education and politics 1900–51*. Oxford: Oxford University Press.

Barnes, C. 1991. *Disabled people in Britain and discrimination*. London: Hurst.

Barnes, J. 1991. Putting power in the hands of the parent. In *Samizdat*, February/March.

Barnett, C. 1986. *The audit of war*. London: Macmillan.

Barr, N. & F. Coulter 1990. Social security: solution or problem? In *The state of welfare*, J. Hills (ed.), 274–337. Oxford: Oxford University Press.

Barton, W. R. 1959. *Institutional neurosis*. Bristol, England: John Wright.

Beck, E., S. Lonsdale, S. Newman, D. Patterson 1992. *In the best of health? The status and future of health care in the UK*. London: Chapman and Hall.

Becker, S. (ed.) 1991. *Windows of opportunity*. London: Child Poverty Action Group.

Bell, D. 1960. *The end of ideology*. Chicago: University of Chicago Press.

Bennett, N. 1975. *Teaching styles and pupil progress*. London: Open Books.

Ben-Tovim, G., J. Gabriel, I. Law, K. Stredder 1986. *The local politics of race*. London: Macmillan.

Bevan, A. 1961. *In place of fear*. London: MacGibbon & Kee.

Beveridge, W. H. 1942. *The pillars of security*. London: Allen & Unwin.

Beveridge, W. H. 1944. *Full employment in a free society*. London: Allen & Unwin.

Beveridge, W. H. 1948. *Voluntary action*. London: Allen & Unwin.

Billis, D. 1993. *Organising public and voluntary agencies*. London: Routledge.

Blom-Cooper, L. 1985. *A child in trust: the report of the panel of inquiry into the circumstances surrounding the death of Jasmine Beckford*. London: Borough of Brent.

Bosanquet, N. 1988. The ailing state of the national health. In *British social attitudes*, R. Jowell, S. Witherspoon, L. Brook (eds), 93–108. Aldershot, England: Gower.

Bosanquet, N. & B. Leese 1989. *Family doctors and economic incentives*. Aldershot, England: Dartmouth/Gower.

Bosanquet, N. & C. Propper 1991. Charting the grey economy in the 1990s. *Policy and Politics* **19**(4), 269–82.

Bouckaert, G. & C. Pollitt (eds) 1994. *Quality improvement in European public services: concepts, cases and commentary*. London: Sage.

Bourdillon, A. (ed.) 1945. *Voluntary social services.* London: Methuen.

Bowen, A. 1991. Labour market policies. In *Labour's economic policies 1974–79*, M. Arbos & D. Cobham (eds), 190–213. Manchester, England: Manchester University Press.

Bowlby, J. 1952. *Maternal care and mental health.* Geneva: World Health Organisation.

Bowling, B. 1990. *Elderly people from ethnic minorities.* London: Age Concern Institute of Gerontology.

Braham, P., A. Rattansi, R. Skellington 1992. *Racism and anti racism.* London: Sage.

Brenton, M. 1985. *The voluntary sector in British social services.* Harlow, England: Longman.

Briggs, A. 1961. The welfare state in historical perspective. *Archives Européennes de Sociologie* **2**, 222–58.

— (ed.) 1962. *William Morris: Selected writings and designs.* Harmondsworth, England: Penguin.

Broadfoot, P. 1991. Review of politics and policy making in education. *British Journal of Sociology of Education* **12**(2), 250–54.

Brooke, S. 1992. *Labour's war: the Labour Party during the Second World War.* Oxford: Clarendon Press.

Brown, C. 1992. "Same difference": the persistence of racial discrimination in the British employment market. In *Racism and anti racism*, P. Braham, A. Rattansi, R. Skellington (eds), 46–63. London: Sage.

Brown, G. & T. Harris 1978. *The social origins of depression.* London: Tavistock.

Brown, J. 1984. *Evidence to the review of benefits for children and young people.* London: Policy Studies Institute.

— 1990. The focus on single mothers. In *The emerging British underclass*, C. Murray (ed.), 43–8. London: Institute of Economic Affairs.

Buchanan, J. & G. Tullock 1992. *The calculus of consent.* Ann Arbor: University of Michigan Press.

Bullock, R., M. Little, S. Millham 1993. *Going home: the return of children separated from their families.* Aldershot, England: Dartmouth.

Burke, J. (ed.) 1989. *Competency based education and training.* Lewes, England: Falmer.

Burton, P. & M. O'Toole 1993. Urban development corporations: post-Fordism in action or Fordism in retrenchment? In *British urban policy and the urban development corporations*, R. Imrie & H. Thomas (eds), 186–99. London: Paul Chapman.

Butler, D. & D. Kavanagh 1992. *The British general election 1992.* London: Macmillan.

Butler, E. 1992. *Long term commitment.* London: Adam Smith Institute.

Butler, E. & M. Pirie 1983. *The future of pensions.* London: Adam Smith Institute.

— 1989. *The health alternatives.* London: Adam Smith Institute.

Butler, J. 1992. *Patients, policies and politics: before and after working for patients.* Milton Keynes, England: Open University Press.

Butler, R. 1982. Control through markets, hierarchies and communes: a transactional approach to organisational analysis. In *Power, efficiency and institutions*, A. J. Francis, J. Turk, P. Willman (eds), 137–58. London: Heinemann.

327

Butler-Sloss, J. 1988. *Report of the inquiry into child abuse in Cleveland.* London: HMSO.

Cabinet Office 1988. *Action for cities.* London: Cabinet Office.

Calder, A. 1991. *The myth of the blitz.* London: Pimlico.

Calnan, M., S. Cant, J. Gabe 1993. *Going private: why people pay for their health care.* Milton Keynes, England: Open University Press.

Campbell, A., C. Macdonald, N. Raynsford, M. Wicks, T. Wright 1993. *A new agenda.* London: Institute for Public Policy Research.

Campbell, J. C. 1992. *How policies change.* Princeton, New Jersey: Princeton University Press

Carter, N. 1991. Learning to measure performance: the use of indicators in organisations. *Public Administration* **69**, 85–101.

Central Advisory Council for Education (England) 1954. *Early leaving.* London: HMSO.

— 1959. *15 to 18.* London: HMSO.

— 1963. *Half our future.* London: HMSO.

— 1967. *Children and their primary schools.* London: HMSO.

Challis, D. & B. Davies 1985. Long-term care for the elderly: the Community Care Schemes. *British Journal of Social Work* **15**(6), 563–80.

Challis, L. 1990. *Organising public social services.* Harlow, England: Longman.

Chitty C. 1986. TVEI: The MSC's Trojan horse. In *Challenging the MSC*, C. Benn & J. Fairley (eds), 76–98. London: Pluto.

— 1988. Central control of the school curriculum. *History of Education* **17**(4), 321–34.

Clarke, M. & J. Stewart 1991. *Choices for local government.* Harlow, England: Longman.

CLES 1990. *First year report of the CLES monitoring project on UDCs.* Manchester, England: Centre for Local Economic Strategies.

Clough, R. 1990. *Practice, politics and power in social services departments.* Aldershot, England: Avebury.

Cm 249 1987. *Promoting better health: the government programme for improving primary health care.* London: HMSO.

— 555 1989. *Working for patients.* London: HMSO.

— 849 1989. *Caring for people: community care in the next decade and beyond.* London: HMSO.

— 1536 1991. *Education and training in the twenty first century.* London: HMSO.

— 1599 1991. *The Citizen's Charter.* London: HMSO.

— 1730 1991. *Competing for quality: buying better public services.* London: HMSO.

— 1986 1992. *The health of the nation, A strategy for health for England.* London: HMSO.

— 2101 1992. *Citizen's Charter first report 1992.* London: HMSO.

— 2207 1993. *Department of the Environment annual report: 1993. The government's expenditure plans 1993–94 to 1995–96.* London: HMSO.

Cmd 6234 1940. *Recommendations of Lord Horder's Committee regarding the conditions in air-raid shelters with special reference to health.* London: HMSO.

— 6404 1942. *Social insurance and allied services.* London: HMSO.

— 6415 1943. *Report of the inter-departmental committee on the rehabilitation and resettle-*

ment of disabled persons. London: HMSO.
— 6527 1944. *Employment policy.* London: HMSO.
— 6922 1946. *Report of the care of children committee.* London: HMSO.
— 8710 1952. *Report of the committee on the law and practice relating to charitable trusts.* London: HMSO.
— 9333 1954. *Report of the committee on the economic and financial problems of the provision for old age.* London: HMSO.
— 9663 1956. *Report of the committee of enquiry into the cost of the NHS.* London: HMSO.
— 9703 1956. *Technical education.* London: HMSO.
Cmnd 2154 1963. *Higher education.* London: HMSO.
— 2605 1965. *Report of the committee on housing in Greater London.* London: HMSO.
— 2838 1965. *The housing programme 1965 to 1970.* London: HMSO.
— 3703 1968. *Report of the committee on local authority and allied personal social services.* London: HMSO.
— 4728 1971. *Fair deal for housing.* London: HMSO.
— 6845 1977. *Policy for the inner cities.* London. HMSO.
— 6869 1977. *Education in schools.* London: HMSO.
— 8173 1981. *Growing older.* London: HMSO.
— 8455 1981. *A new training initiative.* London: HMSO.
— 9469 1985. *Better schools.* London: HMSO.
Cochrane, A. & J. Clarke 1993. *Comparing welfare states.* London: Sage.
Cohen, S. 1973. *Folk devils and moral panics.* London: Paladin.
Commission on Social Justice 1993. *The justice gap.* London: Institute for Public Policy Research.
Conservative Party 1976. *The right approach.* London: Conservative Party.
Cook, J. & S. Watt 1992. Racism, women and poverty. In *Women and poverty in Britain: the 1990s*, C. Glendinning & J. Miller (eds.), 11–26. Brighton, England: Wheatsheaf.
Cooke, P. (ed.) 1986. *Global restructuring: local response.* London: Economic and Social Research Council.
Cooper, J. 1982. *The creation of the British personal social services 1962–1974.* London: Heinemann.
Coulter, A., V. Seagroatt, K. McPherson 1990. Relation between general practices' outpatient referral rates and rates of elective admission to hospital. *British Medical Journal* **301**, 273–6.
Cox, B. 1992. *The great betrayal.* London: Chapmans.
Cox, C. B. & R. Boyson 1975. *Black paper.* London: Dent.
CPAG 1993. *Taxes and benefits: steps to rational reform.* London: Child Poverty Action Group.
Craig, P. 1991. Costs and benefits: a review of research on take-up of income-related benefits. *Journal of Social Policy* **20**(4), 537–65.
Crewe, I. 1993. Parties and electors. In *The developing British political system: the 1990s*, I. Budge & D. McKay (eds), 99–111. Harlow, England: Longman.
Cronin, J. E. 1991. *The politics of state expansion.* London: Routledge.
Crosby, P. 1986. *Quality without tears: the art of hassle-free management.* New York: McGraw-Hill International Edition Management Series.
Crosland, A. 1956. *The future of socialism.* London: Jonathan Cape.

Crosland, C. A. R. 1962. *The Conservative enemy.* London: Jonathan Cape.

Dalley, G. 1991. *Quality management institutions in the NHS: strategic approaches to improving quality.* York, England: Centre for Health Economics.

Dartington, T., E. Miller, G. Gwynne 1981. *A life together.* London: Tavistock.

Davey, B. & J. Popay 1993. *Dilemmas in health care.* Milton Keynes, England: Open University Press.

Davey Smith, G., M. Bartley, D. Blane 1990. The Black Report on socio-economic inequalities in health 10 years on. *British Medical Journal* **301**, 373–8.

Davies, B. 1968. *Social needs and resources in local services.* London: Michael Joseph.

Davies, J. 1993. *Is the family just another lifestyle choice?* London: Institute of Economic Affairs.

Davis, M. 1990. *City of quartz: excavating the future in Los Angeles.* London: Verso.

Dawson, G. 1993. *Inflation and unemployment: causes, consequences, cures.* Cheltenham, England: Edward Elgar.

Day, P. & R. Klein 1987. *Accountabilities.* London: Tavistock.

— 1991. Britain's health care experiment. *Health Affairs*, Fall, 39–59.

Deacon, A. 1982. An end to the means test? Social security and the Attlee Government. *Journal of Social Policy* **11**(3), 289–306.

— 1991. The retreat from state welfare. In *Windows of opportunity*, S. Becker (ed.), 9–21. London: CPAG.

— 1993. Richard Titmuss: twenty years on. *Journal of Social Policy* **22**(2), 235–42.

Deacon, A. & J. Bradshaw 1983. *Reserved for the poor.* Oxford: Blackwell.

— 1986. Social security. In *In Defence of the welfare state*, P. Wilding (ed.), 81–97. Manchester, England: Manchester University Press.

Deakin, N. 1970. *Colour, citizenship and British society.* London: Panther.

— 1988. *In search of the postwar consensus.* London: Welfare State Programme, London School of Economics.

— 1989. Social policy. In *Party ideology in Britain*, L. Tivey & A. Wright (eds), 105–27. London: Routledge.

— 1993. A future for collectivism. In *Social policy review 5*, R. Page & J. Baldock (eds), 12–34. Canterbury, England: Social Policy Association.

Deakin, N. & J. Edwards 1993. *The enterprise culture and the inner city.* London: Routledge.

Dear, M. & A. J. Scott (eds) 1981. *Urbanization and urban planning in capitalist society.* London: Methuen.

Dearing, Sir R. 1994. *The national curriculum and its assessment.* London: SCAA.

Dearlove, J. & P. Saunders 1991. *Introduction to British politics.* Cambridge: Polity.

Deming, W. E. 1986. *Out of the crisis: quality, productivity and competitive production.* Massachussetts: Press Syndicate, University of Cambridge.

Department of Education and Science (DES) 1983. *Curriculum 11–16: towards a statement of entitlement.* London: HMSO.

Department of the Environment (DoE) 1969. *People and planning: report of the committee on public participation in planning.* London: HMSO.

— 1979. *Inner cities policy: statement by Michael Heseltine, Secretary of State for the Environment.* Press notice no. 390. London: DoE.

— 1982. *English house condition survey 1981.* London: HMSO.

— 1993. *John Gummer announces measures to bring a new localism to improved government services*. News Release no. 731. London: DOE.

Department of Health (DOH) 1989. *General practice in the NHS: the 1990 contract*. London: HMSO.

— 1991. *Patterns and outcomes: messages from current research and their implications*. London: HMSO.

— 1992a. *Personal health and social service statistics*. London: Department of Health.

— 1992b. *The Patient's Charter*. London: Department of Health.

— 1993. *Managing the new NHS*. London: Department of Health.

Department of Health and Social Security (DHSS) 1974. *Report of the committee of inquiry into the care and supervision provided in relation to Maria Colwell*. London: HMSO.

— 1976. *Priorities for health and personal social services in England*. London: HMSO.

— 1985. *Social work decisions in child care: recent research findings and their implications*. London: HMSO.

— 1988. *Community care: agenda for action*. London: HMSO.

Department of Health and Social Security and Welsh Office (DHSS) 1978. *A happier old age*. London: HMSO.

Department of Social Security (DSS) 1992. *Households below average income*. London: HMSO.

— 1993. *Income-related benefits: estimates of take-up in 1989*. London: HMSO.

Dex, S. 1988. *Women's attitudes towards work*. London: Macmillan.

Digby, A. 1989. *British welfare policy: workhouse to workfare*. London: Faber & Faber.

Dilnot, A., J. Kay, C. Morris 1984. *The reform of social security*. Oxford: Institute for Fiscal Studies.

Dingwall, R., J. Eekelaar, T. Murray 1988. *The protection of children: state intervention and family life*. Oxford: Blackwell.

Ditch, J. 1993. Next steps: the reorganisation of the DSS. In *The costs of welfare*, N. Deakin & R. M. Page (eds), 64–83. Aldershot, England: Avebury.

Donabedian, A. 1980. *The definition of quality and approaches to its assessment*. Ann Arbor, Michigan: Health Administration Press.

Donnison, D. V. 1967. *The government of housing*. London: Penguin.

— 1983. *Urban policies: a new approach*. London: Fabian Society.

— 1991. *A radical agenda*. London: Rivers Oram Press.

Donoughue, B. 1987. *Prime Minister*. London: Jonathan Cape.

Drucker, P. 1989. Peter Drucker's 1990s: the futures that have already happened. *The Economist*, 21 October, 27–30.

Dunleavy, P. 1991. *Democracy, bureaucracy and public choice: economic explanations in political science*. London: Harvester Wheatsheaf.

Edwards, J. & R. Batley 1978. *The politics of positive discrimination: an evaluation of the Urban Programme 1967–77*. London: Tavistock.

Efficiency Unit 1988. *Improving management in government: the next steps*. London: HMSO.

Ellis, R. (ed.) 1988. *Professional competence and quality assurance in the caring professions*. London: Chapman & Hall.

Employment Department Group. 1993. *Labour market quarterly report*. London: Employment Department.

Enthoven, A. 1985. *Reflections on the management of the NHS.* London: Nuffield Provincial Hospitals Trust.

Evandrou, M., J. Falkingham, H. Glennerster 1991. The personal social services: everyone's poor relation but nobody's baby. In *The state of welfare,* J. Hills (ed.), 206–73. Oxford: Clarendon Press.

Evans, T. 1990. *A friend in need.* London: Adam Smith Institute.

Evers, A. 1993. The welfare-mix approach: understanding the pluralism of welfare systems. Paper presented to the conference: Wellbeing in Europe by strengthening the third sector. Barcelona, May 27–9.

Expert Maternity Group 1993. *Changing childbirth: a report.* London: HMSO.

Falkingham, J., J. Hills, C. Lessof 1993. *William Beveridge versus Robin Hood: social security and redistribution over the lifecycle.* London: London School of Economics Welfare State Programme, London School of Economics.

Falkingham, J. & P. Johnson 1993. *A unified funded pension scheme for Britain.* London: Economic & Social Research Council.

Faludi, A. 1973. *Planning theory.* Oxford: Pergamon.

Fenwick, K. & P. McBride 1981. *The government of education.* Oxford: Martin Robertson.

Ferrara, P. 1982. *Social security reform: the family plan.* Washington D. C.: The Heritage Foundation.

Ferris, J. 1985. Citizenship and the crisis of the welfare state. In *In defence of welfare,* P. Bean, J. Ferris, D. Whynes (eds), 46–73. London: Tavistock.

Field, F. & M. Owen 1993. *Making sense of pensions.* London: Fabian Society.

Finch, J. & D. Groves 1980. Community care: a case for equal opportunities. *Journal of Social Policy* **9**(4), 487–511.

Fitzherbert, L. 1989. *Charity and the national health: a report on the extent and potential of charitable funds within the NHS.* London: Directory of Social Change.

Forrest, R., A. Murie, P. Williams 1990. *Home ownership: differentiation and fragmentation.* London: Unwin Hyman.

Fowler, N. 1990. Speech to Society of Conservative Lawyers, 11.10.90.

Fryer, P. 1984. *Staying power: the history of black people in Britain.* London: Pluto Press.

Fryer, P. 1988. *Black people in the British Empire: an introduction.* London: Pluto Press.

Galbraith, J. K. 1993. *The culture of contentment.* London: Penguin.

Gamble, A. 1983. Thatcherism and Conservative politics. In *The politics of Thatcherism,* S. Hall & M. Jaques (eds), 109–131. London: Lawrence & Wishart.

— 1988. *The free economy and the strong state.* London: Macmillan.

Gaster, L. 1994. *Quality in the public sector: managers' choices.* Milton Keynes, England: Open University Press.

Gaster, L. & M. Taylor 1993. *Learning from consumers and citizens.* Luton, England: Local Government Management Board.

George, V. & S. Miller 1994. *Social policy towards 2000.* London: Routledge.

Gidron, B., R. M. Kramer, L. M. Salamon (eds) 1992. *Government and the third sector: emerging relationships in welfare.* San Francisco: Jossey Bass.

Gilroy, P. 1987. *There ain't no black in the Union Jack: the cultural politics of "race" and nation.* London: Hutchinson.

Gladstone, F. 1979. *Voluntary action in a changing world.* London: Bedford Square Press.

Gleeson, D. 1989. *The paradox of training.* Milton Keynes, England: Open University Press.

Glendinning, C. & J. Millar (eds) 1992. *Women and poverty in Britain,* 2nd edn. Brighton, England: Wheatsheaf.

Glennerster, H. 1990a. Social policy since the Second World War. In *The state of welfare,* J. Hills (ed.), 11–28. Oxford: Clarendon Press.

— 1990b. Education and the welfare state: does it add up? In *The state of welfare,* J. Hills (ed.), 28–87. Oxford: Clarendon Press.

— 1992. *Paying for welfare.* London: Harvester Wheatsheaf.

Glennerster, H., J. Falkingham, M. Evandrou 1990. How much do we care? *Social Policy and Administration* **24**(2), 93–103.

Glennerster, H. & J. Midgley 1991. *The radical right and the welfare state.* Hemel Hempstead, England: Harvester Wheatsheaf

Glennerster, H., M. Matsanganis, P. Owens 1992. *A foothold for fund-holding.* Research Report 12. London: King's Fund Institute.

Goffman, E. 1961. *Asylums: essays on the social situation of mental patients and other inmates.* New York: Anchor Books, Doubleday.

Golby, M. 1985. *Caught in the act: teachers and governors after 1980.* Exeter, England: University of Exeter School of Education.

Golding, P. & S. Middleton 1982. *Images of welfare.* Oxford: Martin Robertson.

Goodlove, C. & A. Mann 1980. Thirty years of the welfare state: current issues in British social policy for the aged. *Aged Care and Services Review* **2**(1), 1–12.

Gordon, P., R. Aldrich, D. Dean 1991. *Education and policy in England in the twentieth century.* London: Woburn Press.

Graham, D. 1993. *A lesson for us all: the making of the national curriculum.* London: Routledge.

Graham, H. 1990. Behaving well: women's health behaviour in context. In *Women's health counts,* II. Roberts (ed.), 195–219. London: Routledge.

Gray, A. & B. Jenkins 1993. Markets, managers and the public service. In *Markets and managers,* P. Taylor-Gooby & R. Lawson (eds), 9–23. Milton Keynes, England: Open University Press.

Green, D. 1992. Liberty, poverty, and the underclass. In *Understanding the underclass,* S. Smith (ed), 68–87. London: Policy Studies Institute.

— 1993. *Families without fatherhood.* London: Institute of Economic Affairs.

Griffith, J. A. G. 1966. *Central departments and local government.* London: Allen & Unwin.

Griffiths, R. 1983. *The NHS management inquiry report.* London: DHSS.

— 1992. Seven years of progress – general management in the NHS. *Health Economics* **1**, 61–70.

Grunow, D. 1991. Customer oriented service delivery in German local administration. In *Local government in Europe,* R. Batley & G. Stoker (eds), 73–88. London: Macmillan.

Gyford, J. & M. James 1983. *National parties and local politics.* London: Allen & Unwin.

Hadley, R. & S. Hatch 1981. *Social welfare and the failure of the state.* London: Allen & Unwin.

Hall, P. 1975. *Urban and regional planning.* London: Penguin.

Hall, P. 1976. *Reforming the welfare: the politics of change in the personal social services.* London: Heinemann.

Hall, S. 1985. Authoritarian populism: a reply. *New Left Review* **151**, 106–13.

Halsey, A. H. 1978. *Change in British society.* Oxford: Oxford University Press.

Ham, C. 1992. *Health policy in Britain,* 3rd edn. London: Macmillan.

Handy, C. 1988. *Understanding voluntary organisations.* London: Penguin.

Hansard 1946. Vol. 414, col. 1222.

— 1946. Vol. 418, col. 1744.

— 1948. Vol. 452, col. 564.

— 1982. Vol. 22 col. 264.

Harding, T. 1992. *Great expectations . . . and spending on social services.* London: National Institute for Social Work.

Harris, A. 1971. *Handicapped and impaired in Great Britain.* London: HMSO.

Harris, J. 1990. Society and the state in twentieth century Britain. In *The Cambridge social history of Britain 1750–1950, vol. 3, Social agencies and institutions,* F. M. L. Thompson (ed.), 63–118. Cambridge: Cambridge University Press.

— 1991. Enterprise and the welfare state: a comparative perspective. In *Britain since 1945,* T. Gourvish & A. O'Day (eds), 39–58. London: Macmillan.

Harris, R. & A. Seldon 1979. *Over-ruled on welfare.* London: Institute of Economic Affairs.

Harrison, S. 1988. *Managing the NHS: shifting the frontier?* London: Chapman & Hall.

Harrison, S., D. Hunter, G. Marnoch, C. Pollitt 1992. *The dynamics of British health policy.* London: Routledge.

Harvey, A. 1960. *Casualties of the welfare state.* London: Fabian Society.

Harwin, J. 1990. Parental responsibilities in the Children Act 1989. In *Social Policy Review 1989–90,* N. Manning & C. Ungerson (eds), 78–96. Harlow, England: Longman.

Haviland, J. 1988. *Take care Mr Baker.* London: Fourth Estate.

Hawkins, K. 1987. *Unemployment,* 3rd edn. Harmondsworth, England: Penguin.

Headey, B. 1978. *Housing policy in the developed economy.* London: Croom Helm.

Health Advisory Service 1983. *The rising tide: developing services for mental illness in old age.* London: HMSO.

Held, D. 1989. Citizenship and autonomy. In *Political theory and the modern state,* D. Held (ed.), 189–213. Cambridge: Polity.

Henderson, J. & V. Karn 1987. *Race, class and state housing.* Aldershot, England: Gower.

Hennessy, P. 1993. Never again. In *What difference did the war make,* B. Brivati & H. Jones (eds), 3–19. Leicester, England: Leicester University Press.

Henney, A. 1984. *Inside local government.* London: Sinclair Browne.

Henwood, M. 1992. Twilight zone. *Health Services Journal* 5th November.

Henwood, M., T. Jowell, G. Wistow 1991. *All things come to those who wait?* London: King's Fund Institute.

Higgins, J. 1989. Defining community care. *Social Policy and Administration,* **23**(1) 3–16.

Hill, M. 1990. *Social security policy in Britain.* Aldershot, England: Edward Elgar.

— 1993. *The welfare state in Britain: a political history since 1945.* Cheltenham,

England: Edward Elgar.

Hills, J. (ed.) 1990. *The state of welfare*. Oxford: Clarendon Press.

Hills, J. 1991. *39 steps to housing finance reform*. York, England: Joseph Rowntree Foundation.

— 1993. *The future of welfare: a guide to the debate*. York, England: Joseph Rowntree Foundation.

Hindess, B. 1987. *Freedom, equality and the market*. London: Tavistock.

Hobhouse, L. T. 1911. *Liberalism*. Oxford: Oxford University Press.

Hogg, Q 1947. *The case for Conservatism*. London: Penguin.

Hoggett, P. 1991. A new management in the public sector. *Policy and Politics* **19**(4), 243–56.

Hogwood, B. W. 1992. *Trends in British public policy: do governments make any difference?* Milton Keynes, England: Open University Press.

Holmans, A. E. 1987. *Housing policy in Britain: a history*. London: Croom Helm.

Holmes, C. 1991. Immigration. In *Britain since 1945*, T. Gourvish & A. O'Day (eds), 209–32. London: Macmillan.

Home Office 1990. *Profiting from partnership: efficiency scrutiny on government funding to the voluntary sector*. London: HMSO.

House of Commons (HC) Social Services Committee 1984. Report on Children in Care, Session 1983–84, HC 360. London: HMSO.

— 1986. Public expenditure on the social services. Session 1985–86, HC 387. London: HMSO.

Howe, G. & C. Jones 1956. *Houses to let*. London: Conservative Political Centre.

Howell, R. 1991. *Why not work?* London: Adam Smith Institute.

Hoyes, L., & R. Means 1992. Markets, contracts and social care services: prospects and problems. In *Community care: a reader*, J. Bornat (ed.), 287–95. London: Macmillan.

— 1993. Quasi-markets and the reform of community care. In *Quasi-markets and social policy*, J. Le Grand & W. Bartlett (eds), 93–124. London: Macmillan.

Hoyes, L., R. Lart, R. Means, M. Taylor 1994. *Community care in transition*. York, England: Rowntree Foundation.

Huby, M. & G. Dix 1992. *Evaluating the social fund*. London: HMSO.

Huws Jones, R. 1952. Old people's welfare – successes and failures. *Social Services Quarterly* **26**(1), 19–22.

Imrie, R. & H. Thomas. 1993. Urban policy and the urban development corporations. In *British urban policy and the urban development corporations*, R. Imrie & H. Thomas (eds), 3–26. London: Paul Chapman.

Jamieson, J & M. Lightfoot 1982. *Schools and industry*. London: Methuen.

Jeavons, T. 1992. When the management is the message: relating values to management practice in nonprofit organisations. *Nonprofit Management and Leadership*, **2**(4), 403–17.

Jeffreys, K. 1991. *The Churchill coalition and wartime politics 1940–1945*. Manchester, England: Manchester University Press.

Johnson, E. 1994. Quality improvement and the demand for N. H. S. services. In *Unhealthy competition: the public-private mix for health*, E. Butler (ed.), 38–41. London: Adam Smith Institute.

Jones, H. 1992. *The Conservative party and the welfare state 1942–55*. PhD thesis,

London School of Economics.

Judd, D. & M. Parkinson (eds) 1990. *Leadership and urban regeneration: cities in North America and Europe.* London: Sage.

Juran, J. 1979. *Quality control handbook.* New York: McGraw Hill.

Kavanagh, D. & P. Morris 1989. *Consensus politics from Attlee to Thatcher.* Oxford: Basil Blackwell.

Kerckhoff, A. C. 1990. *Getting started: transition to adulthood in Great Britain.* London: Westview.

Keynes, J. M. 1936. *The general theory of employment, interest and money.* London: Macmillan.

Kiernan, K. & M. Wicks 1990. *Family change and future policy.* London: Family Policy Studies Centre and The Joseph Rowntree Foundation.

Kiernan, K. & V. Estaugh 1993. *Cohabitation: extra marital childbearing and social policy.* London: Family Policy Studies Centre.

King, D. S. 1987. *The New Right: politics, markets and citizenship.* London: Macmillan.

Klein, R. 1989. *The politics of the National Health Service,* 2nd edn. Harlow, England: Longman.

Knight, B. 1993. *Voluntary action.* London: HMSO.

Knight, C. 1992. *The making of Conservative education policy.* Lewes, England: Falmer.

Kogan, M. (ed.) 1971. *The politics of education.* London: Penguin.

Kogan, M. 1978. *The politics of educational change.* London: Fontana.

Kogan, M. & D. Kogan 1983. *The attack on higher education.* London: Kogan Page.

Laing, W. 1993. *Financing long term care: the crucial debate.* London: Age Concern England.

Lambert, H. & K. McPherson 1993. Disease prevention and health promotion. In *Dilemmas in health care,* B. Davey & J. Popay (eds), 143–63. Milton Keynes, England: Open University Press.

Langan, M. 1990. Community care in the 1990s. *Critical Social Policy* **29**, 58–70.

Lart, R. & R. Means 1993. User empowerment and buying community care: reflections on the emerging debate about charging policies. In *The costs of welfare,* N. Deakin & R. Page (eds), 107–27. Aldershot, England: Avebury.

Lawless, P. 1988. British inner urban policy post-1979: a critique. *Policy and Politics* **16**, 261–75.

— 1989. *Britain's inner cities,* 2nd edn. London: Paul Chapman.

Lawson, N. 1992. *The view from Number 11: memoirs of a Tory radical.* London: Bantam Press.

Lawson, R. 1993. The new technology of management in the personal social services. In *Markets and managers,* P. Taylor-Gooby & R. Lawson (eds), 69–84. Milton Keynes, England: Open University Press.

Lawton, D. 1980. *The politics of the school curriculum.* London: Routledge & Kegan Paul.

Le Grand, J. 1982. *The strategy of equality.* London: Allen & Unwin.

— 1993. Quasi-markets and community care. In *Learning from innovation,* N. Thomas, J. Doling, N. Deakin (eds), 44–65. Birmingham, England: Academic Press.

Le Grand, J., D. Winter, F. Wooley 1990. The National Health Service: safe in whose hands? In *The state of welfare: the welfare state in Britain since 1974*, J. Hills (ed.), 88–134. Oxford: Oxford University Press.

Le Grand, J. & W. Bartlett (eds) 1993. *Quasi-markets and social policy.* London: Macmillan.

Lee, D. (ed.) 1990. *Scheming for youth: a study of YTS in the enterprise culture.* Milton Keynes, England: Open University Press.

Levy, A. and B. Kahan 1991. *The pindown experience and the protection of children.* Stafford, England: Staffordshire County Council.

Lewis, J. 1992. *Women in Britain since 1945.* Oxford: Basil Blackwell.

— 1993. Women, work, family and social policies in Europe. In *Women and social policies in Europe*, J. Lewis (ed.), 1–24. Cheltenham, England: Edward Elgar.

Lewis, J. & D. Piauchaud 1987. Women and poverty in the twentieth century. In *Women and poverty in Britain*, C. Glendinning & J. Millar (eds), 28–52. Brighton, England: Wheatsheaf Books.

Lewis, R. & A. Maude 1949. *The English middle classes.* London: Penguin.

Lilley, P. 1993. *Benefits and costs: securing the future of social security.* The Mais Lecture.

Lipsky, M. 1980. *Street-level bureaucracy: dilemmas of the individual in public services.* New York: Russell Sage Foundation.

Lloyd, C. 1986. *Explanation in social history.* Oxford: Blackwell.

Local Government Management Board 1993. *Survey of organisational change in local government, Interim reports 1 – 4.* Luton, England: Local Government Management Board.

Loney, M. 1983. *Community against government: the British Community Development Project; a study of government incompetence.* London: Heinemann.

Lowe, R. 1990. Welfare policy in Britain 1943–1970. *Contemporary Record* **4**(2), 29–32.

— 1993. *The welfare state in Britain since 1945.* London: Macmillan.

Lowther, C. & J. Williamson 1966. Old people and their relatives. *The Lancet*, 21 March.

Lynn, P. & J. Davis Smith (1991). *The 1991 national survey of voluntary activity in the UK.* Berkhamsted, England: The Volunteer Centre.

Mabbott, J. 1993. *Local authority funding for voluntary organisations: survey report 1993.* London: National Council for Voluntary Organisations.

Macarthy, M. 1986. *Campaigning for the poor.* London: Croom Helm.

Macdowell, L. 1993. Social divisions, income inequality and gender relations in the 1980s. In *Policy and change in Thatcher's Britain*, P. Cloke (ed.), 355–78. Oxford: Pergamon Press.

MacGregor, S. 1990. *Tackling the inner cities: the 1980s reviewed, prospects for the 1990s.* Oxford: Clarendon Press.

Maclean, U. 1989. *Dependent territories: the frail elderly and community care.* London: Nuffield Provincial Hospitals Trust.

Maclure, S. 1983. Profile of Sir James Hamilton. *Times Education Supplement*, April.

— 1992. *Education re-formed*, 3rd edn. London: Hodder & Stoughton.

Madge, J. 1945. *The rehousing of Britain.* London: Pilot Press.

Malpass, P. & R. Means 1993. *Implementing housing policy.* Milton Keynes, England: Open University Press.

Malpass, P. & A. Murie 1994. *Housing policy and practice*, 4th edn. London: Macmillan.

Marks, J. 1983. *Standards in English schools*. London: National Council for Educational Standards.

Marquand, D. 1988. *The unprincipled society*. London: Fontana Press.

Marsh, A. & S. McKay 1993. *Work and benefits*. London: Policy Studies Institute.

Marshall, T. H. 1950. *Citizenship and social class*. Cambridge: Cambridge University Press.

Massey, A. 1993. *Managing the public sector*. Cheltenham, England: Edward Elgar.

Mayo, M. & A. Weir 1993. A future for feminist social policy. In *Social Policy Review* **5**, R. Page & J. Baldock (eds). Canterbury, England: Social Policy Association.

McDonald, C. 1992. *Developing a quality initiative in a social services department*. MSc in Policy Studies dissertation, School for Advanced Urban Studies, University of Bristol.

McFarlane, A. 1990. Official statistics and women's health. In *Women's health counts*, H. Roberts (ed.), 18–62. London: Routledge.

McKeown, T. 1976. *The role of medicine – dream, mirage or nemesis*. London: Nuffield Provincial Hospitals Trust.

McRae, S. 1993. *Cohabiting matters: changing marriage and motherhood*. London: Policy Studies Institute.

Means, R. & R. Smith 1985. *The development of welfare services for elderly people*. London: Croom Helm.

Merrett, S. 1979. *State housing in Britain*. London: Routledge & Kegan Paul.

— 1982. *Owner occupation in Britain*. London: Routledge & Kegan Paul

Millar, J. 1989. Societal security, equality and women in the UK. *Policy and Politics* **17**(4), 311–19.

— 1991. Bearing the cost. In *Windows of opportunity*, S. Becker (ed.), 9–21. London: CPAG.

— 1993. The continuing trend in rising poverty. In *Poverty, inequality and justice*, A. Sinfield (ed.), 11–18. Edinburgh: University of Edinburgh.

Miller, E. & G. Gwynne 1972. *A life apart*. London: Tavistock.

Minford, P. 1993. Welfare reforms at the heart of the Budget. *Daily Telegraph*, 6 December.

Ministry of Health 1951. Circular 32/51.

— 1957. Circular 14/57.

— 1960. Circular 15/60.

Mishra, R. 1984. *The welfare state in crisis*. Brighton, England: Wheatsheaf Books.

Morgan, D. & M. Evans 1993. *The battle for Britain: citizenship and ideology in the Second World War*. London: Routledge.

Morgan, E. V. 1986. *The friendly societies in the welfare state*. London: National Conference of Friendly Societies.

Morgan, K. O. 1984. *Labour in power 1945–1951*. Oxford: Oxford University Press.

— 1990. *The people's peace: British history 1945–1989*. Oxford: Oxford University Press.

Moroney, R. 1976. *The family and the state*. London: Longman.

Morris, J. 1989. *Able lives: women's experiences of paralysis*. London: Women's Press.
— 1993. *Community care or independent living?* York, England: Joseph Rowntree Foundation.
Morris, P., I. Rahal, H. Storey 1993. *Ethnic minorities benefits handbook*. London: CPAG.
Moser, K., H. Pugh, P. Goldblatt 1988. Inequalities in women's health: looking at mortality differences using an alternative approach. *British Medical Journal* **296**, 1221–4.
Mullard, M. 1993. *The politics of public expenditure*. London: Routledge.
Murie, A. 1983. *Housing inequality and deprivation*. London: Heinemann.
Murray, C. 1990. *The emerging British underclass*. London: IEA Health and Welfare Unit.
National Audit Office 1989. *Report of the Comptroller and Auditor General: NHS coronary care*. London: HMSO.
— 1993. *Report on the performance of the second and third generation Urban Development Corporations*. London: HMSO.
National Council for Voluntary Organisations (NCVO) 1991. *Effectiveness in the voluntary sector*. London: NCVO.
Nevitt, D. 1977. Demand and need. In *Foundations of social administration*, H. Heisler (ed.), 113–28. London: Macmillan.
Novak, T. 1988. *Poverty and the state*. Milton Keynes, England: Open University Press.
Nuki, P. 1993. Pension cuts threaten under-40s. *Sunday Times*, 14 November.
Nuttall, S. R. 1993. *Financing long term care in Great Britain*. London: Institute of Actuaries.
Oakland, J. 1989. *Total quality management*. London: Butterworth.
OECD 1992. *The reform of health care: a comparative analysis of 7 OECD countries*. Paris: OECD.
Office of Health Economics 1992. *Compendium of statistics*. London: Office of Health Economics.
Oliver, M. 1989. *The politics of disablement*. London: Free Association Books.
Omega File 1983. London: Adam Smith Institute.
OPCS 1988. *Surveys of disability in Great Britain*. London: HMSO.
Osborne, D. & T. Gaebler 1992. *Reinventing government*. Reading, Mass.: Addison-Wesley.
Owen, D. 1964. *English philanthropy 1660–1960*. London: Oxford University Press.
Owens, P. 1987. *Community care and severe physical disability*. London: Bedford Square Press.
Packman, J. 1975. *The child's generation*. Oxford: Blackwell & Robertson.
Parasuraman, A., V. Zeithaml, A. L. Berry 1988. A conceptual model of service quality and its implications for future research. *Journal of Marketing* **49**, 41–50.
Parker, J. 1965. *Local health and welfare services*. London: Allen & Unwin.
Parker, R. 1986. Child care: the roots of a dilemma. In *Political Quarterly* **57**(3), 305–14.
— 1990. *Away from home: a history of child care*. Ilford, England: Barnardo's.
Parry, R. 1991. The privatisation of welfare under the Thatcher Government.

Business in the Contemporary World, Spring, 41–9.

Parton, N. 1985. *The politics of child abuse.* London: Macmillan.

Perkin, H. 1990. *The rise of professional society.* London: Routledge.

Peters, R. S. (ed.) 1969. *Perspectives on Plowden.* London: Routledge & Kegan Paul.

Peters, T. J. & R. Waterman 1982. *In search of excellence: lessons from America's best run companies.* New York: Harper Collins.

Phillipson, C. 1977. *The emergence of retirement.* Durham, England: University of Durham Working Papers in Sociology.

Piachaud, D. 1993. *What's wrong with Fabianism?* London: Fabian Society.

Pierson, C. 1991. *Beyond the welfare state?* Cambridge: Polity.

Pimlott, B. 1988. The myth of consensus. In *Echoes of greatness,* L. M. Smith (ed.), 129–42. London: Macmillan.

Pirie, M. 1989. *Mind the children.* London: Adam Smith Institute.

— 1991. *The Citizen's Charter.* London: Adam Smith Institute.

— 1993a. *The radical agenda.* London: Adam Smith Institute.

— 1993b. A time for revolutions not for patching. *The Spectator,* 9 October.

Portillo, M. 1993. *Ethics and public finance.* Lecture delivered to the Church at Work in London, 15 September.

Prochaska, F. 1992. *Philanthropy and the hospitals of London.* Oxford: Clarendon Press.

Quick, A. & R. Wilkinson 1991. *Income and health.* London: Socialist Medical Association.

Redcliffe-Maud, Lord 1981. *Experience of an optimist.* London: Hamish Hamilton.

Reeder, D. 1979. A recurring debate: education and industry. In *Schooling in decline,* G. Bernbaum (ed.), 115–48. London: Macmillan.

Reisman, D. 1991. *The political economy of James Buchanan.* London: Macmillan.

Rex, J. 1988. *The ghetto and the underclass: essays on race and social policy.* Aldershot, England: Avebury.

Rex, J. & R. Moore 1967. *Race, community and conflict.* Oxford: Oxford University Press.

Rhodes, R. A. W. 1988. *Beyond Westminster and Whitehall.* London: Unwin Hyman.

Rhodes, R. A. W. & D. Marsh 1992. Policy networks in British politics: a critique of existing approaches. In *Policy networks in British government,* D. Marsh & R. A. W. Rhodes (eds), 1–26. Oxford: Clarendon Press.

Richardson, W. 1993. *The reform of post-16 education and training in England and Wales.* Harlow, England: Longman.

Robb, B. 1967. *Sans everything: a case to answer.* London: Nelson.

Roberts, H. 1990. *Women's health counts.* London: Routledge.

Robinson, R. & K. Judge 1987. *Public expenditure and the NHS: trends and prospects.* London: King's Fund Institute.

Robson, B. 1994. *Assessing the impact of urban policy.* London: HMSO.

Rollings, N. 1988. British budgetary policy 1945–54: a Keynesian revolution? *Economic History Review* **41**, 283–98.

— 1993. *Poor Mr Butskell: a short life wrecked by schizophrenia.* Unpublished paper.

Rowe, J. and L. Lambert 1973. *Children who wait.* London: Association of British Adoption Agencies.

Rowntree, B. S. & G. R. Lavers 1951. *Poverty and the welfare state.* London: Longman.

Rudd, T. 1958. Basic problems in the social welfare of the elderly. *The Almoner* **10**(1), 348–9.

Rutter, M., B. Maugham, P. Mortimore, J. Ouston 1979. *Fifteen thousand hours.* London: Open Books.

Sabin, J. 1992. Mind the gap: reflections of an American health maintenance organisation doctor on the new NHS. *British Medical Journal* **305**, 514–16.

Saggar, S. 1992. *Race and politics in Britain.* London: Harvester Wheatsheaf.

Sainsbury, S. 1970. *Registered as disabled.* London: Bell.

— 1986. *Deaf worlds.* London: Hutchinson.

— 1989. *Regulating residential care.* Aldershot, England: Gower.

— 1993. *Normal life: a study of war and industrially injured pensioners.* Aldershot, England: Avebury.

Salamon, L. M. 1987. Partners in public service: the scope and theory of government-nonprofit relations. In *The nonprofit sector: a research handbook,* W. Powell (ed.), 99–117. New Haven: Yale University Press.

— 1993. The marketisation of welfare: changing nonprofit and for-profit roles in the American welfare state. *Social Service Review* **67**(1), 16–39.

Salamon, L. & H. Anheier 1992. In search of the nonprofit sector. I: The question of definitions. *Voluntas* **3**(2), 125–52.

Samuel, R. 1962. But nothing happens. *New Left Review* **13–14**, 38–71.

Sanderson, I. (ed.) 1992. *Managing for quality in local government.* Harlow, England: Longman.

Sanderson, M. 1991. Social equality and industrial need: a dilemma of English education since 1945. In *Britain since 1945,* T. Gourvish & A. O. Day (eds), 159–82. London: Macmillan.

Seldon, A. 1991. The Conservative Party since 1945. In *Britain since 1945,* T. Gourvish & A. O'Day (eds), 233–62. London: Macmillan.

Self, P. 1993. *Government by the market?* London: Macmillan.

Senker, P. 1992. *Industrial training in a cold climate.* Aldershot, England: Avebury.

Shanas. E., P. Townsend, D. Wedderburn 1968. *Old people in three industrialised societies.* London: Routledge & Kegan Paul.

Sheldon, J. 1948. *The social medicine of old age.* Oxford: Oxford University Press.

Showler, B. 1976. *The public employment service.* Harlow, England: Longman.

Sills, A., G. Taylor, P. Golding 1988. *The politics of the urban crisis.* London: Hutchinson.

Simey, M. 1988. *Democracy rediscovered.* London: Pluto.

Simon, B. 1991. *Education and the social order 1940–1990.* London: Lawrence & Wishart.

Sinfield, A. 1993. Reverse targeting and upside down benefits. In *Poverty, inequality and justice,* A. Sinfield (ed.), 1–11. Edinburgh: University of Edinburgh.

Skelcher, C. 1992. *Managing for service quality.* Harlow, England: Longman.

Skellington, R. 1992. *"Race" in Britain today.* London: Sage.

Slack, K. 1960. *Councils, committees and concern for the old.* London: Codicote Press.

Sly, F. 1993. Women in the labour market. *Employment Gazette,* November, 483–91.

Smith, D. J. & S. Tomlinson 1989. *The school effect*. London: Policy Studies Institute.

Smith, H. L. (ed.) 1986. *War and social change*. Manchester, England: Manchester University Press.

Smith, R., L. Gaster, L. Harrison, L. Martin, R. Means, P. Thiselthwaite 1993. *Working together for better community care*. Bristol, England: School for Advanced Urban Studies.

Smith, S. J. 1989. *The politics of "race" and residence: citizenship, segregation and white supremacy in Britain*. Cambridge: Polity.

Smithers, A. 1993. *All our futures*. Manchester: Centre for Education and Employment Research, University of Manchester.

Social Trends 21. 1991. London: HMSO.

— 23. 1993. London: HMSO.

Solomos, J. 1989. *Race and racism in contemporary Britain*. London: Macmillan.

— 1993. *Race and racism in Britain*, 2nd edn. London: Macmillan.

Squires, P. 1990. *Anti-social policy*. Brighton, England: Harvester Wheatsheaf.

Stevenson, J. 1984. *British Society 1914–45*. London: Penguin.

— 1986. Planner's moon? The Second World War and the planning movement. In *War and social change*, H. L. Smith (ed.), 58–77. Manchester, England: Manchester University Press.

Stewart, J. & K. Walsh 1989. *The search for quality*. Luton, England: Local Government Management Board.

Stoker, G. 1988. *The politics of local government*. London: Macmillan.

Stoleru, L. 1991. *The European*. Paris: OECD.

Sullivan, M. 1992. *The politics of social policy*. London: Harvester Wheatsheaf.

Taylor, M. 1983. Shifting emphases in community work. In *Community work in the 1980s*, D. Thomas (ed.), 21–6. London: National Institute for Social Work.

— 1992a. The changing role of the nonprofit sector in Britain: moving towards the market. In *Government and the third sector: emerging relationships in welfare states*, B. Gidron, R. M. Kramer, L. M. Salamon (eds), 147–75. San Francisco: Jossey-Bass.

— 1992b. *Signposts to community development*. London: Community Development Foundation.

Taylor, M. & J. Lansley 1992. Ideology and welfare in the UK: the implications for the voluntary sector. *Voluntas* 3(2), 153–74.

Taylor, M., J. Kendall, A. Fenyo 1993. The survey of local authority payments to voluntary organisations and charitable organisations. In *Charity trends*, 16th edn. Tonbridge, England: Charities Aid Foundation.

Taylor, P. 1993. Changing political relations. In *Policy and change in Thatcher's Britain*, P. Cloke (ed.), 33–54. Oxford: Pergamon Press.

Taylor-Gooby, P. & R. Lawson (eds) 1993. *Markets and managers*. Milton Keynes, England: Open University Press.

Thane, P. 1988. A woman's place. In *Echoes of greatness*, L. M. Smith (ed.), 71–84. London: Macmillan.

Thomas, D. 1983. *The making of community work*. London: Allen & Unwin.

Thomas, N., J. Doling, N. Deakin (eds) 1993. *Learning from innovation: housing and social care in the 1990s*. Birmingham, England: Academic Press.

Thompson, A. P. 1949. Problems of ageing and chronic sickness. *British Medical Journal*, 30 July, 243–50.

Timmins, N. 1989. Is the health service safe in their hands? *The Independent*, 9 February.

— 1993. Extra cost of NHS changes challenged. *The Independent* 20 November.

Tiratsoo, N. & J. Tomlinson 1993. *Industrial efficiency and state intervention: Labour 1939–51*. London: Routledge.

Titmuss, R. M. 1950. *Problems of social policy*. London: HMSO.

— 1958. *Essays on the welfare state*. London: Allen & Unwin.

— 1968. *Commitment to welfare*. London: Allen & Unwin.

— 1974. *Social policy: an introduction*. London: Allen & Unwin.

Tomlinson, J. 1987. *Employment policy: the crucial years 1939–1955*. Oxford: Clarendon Press.

— 1993. Mr Attlee's supply-side socialism. *Economic History Review* **46**, 1–22.

Tomlinson, S. 1989. The schools. In *The Thatcher effect*, D. Kavanagh & A. Seldon (eds), 183–97. Oxford: Oxford University Press.

Topliss, E. & B. Gould 1981. *A charter for the disabled*. Oxford: Basil Blackwell & Martin Robertson.

Townsend, P. 1952. *Poverty: ten years after Beveridge*. Planning 344.

— 1962. *The last refuge*. London: Routledge & Kegan Paul.

— 1963. *The family life of old people*. London: Penguin.

— 1976a. Seebohm and family welfare. In *Sociology and social policy*, P. Townsend (ed.), 202–6. London: Penguin.

— 1976b. *The difficulties of policies based on the concept of area deprivation*. London: University of London, Queen Mary College.

— 1979. *Poverty in the United Kingdom*. London: Allen Lane Press.

— 1980. Social planning and the Treasury. In *Labour and equality*, N. Bosanquet & P. Townsend (eds), 3–23. London: Heinemann.

Townsend, P. & N. Davidson 1982. *Inequalities in health*. London: Penguin.

Tritter, J. 1994. The Citizen's Charter: opportunities for users' perspectives. *Political Quarterly* **65**(4), 397–414.

Turner, B. S. 1986. *Citizenship and capitalism: the debate over reformism*. London: Allen & Unwin.

Veit-Wilson, J. 1986. Paradigms of poverty: a rehabilitation of B. S. Rowntree. *Journal of Social Policy* **15**(1), 55–99.

Venables, Sir P. 1955. *Technical education, its aims, organisation and future development*. London: Bell.

Waine, B. 1992. The voluntary sector – the Thatcher years. In *Social Policy Review 4*, N. Manning & R. Page (eds), 70–89. Canterbury, England: Social Policy Association.

Waldegrave, W. 1993. *The reality of reform and accountability in today's public service*. London: Public Finance Foundation.

Walker, C. 1983. *Changing social policy*. London: Bedford Square Press.

Walker, M. 1993. *Reforming welfare states: lessons from recent Canadian experience*. Stockholm: Atlas Foundation.

Walker, R. & D. Lawton, 1988. Social assistance and territorial justice: the example of single payments. *Journal of Social Policy* **17**(4),437–76

Ware, A. (ed). *Charities and government.* Manchester, England: Manchester University Press.

Waring, M. 1988. *Counting for nothing.* New Zealand: Port Nicholson Press.

Webb, A. & G. Wistow 1987. *Social work, social care and social planning: the personal social services since Seebohm.* Harlow, England: Longman.

Webster, C. 1988. *The health services since the war: Volume 1.* London: HMSO.

— (ed.) 1991. *Aneurin Bevan on the National Health Service.* Oxford: Wellcome Unit for the History of Medicine, University of Oxford.

Whitehead, M. 1988. *The health divide: inequalities in health in the 1980s.* London: Penguin.

Whiteside, N. 1995 forthcoming. Aiming at consensus: social welfare and industrial relations 1939–79. In *A History of British Industrial Relations Vol. III: the era of economic decline,* C. J. Wrigley (ed.). Cheltenham, England: Edward Elgar.

Wicks, M. 1987. *A future for all: do we need a welfare state?* London: Penguin.

— 1994. Community care costs. *The Mixed Economy of Care Bulletin* **3**, 14–15.

Wilcock, S. 1993. *Local housing companies: new opportunities for council housing.* York, England: Joseph Rowntree Foundation.

Wilding, P. 1992. The public sector in the 1980s. In *Social Policy Review 4,* N. Manning & R. Page (eds), 8–25. Canterbury, England: Social Policy Association.

Wilkinson, R. 1992. Income distribution and life expectancy. *British Medical Journal* **304**, 165–8.

Williams, F. 1989. *Social policy: a critical introduction.* Cambridge: Polity.

— 1993. Gender "race" and class in British welfare policy. In *Comparing welfare states,* A. Cochrane & J. Clarke (eds), 77–104. London: Sage.

Williamson, B. 1990. *The temper of the times.* Oxford: Basil Blackwell.

Wistow, G., M. Knapp, B. Hardy, C. Allan 1992. From providing to enabling: local authorities and the mixed economy of social care. *Public Administration* **70**(1), 25–46.

Wolfenden, J. 1978. *The future of voluntary organisations.* London: Croom Helm.

Woodfield, P. 1987. *Efficiency scrutiny of the supervision of charities.* London: HMSO.

Wright, A., J. Steward, N. Deakin 1984. *Socialism and decentralisation.* London: Fabian Society.

Yarrow, G. 1993. *Social security and friendly societies: options for the future.* London: National Conference of Friendly Societies.

Younghusband, E. 1978. *Social work in Britain: 1950–75,* vol. I. London: Allen & Unwin.

Index